OXFORD CLINICAL NEPHROLOGY SERIES

Complications of Long-term Dialysis

Complications of Long-term Dialysis

Edited by

EDWINA A. BROWN

Consultant Nephrologist,
Charing Cross Hospital, Imperial College School of Medicine, London, UK

and

PATRICK S. PARFREY

University Research Professor (Medicine),
Division of Nephrology and Clinical Epidemiology Unit,
Memorial University of Newfoundland, St. John's, Canada

Oxford   New York   Tokyo
OXFORD UNIVERSITY PRESS
1999

Oxford University Press, Great Clarendon Street, Oxford OX2 6DP

Oxford New York

Athens Auckland Bangkok Bogotay Buenos Aires Calcutta
Cape Town Chennai Dar es Salaam Delhi Florence Hong Kong Istanbul
Karachi Kuala Lumpur Madrid Melbourne Mexico City Mumbai
Nairobi Paris São Paolo Singapore Taipei Tokyo Toronto Warsaw

and associated companies in
Berlin Ibadan

Oxford is a trade mark of Oxford University Press

Published in the United States
by Oxford University Press, Inc., New York

First published 1999

British Library Cataloguing in Publication Data
Data available

Library of Congress Cataloging in Publication Data
(Data applied for)

1 3 5 7 9 10 8 6 4 2   H/b

ISBN 0 19 262829 1

Typeset by Jayvee, Trivandrum, India
Printed in Great Britain on acid free paper by Bookcraft Ltd.,
Midsomer Norton, Avon

CONTENTS

CONTRIBUTORS

Edwina A. Brown Charing Cross Hospital, Fulham Palace Rd, London W6 8RF, UK

Graeme R. D. Catto, Faculty of Medicine, Unversity of Aberdeen, Aberdeen, AB2S 2ZO, Scotland

Bernard Charra Centre de Rein Artificiel de Tassin, 69160-Tassin, France

Peter J. Conlon Beaumont Hospital, Dublin 9, Ireland; and Duke University Medical Center, Durham, NC, USA

John Cunningham, Royal London Hospital, Whitechapel, London, E11BB, UK

Marc E. De Broe Department of Nephrology-Hypertension, University Hospital of Antwerp, Wilrijkstraat 10, B-2650 Edegem, Belgium

Patrick C. D'Haese Department of Nephrology-Hypertension, University Hospital of Antwerp, Wilrijkstraat 10, B-2650 Edegem, Belgium

Fredric O. Finkelstein Department of Medicine, Yale University and Section of Nephrology, Hospital of St Raphael, Renal Research Institute, New Haven, Connecticut, USA

Susan H. Finkelstein Department of Social Work in Psychiatry, Yale University and Department of Social Work, Southern Connecticut State University, Renal Research Institute, New Haven, Connecticut, USA

Robert N. Foley Division of Nephrology and Clinical Epidemiology Unit, The Health Sciences Centre, Memorial University, St John's, Newfoundland, Canada.

Frank Gotch Artificial Kidney Center, Franklin Hospital, San Francisco and University of California, San Francisco, USA

Susan Harris, Charing Cross Hospital, Fulham Palace Rd, London W6 8RF, UK

Isao Ishikawa Division of Nephrology, Department of Internal Medicine, Kanazawa Medical University, Uchinada, Kahoku, Ishikawa, 920-0293 Japan

Michel Jadoul University of Louvain Medical School, Department of Nephrology, Cliniques Universitaires St-Luc, 1200 Bruxelles, Belgium

Izhar H. Khan, Aberdeen Royal Hospitals NHS Trust, Aberdeen, Scotland

Guy Laurent Centre de Rein Artificiel de Tassin, 69160-Tassin, France

Norbert Lameire Renal Division, Department of Internal Medicine, De Pintelaan 185, B-9000 Gent, Belgium

Nathan W. Levin Division of Nephrology and Hypertension, Beth Israel Medical Center, New York and Albert Einstein College of Medicine of Yeshiva University, New York, USA

Patrick S. Parfrey Division of Nephrology and Clinical Epidemiology Unit, The Health Sciences Centre, Memorial University, St John's, Newfoundland, Canada

Brian J. G. Pereira Division of Nephrology, New England Medical Center, Tufts University School of Medicine, Massachusetts 02111, USA

David Reaich South Cleveland Hospital, Middlesbrough, Cleveland TS4 3BW, UK

Steve J. Schwab Division of Nephrology, Duke University Medical Center, Durham, North Carolina 27705, USA

Wim Van Biesen Renal Division, Department of Internal Medicine, De Pintelaan, 185, B-9000 Gent, Belgium

Charles van Ypersele de Strihou University of Louvain Medical School, Department of Nephrology, Cliniques Universitaires St-Luc, 1200 Bruxelles, Belgium

ABBREVIATIONS

$1\alpha(OH)D_2$	1α-hydroxyvitamin D_2
AAMI	(?chapter 10)
ACE	angiotensin converting enzyme
AFP	alpha-fetoprotein
AGE	advanced glycosylation end product
AIDS	acquired immune deficiency syndrome
ALT	alanine aminotransferase
APD	automated peritoneal dialysis
ARBD	aluminum-related bone disease
AS	aortic stenosis
AV	arteriovenous
ß2m	$ß_2$-microglobulin
ß2mA	$ß_2$-microglobulin amyloidosis
BCAA	branched chain amino acid
BDI	Beck Depression Inventory
bDNA	branched-chain DNA
bFGF	basic fibroblast growth factor
BIA	bioelectrical impedance
BUN	blood urea nitrogen
C	basic nucleocapsid
c.f.u.	colony-forming units
CA	cancer antigen
CANUSA	Canada and USA
CAPD	continuous ambulatory peritoneal dialysis
CCPD	continuous cyclic peritoneal dialysis
CDC	Center for Disease Control and Prevention
CEA	carcinoembryonic antigen
CHF	congestive heart failure
CHX	Charing Cross hospital
Co	predialysis BUN
CRF	chronic renal failure
Ct	postdialysis BUN
CT	computed tomography
Ct'	equilibrated BUN
CTS	carpal tunnel syndrome
CVD	cerebrovascular disease
D/P	dialysate/plasma
DEXA	dual-energy, X-ray absorptiometry

DFO	desferrioxamine
DI	dialysis index
DRA	dialysis-related amyloidosis
DTPA	diethylenetriaminepentaacetic acid; pentetic acid
E1	first envelope structural region of virus
E2/NS1	second envelope/non-structural-1 region of virus
ECF	extracellular fluid
ECV	extracellular volume
EDTA	ethylenediaminetetraacetic acid
EDTA	European Dialysis and Transplantation Association
EEG	electroencephalogram
EGF	epidermal growth factor
EGFR	epidermal growth factor receptor
eKt/Vd	equilibrated Kt/Vd
ELISA	enzyme-linked immunosorbent assay
eNPCR	equilibrated NPCR
EPO	erythropoietin
ERA	European Renal Association
ESRD	end-stage renal disease
Fc	crystallizable fragment (of immunoglobulin)
FDA	Food and Drug Administration (USA)
FNC	femoral neck capsule
FSH	follicle-stimulating hormone
GBV	GB virus
GFR	glomerular filtration rate
Hb	hemoglobin
HBsAg	hepatitis B surface antigen
HBV	hepatitis B virus
HCFA	Health Care Financing Administration
Hct	hematocrit
HCV	hepatitis C virus
HD	hemodialysis
HDL	high-density lipoprotein
HGV	hepatitis G virus
HLA	human leukocyte antigen (system)
HMG-CoA	hydroxymethylglutary co-enzymeA
HTGL	hepatic triglyceride lipase
ICTP	(type) I, carboxy-terminal telopeptide
IDPN	intradialytic parenteral nutrition
IFN-α	interferon-alpha
IFN-γ	interferon-gamma
IGF	insulin-like growth factor
IHD	ischemic heart disease
IL	interleukin

IV	intravenous
IVDA	intravenous drug abuse
IVNAA	*in-vivo* neutron activation analysis
Kt/V	dialyzer clearance (K) multiplied by the treatment time (t) divided by the solute distribution volume (V)
*Kt/V*d	delivered *Kt/V*
KUF	ultrafiltration coefficient
LCAT	lecithin—cholesterol aminotransferase
LDL	low-density lipoprotein
LGR	large granular lymphocytes
LH	luteinizing hormone
LRH	luteinizing releasing hormone
MAACL	Multiple Adjective Check List
MAP	mean arterial pressure
MDRD	Modification of Diet in Renal Disease
MHC	major histocompatibility complex
MI	myocardial infarct
MR	mortality rate
N.S.	not significant
NANBH	non-A, non-B hepatitis
NCDS	National Cooperative Dialysis Study
NCR	non-coding region
NIH	National Institutes of Health
NIPD	nightly intermittent peritonal dialysis
NK	natural killer (cell)
NKF-DOQI	National Kidney Foundation-Dialysis Outcomes Quality Initiative
nPCR	normalized protein catabolic rate
NPD	nightly peritoneal dialysis
nRR	normalized relative risk
NS	non-structural (region of virus)
NTPD	nocturnal tidal peritoneal dialysis
PBMC	peripheral blood mononuclear cells
PCKD	polycystic kidney disease
PCR	polymerase chain reaction
PCR	protein catabolic rate
PD	peritoneal dialysis
PDGF	platelet-derived growth factor
PF	probability of failure
P_i	inorganic phosphate
PICP	(type) I carboxy-terminal extension peptide (query to author)
PNA	protein nitrogen appearance
PPV	positive predictive value
PSA	prostate-specific antigen
PTFE	polytetrafluoroethylene
PTH	parathyroid hormone

PVD	peripheral vascular disease
RDA	representational difference analysis
RFLP	restriction fragment length polymorphism
rHEPO	recombinant human erythropoietin
rHGH	recombinant human growth hormone
rHIGF-1	recombinant human insulin–like growth factor-1
RIBA	recombinant immunoblot assay
RR	relative risk
RR/D	relative risk/dose
RRF	residual renal function
RRT	renal replacement therapy
Sal	serum aluminum
SAP	serum amyloid P component
SMR	standardized mortality ratio
spKt/Vd	single-pool Kt/Vd
spNPCR	single-pool NPCR
SST	supraspinatus shoulder tendon
TAC	time-averaged concentration
TGF-α	transforming growth factor-α
TNF-α	tumor necrosis factor-α
TP	transplantation
URR	urea reduction ratio
US	ultrasonography
USRDS	United States Renal Data System
VDP	venous dialysis pressure
VDR	vitamin D receptor

PART I
Introduction

1

Long-term complications of dialysis: an introductory chapter

Susan Harris and Edwina A. Brown

Introduction

Charing Cross hospital (CXH) was one of the first centers in the UK to begin a maintenance hemodialysis program. Encouraged by the work of Scribner and his colleagues in the USA, Professor de Wardener sent a team of doctors and nurses to Seattle in 1964 to learn the technique. It was decided to start with just one patient. This patient was carefully selected to have the best chance of a successful outcome, such that the result of the treatment would be most likely to encourage other centers to take an interest in chronic dialysis. In 1964, watched by all 15 members of the renal team, this patient began his first treatment on a schedule of long-term hemodialysis (this patient survived for 27 years). Teething problems were expected, difficulties with fluid and electrolyte balance were anticipated and tackled as they arose. But the expectation was that this would be a complete renal replacement therapy, and that once patients were established on hemodialysis they would return to work and live a full and happy life. For, apart from the problems of vascular access which were fully recognized and described as 'the Achilles heel' of long-term dialysis (de Wardener, 1966) the other long-term complications such as amyloidosis and cardiovascular disease could not have been foreseen.

The purpose of this chapter is to introduce the subject of the long-term complications of hemodialysis (HD) by looking at those patients who survived for longer than 10 years on renal replacement therapy (RRT) at the CXH up to 1st January 1996. These patients were, by definition, started on HD prior to 1st January 1986.

Up to this time 530 patients had commenced HD at the CXH; details of 423 of these patients are still available on the renal unit computer. Of these 423 there were 251 men (59%): at the start of dialysis the ages ranged from 10 years to 83 years (mean 45 years). In all, 199 of these patients survived for at least 10 years; 43 are known to have survived for 20 years (40 patients moved away) and 4 patients have survived for 30 years, 3 of whom currently have functioning transplants. Of those 199 patients followed for at least 10 years, 111 were men (56%) and the mean age at the start of dialysis was 36 years (range 11 to 69 years).

This chapter will not be concerned with those patients who had transplants after less than 10 years on maintenance dialysis and in whom the transplants were still functioning at death or at the end of the study period. Patients who have had a functioning transplant for the majority of the time but, who after transplant failure, have returned to maintenance dialysis will be included as these patients are now known to have their own set of problems, which again were unforeseen when maintenance dialysis was begun (Cattran and Fenton, 1993). In all, 116 patients are described. At Charing Cross hospital, Kiil dialyzers were used until disposable dialyzers were phased in during 1980/81. The number of hours of dialysis has been gradually reducing, from two 14-hour sessions per week for the first patients to two 6-hour sessions in the early 1980s for those on disposable dialyzers. Thrice-weekly dialysis (4- or 5-hour sessions) was introduced in the late 1980s. However, thrice-weekly dialysis has only been very slowly phased in, and many of the long-term patients included in this study were reluctant to change and, in fact, never changed to this regime. Continuous ambulatory peritoneal dialysis (CAPD) was introduced at the CXH in 1980; most patients have used a disconnect system since 1991 and are performing four 2- or 2.5-liter exchanges a day.

Method

This is a retrospective study using information obtained from the renal unit computer and from medical records.

Patients who had been on renal replacement therapy at the CXH for longer than 10 years were identified from the renal unit computer. They were grouped according to the RRT modalities they had received (Table 1.1). Patients in group 1 had, for the purpose of discussing long-term complications, effectively received no other form of renal replacement therapy, other than hemodialysis, for more than 3 months in succession, i.e. if they had received a renal allograft it had either failed within 3 months or the patient had died within 3 months of transplantation, likewise they had not been on peritoneal dialysis for more than 3 months at any one time. Patients in group 2, in addition to HD, also had a period of time on peritoneal dialysis. Group 3 includes those patients who were successfully transplanted, but not until they had been on dialysis for more than 10 years. These patients had a working renal allograft at death or at the end of the study period. Patients in group 4 had received at least one renal transplant that had lasted for more than 3 months, but the transplant had failed and they had returned to dialysis—either PD or HD. Only the patients in this last group may have been on dialysis for less than a total of 10 years; and indeed one patient in this group never received hemodialysis but returned to CAPD when her renal transplant failed after 27 years.

The notes for each of these patients were reviewed and data collected with respect to age, sex, cause of end-stage renal disease (ESRD), modality of treatment, mortality, and morbidity related to dialysis.

The characteristics of the patients studied, including the length of time for which they have been on each RRT modality, are shown in Table 1.2.

Morbidity data was obtained from the case records and the renal unit computer rather than from death certificates, in order to learn as accurately as possible the problems leading to death rather than the final diagnosis. If a patient died of bronchopneumonia but that illness was contracted in hospital where he/she was immobilized by severe peripheral vascular disease (PVD), then PVD is the recorded cause of death for the purpose of this study.

Table 1.1 Categorization of patients

Group	Notation	Modalities and sequence of renal replacement therapy
1	HD	Hemodialysis only. No transplant successful for > 3 months
2	HD + PD	Hemodialysis and peritoneal dialysis with no successful transplants
3	HD/Tx	Hemodialysis ± PD for longer than 10 years followed by transplantation
4	HD/Tx/HD	HD ± PD with subsequent transplant(s) which failed and the patient restarted HD

Morbidity related to long-term dialysis was measured by collecting detailed data which, for the purpose of explanation, was divided in to five categories:

1. *Morbidity related to access surgery and transplantation.* The number and type of procedures required by each patient to maintain access for both HD and PD were totaled for each 5-year treatment period. The number and success of transplant attempts and any morbidity resulting from a transplant operation or transplant failure was recorded. The incidence of technique failure on both HD and PD was recorded, together with the reason for this failure.

2. *Cardiovascular morbidity.* Hypertension was assessed at 5-year intervals. The patient was recorded as being hypertensive if their blood pressure was greater than 165 mmHg systolic or 90 mmHg diastolic for more than one year out of the preceding 5 years, or if they had required antihypertensive treatment for more than one year out of the last five. The development of vascular disease was recorded, noting the time from the start of RRT to the first signs or symptoms of: ischemic heart disease (IHD); angina, or breathlessness on exertion not related to underlying lung disease, cerebrovascular disease (CVD); transient ischemic attacks, a diagnosis of multi-infarct dementia or a finding of changes suggestive of previous cerebral infarcts on a computed tomographic brain scan and peripheral vascular disease determined by claudication, the finding of cool extremities with absent peripheral pulses, ischemic ulceration, and also a diagnosis of ischemic bowel disease. The age of the patient and their smoking status at the onset of these signs or symptoms and whether they progressed to having a myocardial infarction, a disabling stroke, or needing surgical treatment such as bypass or amputation for peripheral vascular disease was also recorded. Development of aortic stenosis was recorded as positive if the patient had had an echocardiogram showing significant stenosis or if stenosis was recorded at postmortem; a negative answer was recorded if the patient had no ejection systolic murmur or a negative echocardiogram. If the patient had an ejection systolic murmur but the presence of a significant stenosis of the valve was never confirmed, then 'don't know' was recorded—an ejection murmur can be a very non-specific sign especially in patients who are likely to have been anemic.

Table 1.2 Characteristics of patients surviving over 10 years on RRT at the CXH by treatment group

Group	No.	Sex No. male (%)	Age ESRD Mean, range (years)	RRT mean, range (years)	HD mean, range (years)	PD mean, range (years)	Transplant mean, range (years)	>20 years RRT No. of patients	Still alive No. of patients
HD	50	36 (72)	43 (19–61)	14.5 (10–23)	14.5 (10–23)	NA	NA	4	15
HD+PD	15	2 (13)	42 (22–68)	13.4 (11–20)	11.3 (4.1–19.5)	2.0 (0.3–6.8)	NA	1	5
HD/Tx	18	11 (61)	28 (17–44)	23.5 (16–29)	14 (10.3–21.4)	0	9.5 (0.3–18.3)	14	11
HD/Tx/HD	33	19 (58)	32 (18–57)	17.2 (10–30)	10.2 (0*–22.3)	1.0 (0–6.3)	6.3 (0.3–28.1)	9	19
All	116	68 (59)	37	16.50				28	50

*One patient never received HD, returning to PD when her transplant failed after 27 years. ESRD, end-stage renal disease; RRT, renal replacement therapy; HD, hemodialysis; PD, peritoneal dialysis.

3. *Hyperparathyroidism and dialysis-related amyloidosis.* The first indication of significant morbidity from musculoskeletal disease was recorded as the time the patient first complained in the clinic of joint pains: either pains in large joints, suggestive of amyloidosis, or pains in peripheral joints, suggestive of hyperparathyroidism. Whether they later developed disabling joint disease (i.e. joint disease that made them dependent on others for any activities of daily living or which caused them to give up employment) was also noted. With respect to hyperparathyroidism, it was only possible to record whether patients had undergone parathyroidectomy and not to differentiate secondary from tertiary disease. If parathyroidectomy was performed, any recurrent disease following surgery and how many operations they had altogether was recorded. Amyloidosis was assessed by recording the time when the patients developed carpal tunnel syndrome (CTS): whether it was bilateral and if symptoms recurred following carpal tunnel release. Any other symptoms or signs suggestive of renal amyloidosis, such as trigger finger and cervical spondyloarthropathy, were also noted.

4. *Morbidity related to compromise of the immune system.* The number of infections occurring in each patient for each 5 years of RRT was counted; these were classified according to the type of infection: viral, bacterial, fungal, and protozoal. Urinary tract and respiratory tract infections were totaled separately and any existing predisposition to these infections, such as underlying chronic obstructive airways disease, recorded. Each episode of infection was also classified according to whether it was community- or hospital-acquired, or if the patient was taking immunosuppressive drugs at the time. Infections related to a breach of the normal mechanical barriers—such as fistula or neckline infections, peritonitis and exit-site infections, and blood-borne infections notably hepatitis B (HBV) and hepatitis C virus (HCV) infection—were recorded separately. Development of any malignant disease including the primary site of malignancy was recorded.

5. *Chronic liver disease.* The presence of chronic liver disease was recorded if clinical signs were present and not on biochemical indices alone. This will be mainly discussed in terms of its association with HCV infection below.

Data on patients still alive on 1st January 1996

The patients who were alive at the end of the study were separately assessed. The mean of three hemoglobin and albumin levels (taken not less than 3 months apart) were determined retrospectively by using predialysis blood tests taken over a period of one year (1995), using as a starting point the last blood test taken in 1995.

Blood pressure control was assessed, when possible, by taking the mean systolic and diastolic values from three 2-week blocks of predialysis blood pressure measurements, the 2-week blocks being at least 3 months apart but less than 6 months apart. In the case of some of the home dialysis patients it was only possible to obtain random BP measurements, rather than predialysis. The minimum number of separate readings from which a mean was calculated was four, particularly in CAPD patients who only have a BP check at 3-monthly, out-patient appointments. Other information collected was the modality of RRT and regimen used, the use of erythropoietin, and employment status at 01/01/96.

Results

Causes of end-stage renal disease

The causes of ESRD in those patients who have survived for longer than 10 years on hemodialysis are shown in Table 1.3. The most commonly diagnosed causes of renal failure in these patients are glomerulonephritis and polycystic kidney disease (PCKD). Only one patient whose renal failure was secondary to diabetes mellitus has survived longer than 10 years; one other patient who has been diabetic from the start of RRT is included in this study, but his ESRD was due to interstitial nephritis not to diabetic nephropathy: at the time of this study he had developed no complications related to his diabetes. Although hypertension and renovascular disease are relatively common causes of ESRD, they account for only 6% of those patients who have survived for more than 10 years of dialysis in our unit.

Table 1.3   Causes of end-stage renal disease in long-term patients

Cause of renal disease	Number of patients
Glomerulonephritis (biopsy proven)	36 (26)
Polycystic kidney disease	18
Reflux/obstructive nephropathy	10
Chronic pyelonephritis ± renal stones	9
Hypertension and renovascular disease	7
Diabetic nephropathy	1
Other	14
Unknown	21
Total	116

Causes of death

Of the 116 patients studied, 65 are known to have died (one patient was lost to follow-up). The causes of death are given in Table 1.4. The majority of deaths were secondary to vascular disease; only 2 out of the 36 deaths related to cardiac or other vascular deaths are attributable to transplant-related causes, in that these two patients suffered a fatal myocardial infarction within 1 month of transplant failure. The second most frequent cause of death was infection; although of the 14 patients for whom this was the given cause of death six were immunosuppressed at the time they contracted the infection, usually because of a functioning renal transplant. A further three patients died indirectly as a result of infection: one died after severe hemorrhage from esophageal varices caused by hepatitis C virus infection and two patients withdrew from dialysis, at least in part, as a result of chronic infection. Only three patients died of cancer: the primary disease was known in two, namely endometrium and breast. Another transplant patient died of adenocarcinoma of unknown primary origin. Of the long-term dialysis patients, five eventually withdrew from dialysis: the reasons for withdrawal are given in Table 1.5.

Table 1.4 Causes of death in long-term patients

Cause of death	No. of patients
Infection	14 (6)
Sudden	11
Myocardial infarct (MI)	10 (2)
Cardiac cause *not* MI	5
Cerebrovascular disease	7
Other vascular disease	3
Withdrawal from dialysis	5
Cancer	3 (1)
Other*	6 (2)
Unknown	1
Total number of deaths	65

*Other includes: transplant surgery (2), hemorrhage during dialysis, hemorrhage from esophageal varices, gradual deterioration with multisystem disease, and suicide.
Numbers in parentheses indicate the number of deaths from that cause which were related to a current or recent transplant.

Table 1.5 Reasons for withdrawal from RRT

Severe cardiac and peripheral vascular disease
Poor access and ischemic heart disease
Chronic diarrhea, debilitation
Chronic sepsis
Unknown

Those patients still surviving on 1st January 1996 (Table 1.6)

At the end of the study 50 patients were still alive, and more detailed information was available for these patients. In all 11 patients had a functioning transplant. No further information was available for one patient who had moved away.

Of the 15 patients still alive in the hemodialysis–only group, nine were on home haemodialysis and three had transferred from home to hospital dialysis within the last year. The average dialysis time was 14.7 hours per week; only two patients were still dialyzing twice a week. The average length of time for which these patients had been on dialysis was 16 years. The mean hematocrit (Hct) and hemoglobin (Hb) levels for these patients in 1995 were respectively, 33% (range 27 to 40) and 10.8 g/dl (range 8.2 to 13.8). In 1990 we began using erythropoietin (EPO) routinely for patients in CXH with low hemoglobin levels. Only eight of these patients needed EPO treatment; their hemoglobin levels on EPO were slightly lower than those of patients who did not require it, 10.2 g/dl compared to 11.8 g/dl. The mean serum albumin was 34 g/l (range 27 to 37). Blood pressure (BP) control in these patients for the last year of the study was variable: mean predialysis systolic pressure was 144 mmHg (range 101 to 170) and diastolic pressure was 82 mmHg (range 63 to 102). The average age of these patients on

Table 1.6 Data on patients still alive and on dialysis at the end of the study

Group	No. of patients	Time on RRT (range) (years)	Age at 1/1/96 (range) (years)	Hct (%) (range)	Hb (g/dl) (range)	No. patients on EPO (%)	Albumin (g/l) (range)	SBP (mmHg) (range)	DBP (mmHg) (range)
HD	15	16.1 (10.8–23.4)	55.1 (40–76)	33 (27–40)	10.8 (8.2–13.8)	8 (53)	34 (27–37)	144 (101–170)	82 (63–102)
HD/PD	5	13.5 (10.6–20.2)	48.8 (34–81)	32 (28–37)	10.8 (9.5–12.3)	4 (80)	33 (21–36)	146 (117–173)	80 (71–107)
HD/Tx/HD	18	16.3 (10.1–29.6)	45.3 (29–59)	30 (25–35)	10.2 (7.7–12.1)	17 (94)	32 (22–40)	144 (99–179)	81 (55–101)

RRT, renal replacement therapy; HCT, hematocrit; Hb, hemoglobin; EPO, erythropoietin; SBP, systolic blood pressure; DBP, diastolic blood pressure.

1st January 1996 was 55.1 years. Of the ten patients under retirement age, five were currently in paid employment.

Of the 15 patients who had been treated with both HD and PD, five were alive at the end of the study. These five had been on dialysis for an average of 13.5 years; one had been on peritoneal dialysis for $5\frac{1}{2}$ years and the other four had received PD for less than 2 years. Only two out of the four patients who were under retirement age were currently working, the other patient was 81 years old on 01/01/96. The average values for hemoglobin, albumin, and blood pressure for 1995 were comparable to the hemodialysis-only survivors.

From the group who returned to dialysis after failure of a transplant which had functioned for at least 3 months, 18 were alive on 01/01/96. These patients received RRT for an average of 16 years: 9 years HD, 6 years with a functioning transplant, and 1 year PD. The average age on 01/01/96 was 45.3 years; eight were in paid employment, one was a part-time student, and two, aged 55 years, had recently retired. The other seven were unemployed. Blood parameters are given in Table 1.6.

Access surgery

In the 116 long-term patients studied, a total of 961 procedures were performed to create access for dialysis; in 1484 patient-years of hemodialysis, 885 procedures were undertaken, an average of one for every 1.7 years of treatment. For patients who had peritoneal dialysis the frequency of operations to insert PD catheters was even greater, 76 in 62 patient-years of treatment. The timing, type, and frequency of access attempts for patients who only received hemodialysis are shown in Fig. 1.1. From this it can be seen that even in these patients who were successful in surviving longer than 10 years

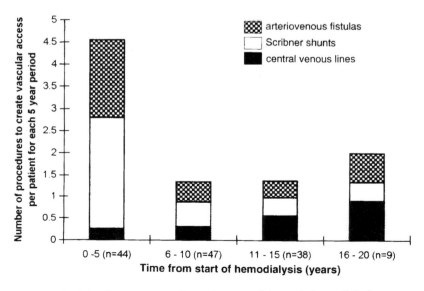

Fig. 1.1 Access surgery for patients receiving only hemodialysis.

on haemodialysis, there were often early problems with vascular access—patients required an average of one new attempt at access every year for the first 5 years. Access then became less of a problem, with patients requiring an average of one procedure every 5 years. When we subdivided the patients who only received hemodialysis into those who had mainly home hemodialysis (37 patients) and those who had mainly in-center treatment (13 patients), we found that the operation rate after the first 5 years was lower for home patients— one procedure every 7.6 years compared to 2.4 years for patients on hospital HD. Figure 1.1 also shows the trends in types of access, with diminishing use of the Scribner shunt as central venous lines became available.

Technique failure (Table 1.7)

Technique failure on hemodialysis in these patients was infrequent (11%) and tended to be late. In most cases failure was due to the exhaustion of sites for vascular access; for one patient this was the reason for withdrawal from dialysis (see Table 1.5). There was only one case of early technique failure on HD: the patient suffered intolerable headaches and nausea during the dialysis procedure which could not be overcome. (It is recognized that in any study of long-term survivors on hemodialysis, patients with early technique failure will, in   general, have been excluded.) Technique failure on PD was more frequent, affecting 42% of patients treated with this modality, and it occurred earlier; most often it was due to repeated or severe peritonitis, which one may expect to occur most commonly in the first year before the patient is very familiar with the technique and when hitherto undiagnosed gastrointestinal tract problems, such as diverticulitis, may present with recurrent peritonitis.

Table 1.7   Dialysis technique failure in patients on long-term RRT

Dialysis modality	No. of patients	Patient-years observed	Technique failure No. of patients (%)	Time to technique failure Mean (range) (years)	Reason for technique failure No. of patients	Reason
PD	36	62	15 (42)	2 (0–6.8)	12	peritonitis
					1	fluid leakage
					1	inadequate dialysis
					1	poor drainage
HD	115	1484	13 (11)	10.8 (4.1–19.5)	10	Poor vascular access
					1	unable to tolerate HD
					1	death of carer *
					1	unknown

*Patient on home HD who would not consider in center treatment so changed to PD on death of carer.
For abbreviations, see Table 1.2.

Transplantation

As stated earlier, 199 patients treated at the CXH have survived for more than 10 years after developing ESRD. Of these patients 83 received successful transplants which were still functioning at death or at the end of the study period, within 10 years of commencing treatment; these patients are not included in this study. Out of the 116 remaining patients studied, 77 received at least one renal allograft, and between these patients a total of 106 transplant operations were performed up to 01/01/96, 86 of which eventually failed and a further two when the patients died acutely following transplant surgery. We had one patient who received four grafts during her time on RRT. Groups 1 and 2 also include 23 patients who had transplant surgery, i.e. they are recorded as having had only HD or PD because their grafts, if they functioned at all, did so for less than 3 months. The deaths of 10 of these long-term patients are linked to renal transplantation (see Table 1.4), two died as a direct result of the surgery, six died of infections which developed while they were immunosuppressed, and two patients died of myocardial infarctions within 1 month of transplant failure. All the patients at the CXH who have survived for more than 25 years on RRT have had a successful renal transplant for at least part of the time. The longest survivor on dialysis alone up to 01/01/96 had undergone 23 years of haemodialysis.

Cardiovascular morbidity

The incidence of cardiovascular morbidity and its relationship to dialysis modality and the length of time on RRT are shown in Figs 1.2 and 1.3.

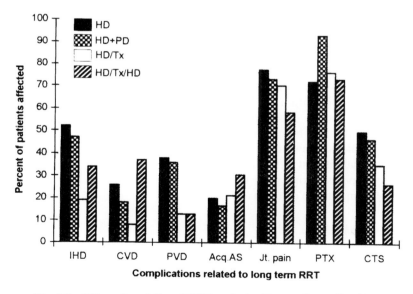

Fig. 1.2   Effect of modality of RRT on the incidence of complications.

Risk factors for cardiovascular morbidity

Hypertension and cigarette smoking were very common among the long-term patients. At the time of starting RRT, 81 of the patients were known to be hypertensive,

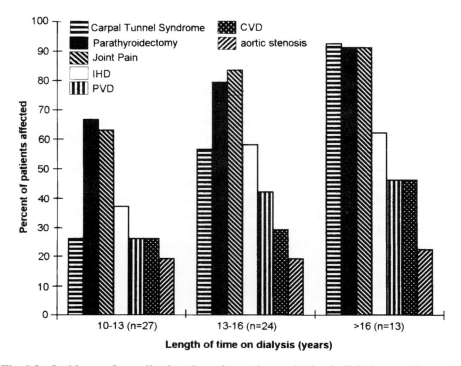

Fig. 1.3 Incidence of complications in patients who received only dialysis according to the length of time on dialysis. IHD, ischemic heart disease; PVD, peripheral vascular disease; CVD, cerebrovascular disease.

84% of those for whom information is available. After 5 years on treatment this number fell, but 56% of patients were still either hypertensive or required regular antihypertensive medication; at 10 years this dropped to 43%. Hypertension was slightly more prevalent in the transplanted patients, but the difference was not statistically significant. There were 64 patients who were recorded as regular smokers, 50 as non-smokers. However, one-third of smokers (21) had given up prior to commencing dialysis, but a further 22 patients never stopped smoking. Other than those who stopped smoking prior to dialysis, the most common time to stop was at the onset of symptoms of cardiovascular disease.

Incidence of vascular disease

Vascular morbidity was present in 62 patients (56% of those for whom data is available) (Table 1.8.). Ischaemic heart disease (IHD) was present in 45 patients, 24 patients had cerebrovascular disease (CVD), and 29 had peripheral vascular disease (PVD), 5 patients had evidence of all three of these pathologies. There was no significant difference in the length of time for which the patients who developed vascular disease compared with those who did not were observed on RRT. However, 66% of those patients who showed no evidence of vascular disease were alive at the end of the study time, compared to 26% of those with vascular disease. Patients developing vascular disease were significantly older at the start of RRT. There was no statistically significant difference between the percentage of men and women affected, 56% and 55%, respectively. Smokers were significantly more likely to develop vascular disease than those who had never smoked; 69% of smokers being affected compared with 43% of non-smokers ($p = 0.005$). Blood pressure control tended to be worse at 0, 5, and 10 years in affected patients, but this trend was only statistically significant for hypertension at the start of RRT; 77% of patients who subsequently developed vascular disease being hypertensive at the start compared to 59% of those who did not develop clinical evidence of vascular disease ($p = 0.04$). Vascular disease was more prevalent in those patients who never received a successful transplant, i.e. those in groups 1 and 2, and least prevalent in patients in group 3 who still had a functioning graft at the end of the study ($p = 0.005$), but there was no significant difference between those patients in group 4 who had returned to dialysis after a failed transplant and the incidence of vascular disease in any of the other groups.

Table 1.8   Vascular morbidity in long-term patients

Vascular disease present	Yes	No
No. of patients (%)	62 (56%)	49 (44%)
Years of RRT observed, mean (range)	16.3 (10.1–29.1)	16.7 (10.1–29.6)
Patients alive at end of study (%)	16 (26)	33 (67), $p < 60; 0.001$
Age ESRD, mean (range)/years	41.0 (21.3–68.0)	32.8 (17.3–57.8) $p < 0.001$
No. of men	36	28
Smokers (%)	43 (69)	21 (43), $p = 0.005$
Hypertension		
At start RRT, No. (%)	48 (77)	29 (59), $p = 0.04$
At 5 years, No. (%)	33 (53)	21 (43)
At 10 years, No. (%)	28 (45)	17 (35)
Treatment modalities		
HD, No. (% of patients in that group)	31 (63)	18 (37)
HD/PD	9 (60)	6 (40)
HD/Tx	6 (38)	10 (62)
HD/Tx/HD	16 (52)	15 (48)

HD, hemodialysis; PD, peritoneal dialysis; Tx, transplant; ESRD, end-stage renal disease; RRT, renal replacement therapy.

Ischemic heart disease   Of the 45 patients who developed ischemic heart disease, 19 had a myocardial infarction, directly resulting in death for 10 of these patients. The average age of onset of IHD was 50.6 years (range 20 to 69 years) and for myocardial infarction it was 58 years; 14 patients were aged less than 60 years when they had a myocardial infarction.

Cerebrovascular disease   In this study cerebrovascular disease appeared to affect more women than men, 28% compared with 19% (not significant). Smokers were not significantly more affected than non-smokers, but in those patients for whom data is available 100% were hypertensive at the start of RRT and were more likely to have remained hypertensive throughout treatment, although with the small numbers involved the only significant effect of hypertension was at the start of RRT, $p = 0.04$. A total of 11 patients had a cerebrovascular accident causing permanent disability, 8 of whom were under 60 years when this occurred. (From the information available in the case records it has not been possible to distinguish ischemic from hemorrhagic strokes.)

Peripheral vascular disease   Peripheral vascular disease (PVD) was evident in 29 patients, but in four of these patients the peripheral vascular disease was secondary to surgery either for vascular access or for transplantation, one patient required a femoral bypass after a failed renal allograft. Where there was no surgical cause for PVD, four patients developed severe disease in that they developed ischemic ulceration or required bypass surgery (three patients) or amputation (one patient). In three cases the main cause of death was given as PVD, and in one other it was a contributing factor in the decision to withdraw from dialysis.

Calcific aortic valve disease   Reliable data on the presence or absence of calcific aortic valve disease was only available for 93 patients, 21 of whom had a gradient across the aortic valve. It was more common in older patients; the average age at the start of dialysis of those who had aortic stenosis (AS) was 42 years compared with 31 years for those who did not ($p = 0.001$). Aortic stenosis was a late complication, the average duration of RRT prior to a confirmed diagnosis being 13 years, range 6 to 23 years.

Musculoskeletal disease (Table 1.9)

The incidence of problems related to musculoskeletal disease and their relationship to dialysis modality and length of time on RRT are shown in Figs 1.2 and 1.3.

Parathyroid surgery

Parathyroidectomy was performed in 82 patients (75% of those for whom information is available), with no significant difference between the different treatment groups. The patients who required parathyroidectomy tended to be younger at the start of RRT than those who did not, but this is only statistically significant for patients in group one, 40.8 years compared to 48.7 ($p = 0.01$). The average duration of RRT prior to parathyroid surgery was approximately 8 years, but the need increased with increasing time on dialysis; in the patients who survived longer than 15 years 90% required surgery compared to 66% of those who survived between 10 and 12 years. Recurrent disease occurred in 26 patients (32%), 16 of whom had further surgery, 4 patients having three operations each.

Table 1.9 Complications related to renal osteodystrophy in long-term patients

	All patients		HD group	
	Yes	No	Yes	No
Parathyroidectomy (PTX)				
No. of patients (%)	82 (75)	27 (25)	34 (72)	13 (28)
ESRD diagnosed, mean age (years)	36.6	39.5	40.8	48.7 ($p = 0.01$)
Duration RRT to 1/1/96, mean (years)	16.6	17.5	15.0	12.9 ($p = 0.01$)
Duration RRT pre-PTX, mean (years)	7.9 (0–20)	—	7.8 (3–17)	—
Recurrent hyperparathyroidism, No. (%)	26 (32)	—	12 (35)	—
Joint pain complained of in clinic				
No. of patients (%)	78 (71)	32 (29)	38 (78)	11 (22)
ESRD diagnosed, mean age (years)	37.7	36.4	43.2	41.9
Duration RRT to 1/1/96, mean (years)	16.9	15.8	15.1	12.8 ($p = 0.01$)
Duration RRT pre-joint pain, mean (years)	8.4 (0–22)	—	7.7 (2–12)	—
Disabling joint disease, No. (%)	17 (22)	—	6 (16)	—
Carpal tunnel syndrome (CTS)				
No. of patients (%)	44 (40)	64 (60)	23 (50)	23 (50)
ESRD diagnosed, mean age (years)	40.3	35.6	44.1	43.1
Duration RRT to 1/1/96, mean (years)	17.7	15.8	16.0	12.7 ($p < 0.001$)
Duration RRT pre-CTS, mean (years)	11.3 (3–20)	—	11.1 (4–18)	—
Bilateral CTS, No. (%)	31 (70)	—	18 (78)	—
Recurrent CTS, No. (%)	13 (30)	—	8 (35)	—

Total no. patients vary in each group as records are not all complete.

Joint pain and disability

In all, 78 patients (71%) complained of joint pain such that it was recorded in their clinic notes. The average time to develop joint pains was 8.4 years, and again incidence increased with increasing duration of treatment so that 90% of patients surviving longer than 15 years were affected. A total of 17 patients developed such severe disabling joint disease that they were unable to continue their activities of daily living unaided. In two patients there was regression of joint disease following transplantation and they were able to go back to work. The most common example of disabling joint disease was bilateral frozen shoulder, but severe cervical spondylosis was also recorded.

Amyloidosis

Carpal tunnel syndrome occurred in 44 patients (40%); it rarely became evident within the first 5 years of treatment, developing on average after about 11 years. Risk increased with increasing time on dialysis. In those patients who received only hemodialysis, more than 90% of patients were affected if they survived longer than 15 years. CTS was bilateral in 70% of patients, and recurred after surgery in 13 patients (30%). Patients who developed carpal tunnel syndrome tended to be older at the start of RRT than those who did not; this was most notable in group 2, 52.2 years compared to 33.4 years ($p = 0.01$). No comment can be made about any protective effect of PD compared to HD with respect to the development of amyloidosis as only four of the patients in this study were on PD for longer than 5 years.

Infections in chronic dialysis patients

In this successful group of long-term survivors on RRT, 868 episodes of infection in 1918 patient-years of treatment were recorded in the patient notes. Of these infections 243 occurred in patients on immunosuppression therapy, usually for a functioning renal transplant, but a small number were on steroid therapy for control of their underlying disease. The focus for the remaining 625 episodes of infection is shown in Table 1.10. As can be seen, nearly half of the recorded episodes related to breach of the mechanical barriers to infection; infected vascular access sites accounted for 19% of all infections and infections directly related to peritoneal dialysis accounting for 29% of all infections. In 62 patient-years of peritoneal dialysis 180 episodes of either peritonitis or exit-site infection were recorded; 121 episodes of respiratory tract infection were recorded, 33 of which were hospital-acquired. Of the 88 community-acquired, respiratory tract infections 43 occurred in patients who were currently smoking or had an underlying diagnosis of chronic obstructive airways disease. In addition, 31 urinary tract infections were recorded, more than a third of which were hospital-acquired.

The infection rates for each 5 years of RRT are shown in Fig. 1.4. There are approximately two episodes of infection recorded for every 5 years on dialysis; this rate does not increase with increasing time on dialysis. Less than half of all recorded infections in the long-term dialysis patients were community-acquired, i.e. less than one infection every 5 years.

Only six episodes of infection were recorded which might be classified as opportunistic infection: episodes of esophageal candidiasis, widespread cutaneous candidiasis, severe fungal nail infection, xanthomonal discitis, and a patient with multiple viral warts who had not to that date been transplanted. We found six dialysis patients who developed herpes zoster. Tuberculosis did not occur in any of the patients on dialysis, although it was found in patients who had a functioning transplant and were consequently immunosuppressed.

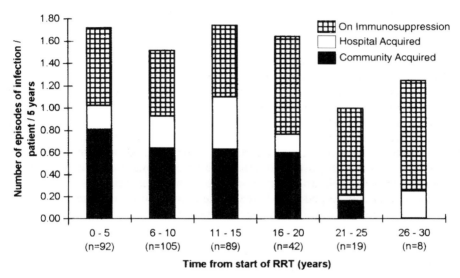

Fig. 1.4 Incidence of all infections, excluding those related to dialysis access.

Table 1.10 Causes of infection in long-term patients

	No. of episodes	% of total
Related to breach of mechanical barriers to infection		
Vascular access	118	19
Peritonitis and exit site	180	29
Other infections		
Respiratory tract	121	19
Urinary tract	31	5
Other bacterial	138	22
Other viral	27	4
Other fungal	10	2
Total	625	100

Mortality from infection

In 14 patients death was directly attributed to infection, two others withdrew from dialysis because of chronic infection; six of the deaths were in patients with a functioning renal transplant: three from pneumonia, two from septicemia, and one from septic pericarditis. In the dialysis patients there were five deaths from pneumonia; in four of these patients community-acquired pneumonia was the primary illness that led to death. The fifth death from pneumonia was in a smoker with severe ischemic heart disease. Of the remainder, one patient died of septicemia and two patients on peritoneal dialysis died of peritonitis.

Chronic liver disease and viral hepatitis

Infections with hepatitis B and C virus have not been included in the discussion so far as they are rarely recorded as episodes of infection at the time they occur, but rather are identified later on routine testing. While testing for hepatitis B status has been available since the start of the chronic hemodialysis program at the CXH, routine testing for hepatitis C has only been available since 1990. As a result of ignorance about this blood-borne virus, many hemodialysis patients were infected from contaminated blood transfusions before 1990. HCV status is known in only 67 of these patients, 27 of whom were positive for HCV antibody; five of these patients developed chronic liver disease. We found that one patient with portal hypertension as a result of HCV infection died secondary to hemorrhage from esophageal varices. A record of HBV status was obtainable for 104 patients, three of whom were positive; none of these patients had evidence of chronic liver disease. Chronic liver disease was present in 11 patients; five, as stated above, were known to be HCV-antibody positive, the remaining six died before 1990 so their HCV status is unknown, HBV status is unknown in two. The recorded diagnoses of chronic liver disease in these six patients are: 'cirrhosis ? cause'; 'lobular hepatitis'; 'hemosiderosis' (two); and 'unknown cause' (two). It is, of course, possible that many of these patients had hepatitis C.

Cancer

A diagnosis of cancer was made in 12 patients, of whom six had not been transplanted. In the six patients who had only received HD and PD, seven primary malignancies were recorded: breast (two); thyroid (two); lung; uterus; and bladder. In the transplanted patients the primary cancers were squamous cell carcinoma (three), breast (two), and adenocarcinoma of unknown primary. Only three of these malignancies were the cause of death in the affected patient. The dialysis patient who had two separate primary cancers—thyroid and bladder—eventually died of a myocardial infarction.

Discussion

The data collected for this study on complications of long-term dialysis is retrospective data obtained mainly from medical case records, and as such may be incomplete compared with prospective data. Even so, useful information about the effects of more than 10 years on dialysis can be obtained.

The patients who have survived more than 10 years' dialysis are a selected group. It is therefore not surprising that the majority of the patients studied had a primary renal disease, such as chronic glomerulonephritis or polycystic kidney disease, rather than a disease associated with a high level of comorbidity, such as diabetes or hypertension. The lack of diabetic patients in these long-term survivors reflects not only the reduced life expectancy of diabetic dialysis patients, shown to be less than half that of non-diabetic dialysis patients (Port *et al.*, 1994) but also the reluctance to accept diabetic patients on to dialysis programs in the UK until the mid-1980s.

The most common cause of death in dialysis patients is from cardiovascular disease (USRDS, 1991). It is unclear whether vascular complications are a complication of the dialysis process or are related to pre-existing vascular disease. Recently, the increasing amount of data emerging about patients who have been on RRT for longer periods has suggested that cardiovascular problems are related to pre-existing disease, i.e. long-standing hypertension and renal failure, and therefore that is the most common cause of death only in those patients who die within a few years of starting dialysis. Thus, in a study by Mailloux *et al.* (1991) the most common causes of death in their patients who had been on dialysis for longer than 10 years were infection and withdrawal from dialysis, compared with their patients who died within 4 years of starting dialysis in whom cardiovascular mortality was more common. In contrast, in our long-term patients the majority of deaths are due to cardiovascular causes, with infections taking second place. This is also the case for the Tassin patients (Chapter 11), although in their patients surviving over 10 years, cardiovascular mortality, while being most common, is less prevalent than it is in our patients, accounting for 33% of deaths compared to 55%.

Vascular disease was common in our patients, especially in those who received only dialysis. This must, in part, reflect the avoidance of patients with pre-existing vascular disease when selecting for transplantation. However, there is some evidence from this study that a working transplant may, in fact, reduce the risk of vascular disease compared to being on dialysis. Over a third of the patients included in the dialysis-only group were transplanted (though unsuccessfully). Second, vascular disease was more common in the group of patients in whom a working transplant failed, affecting 52% compared with 38% of those in whom the graft continues to work, although this difference is not statistically significant.

The prevalence of risk factors for cardiovascular disease was high in our long-term patients. The 1994 NIH consensus statement (Consensus Development Panel, 1994) recommends that the biggest reductions in cardiovascular morbidity in dialysis patients can be made by reducing smoking and controlling blood pressure. Many of our patients were smokers, although a third of them gave up smoking when they became symptomatic with renal failure. Blood pressure control was generally quite poor, about 50% of patients remaining hypertensive or requiring antihypertensive medication throughout their time on dialysis. This is in marked contrast to the patients dialyzed in Tassin described later in this book, where only 2% of dialysis patients require antihypertensive treatment after the first 3 months on dialysis. This may, in part, explain the lower cardiovascular mortality in the Tassin patients who survived for more than 10 years on dialysis. The majority of the patients in this study were chronically anemic because they were dialyzed before the development and widespread use of erythropoietin. Reduction of anemia with the use of erythropoietin has been shown to cause a regression in the elevated left ventricular mass of dialysis patients (Harnett *et al.*, 1995), and may result in reduced cardiac failure and cardiac mortality including sudden deaths.

Only five patients in this sample withdrew from dialysis. In agreement with the findings in the nephrology forum (Port *et al.*, 1994) the reasons for withdrawal have been chronic deterioration in health with severe failure to thrive. In other samples single major events, such as a disabling stroke, have prompted withdrawal in patients who have been on dialysis for many years.

Maintenance hemodialysis was made possible by the invention of Teflon and silastic from which Scribner constructed the external arteriovenous shunt. Despite this, with problems of clotting and infection, vascular access was the Achilles' heel of treatment for the early dialysis patients. Even with the innovation of the Cimino–Brescia fistula, and, more recently, the introduction of synthetic arteriovenous grafts and the development of short- and long-term, in-dwelling central venous catheters, vascular access is still a major cause of morbidity for hemodialysis patients (Hung *et al.*, 1995; Rocco *et al.*, 1996). For reasons of infection or poor drainage, PD catheters, likewise, do not have an infinite life span and also represent a cause of morbidity for PD patients. In this study, operations to create access for dialysis necessitating hospital admission were particularly frequent in the first 5 years of dialysis, and then about once every 5 years. This is in agreement with studies showing that the average life expectancy of a working arteriovenous fistula is around 5 years (Chazzan *et al.*, 1995). However, in the report from Tassin (Chapter 11) the authors state that their mean patency rate for AV fistulas is 7.5 years. In our patients, this good fistula patency rate was only achieved in the home hemodialysis patients. It is clear that throughout their time on hemodialysis patients are often subjected initially to temporary forms of access, because dialysis may be urgently required or because of insufficient resources to create more permanent arteriovenous fistulas in time. As peripheral sites are used up for access and peripheral vessels become stenosed, sites for vascular access become limited to the central veins. Exhaustion of all possible sites for vascular access was the main cause for failure of hemodialysis (Table 1.7) and conversion to peritoneal dialysis. To reduce the morbidity caused by repeated access attempts, the most effective measure would be to ensure that all patients have permanent access functioning at the time they start chronic dialysis. This can only be achieved if patients are referred early to a nephrologist and if there are sufficient operating resources available for access surgery (Rocco *et al.*, 1996). It is also vitally important to take good care of fistulas, since, as shown in our patients, those on home dialysis who needle their own fistulas have less access problems.

In this group of patients there were many attempts at transplantation, half of which failed acutely and a further third that failed after anything from 4 months to 27 years. Cattran and Fenton (1993) describe the poor outcome for patients after a failed renal transplant, with a doubling of mortality for both diabetic and non-diabetic patients.

This study demonstrated that the effects of early failure were worse than those of late graft failure. While renal transplantation can be a source of morbidity for patients on RRT it is also the means of achieving longer survival. It is particularly notable from our patients that all those who survived for more than 25 years have had a working graft for at least part of the time, and in most cases have a currently functioning graft.

Musculoskeletal disease is another major cause of morbidity. The most important pathogenetic factors involved are hyperparathyroidism and dialysis-associated, beta2-microglobulin amyloid deposition. Also involved are abnormal vitamin D metabolism, aluminum toxicity, and age-related osteoporosis (Drüeke, 1995). The manifestations of hyperparathyroidism, both appropriate and autonomous, are joint pains, bony destruction, and pathological fractures. Despite the increasing use of phosphate-binding agents, vitamin-D analogs, and calcium-adjusted dialysis fluid it is still common for the patients to require parathyroidectomy. It is now also recognized that if a patient has developed tertiary hyperparathyroidism, even after total parathyroidectomy, hyperparathyroidism may recur, probably due to seeding of autonomous cells at the time of surgery (Ljutić *et al.*, 1994). Our four patients had three parathyroidectomies, all of which at the time of surgery were judged to be 'total parathyroidectomies'.

Dialysis-related amyloidosis is most commonly manifest as large joint pain, especially of the shoulders, or as carpal tunnel syndrome later progressing to destructive arthropathy and fractures. In this study and in others (Aoike *et al.*, 1995; Bazzi *et al.*, 1995) joint pains were almost ubiquitous after more than 15 years of dialysis. The prevalence of carpal tunnel syndrome also increased with increasing time on dialysis, until it also was ubiquitous after more than 15 years. The development of more 'bio-compatible' dialysis membranes may provide a means of reducing the severity of dialysis amyloid, but this is not yet fully established (Zingraff and Drüeke 1991; Aoike *et al.*, 1995).

Another recognized complication of the hypercalcemia associated with autonomous hyperparathyroidism is calcific valvular heart disease. Studies have shown that a significant gradient across the aortic valve may be demonstrated in up to 10% of dialysis patients. Accelerated aortic stenosis has been described in dialysis patients, and this diagnosis should be considered in any dialysis patient with rapidly worsening angina (Maher *et al.*, 1987; Raine, 1994). In our patients, aortic stenosis was a late complication occurring after more than 10 years on dialysis, affecting 20% of patients for whom information, mainly echocardiographic, was available.

There is good clinical and *in-vitro* evidence that dialysis patients are chronically immunosuppressed (Descamps-Latscha and Herbelin, 1993), but, as discussed in the chapter by Khan, in practice dialysis patients in many ways do not behave as if they are immunosuppressed. They do not appear to develop more infections with increasing time on dialysis, nor do they frequently suffer from infections that would normally be classed as opportunistic. There is no doubt that they are prone to episodes of infection, but, as Khan states, this might easily be explained by the fact that the normal mechanical barriers to infection are frequently breached in these patients and that they are more frequently exposed to pathogens by virtue of their spending so much time in hospital. Indeed, nearly half of the infections recorded in our long-term patients were infections related to dialysis access, and thus breach of the normal mechanical barriers to infection. Of the remainder, more than half of the infections were in patients who were concomitantly receiving immunosuppressive treatment or who were in hospital at the time. The incidence of infections which would normally be described as opportunistic was very low, and the only episodes of tuberculosis recorded in these long-term survivors were in patients on immunosuppressive drugs with a functioning renal allograft. In agreement with Chapter 3, it seems that while infections contribute significantly to the morbidity and mortality of chronic dialysis patients there is scope for reducing this morbidity and mortality by reducing the time spent in hospital and by improving the aseptic techniques used when dialyzing patients. Many improvements have already occurred since these patients started treatment, especially with respect to peritoneal dialysis and the development of disconnect systems (Bazzato *et al.*, 1984).

Hepatitis remains a problem in long-term dialysis. HCV is a major cause of chronic liver disease in dialysis patients (Knudsen, 1993). Half of the patients in this study who developed chronic liver disease were HCV-antibody positive and in the remainder it is possible that HCV was the causative agent, although this cannot be proven. It is clear that prior to the ability to test for HCV, its spread was unchecked. The principal route of spread was by blood transfusion, but there is also evidence of nosocomial spread (Jadoul, 1996; Pinto dos Santos *et al.*, 1996). This is discussed in greater detail in Chapter 14.

Cancer was relatively rare in these patients. There were only 13 primary cancers in nearly 2000 patient-years on RRT, and notably none of these primary cancers were diseases of the urogenital tract, e.g. renal cell carcinoma.

It is clear that for long-term surviving patients on renal replacement therapy a successful transplant can reduce the incidence of some dialysis-associated complications, and that morbidity related to renal osteodystrophy and amyloidosis at present represent a virtual certainty for patients on hemodialysis for longer than 15 years. It is possible that by measuring the adequacy of dialysis together with evidence from centers like that in Tassin, where a very high level of dialysis adequacy is achieved, may encourage the use of practices that reduce the incidence of even these seemingly inevitable complications. From looking at the long-term survivors who are still alive, it is evident that most of the patients who do so well on dialysis are a select group with near-normal albumin and hemoglobin values and generally with good blood pressure control even if this requires regular medication. However, it is testimony to the success of dialysis that even after more than 10 years of treatment some patients continue to work and do indeed lead a 'full and happy life'.

References

Aoike, I., Gejyo, F., Arakawa, M., and Niigata Research Programme for β_2-M Removal Membrane (1995). Learning from the Japanese registry: how will we prevent long-term complications? *Nephrology, Dialysis, Transplantation*, **10** (Suppl. 7), 7–15.

Bazzato, G., Coli, U., Landini, S., *et al.* (1984). The double bag system for CAPD reduces the peritonitis rate. *Trans-American Society of Artificial Internal Organs*, **30**, 690–2.

Bazzi, C., Arrigo, G., Luciani, L., *et al.* (1995). Clinical features of 24 patients on regular hemo-dialysis treatment (RDT) for 16–23 years in a single unit. *Clinical Nephrology*, **44**, 96–107.

Cattran, D. C., and Fenton, S. S. A. (1993). Contemporary management of renal failure: outcome of the failed allograft recipient. *Kidney International*, **43** (Suppl. 41), S36–S39.

Chazzan, J. A., London, M. R., and Pono, L. M. (1995). Long-term survival of vascular accesses in a large chronic hemodialysis population. *Nephron*, **69**, 228–33.

Consensus Development Conference Panel (1994). Morbidity and mortality of renal dialysis: an NIH consensus conference statement. *Annals of Internal Medicine*, **121**(1), 62–70.

de Wardener, H. E. (1966). Some ethical and economic problems associated with intermittent haemodialysis. *Ciba Foundation Symposium on Ethics in Medical Progress*, Ed. Wolstenholme, G.E.W. and O'Connor, M. published by Jr A Churchill, London, pp. 104–18.

Descamps-Latscha, B. and Herbelin, A. (1993). Long-term dialysis and cellular immunity: a critical survey. *Kidney International*, **43** (Suppl. 41), S135–S142.

Drüeke, T. B. (1995). Will bone disease still remain one of the most serious complications in dialysis patients. *Nephrology, Dialysis, Transplantation*, **10** (Suppl. 7), 16–19.

Harnett, J. D., Kent, G. M., Foley, R. N., and Parfrey, P. S. (1995). Cardiac function and hematocrit level. *American Journal of Kidney Diseases*, **25** (Suppl. 1), S3–S7.

Hung, K. Y., Tsai, T. J., Yen, C. J., and Yen, T. S. (1995). Infection associated with double lumen catheterization for temporary haemodialysis: experience of 168 cases. *Nephrology, Dialysis, Transplantation*, **10**, 247–51.

Jadoul, M. (1996). Transmission routes of HCV infection in dialysis. *Nephrology, Dialysis, Transplantation*, **11** (Suppl. 4), 36–8.

Knudsen, F., Wantzin, P., Rasmussen, K., *et al.* (1993). Hepatitis C in dialysis patients: relationship to blood transfusions, dialysis and liver disease. *Kidney International*, **43**, 1353–6.

Ljutić, D., Cameron, J. S., Ogg, C. S., Turner, C., Hicks, J. A., and Owen, W. J. (1994). Long-term follow-up after parathyroidectomy without parathyroid reimplantation in chronic renal failure. *Quarterly Journal of Medicine*, **87**, 685–92.

Maher, E. R., Young, G., Smyth-Walsh, B., Pugh, S., and Curtis, J. R. (1987). Aortic and mitral valve calcification in patients with end-stage renal disease. *Lancet*, **2**, 875–7.

Mailloux, L. U., Bellucci, A. G., Wilkes, B. M., *et al.* (1991). Mortality in dialysis patients: analysis of the causes of death. *American Journal of Kidney Diseases*, **18**, 326–35.

Pinto dos Santos, J., Loureiro, A., Cendroroglo Neto, M., and Pereira, B. J. G. (1996). Impact of dialysis room and reuse strategies on the incidence of hepatitis C virus infection in haemodialysis units. *Nephrology, Dialysis, Transplantation*, **11**, 2017–22.

Port, F. K., Cohen, J. J., Harrington, J. T., Madias, N. E., and Zusman, C. J. (1994). Nephrology forum: morbidity and mortality in dialysis patients. *Kidney International*, **46**, 1728–37.

Raine, A. E. G. (1994). Acquired aortic stenosis in dialysis patients. *Nephron*, **68**, 159–68.

Rocco, M. V., Bleyer, A. J., and Burkart, J. M. (1996). Utilization of inpatient and outpatient resources for the management of hemodialysis access complications. *American Journal of Kidney Diseases*, **28**, 250–6.

USRDS (1991). *US Renal Data System: Annual Data Report*, August 1991, National Institute of Diabetes and Digestive and Kidney Diseases. National Institutes of Health, Bethesda, MD.

Zingraff, J., and Drüeke, T. (1991). Can the nephrologist prevent dialysis-related amyloidosis? *American Journal of Kidney Disease*, **18**, 1–11.

PART II
Medical complications

2

Complications of long-term dialysis: cardiovascular complications and cardiac risk-factor interventions

Robert N. Foley and Patrick S. Parfrey

Introduction—the burden of disease

Pericarditis frequently heralded the demise of patients with end-stage renal disease (ESRD), before the advent of renal replacement therapy (Schreiner and Maher, 1961). Cardiomyopathy, which was remarked on less frequently, was felt to reflect hypertension and underlying vascular disease; some authors speculated on the existence of a specific uremic cardiomyopathy, a concept that has since gained widespread acceptance (Schreiner and Maher, 1961). In the early days of chronic dialysis it became evident that perhaps 30–40% of all deaths were due to cardiac disease (Drukker *et al.*, 1966; Brunner *et al.*, 1972), a noteworthy burden of disease, considering that in this era patients selected for maintenance dialysis therapy were young and largely free of comorbid illness. In 1974 the Seattle group reported that 60% of deaths in their dialysis program were due to cardiovascular disease, and proposed that uremia led to accelerated atherosclerosis (Lindner *et al.*, 1974). This latter contention remains to be proved or refuted with any degree of finality.

Even now, cardiovascular disease accounts for approximately half of all deaths in dialysis patients. This figure is remarkably stable in different reports and seems to apply to almost all groups of dialysis patients, regardless of age, gender, ethnicity, nationality, or primary renal disease (Agadoa and Eggers, 1995; Disney, 1995; Fenton *et al.*, 1995; Jacobs and Selwood, 1995; Mallick *et al.*, 1995; Teraoka *et al.*, 1995). Cardiac morbidity is also common in end-stage renal disease; in the Canadian Hemodialysis Morbidity Study, the likelihood of admission was approximately 10% per year for both ischemic heart disease and cardiac failure (Churchill *et al.*, 1992). Cardiovascular disease is a major consumer of resources in dialysis programs. In a recent study of 1572 dialysis patients, peripheral vascular disease, angina pectoris, and congestive heart failure were all independent predictors of the number of days patients spent in hospital (Rocco *et al.*, 1996). The psychosocial impact of cardiovascular disease in dialysis patients has never been formally evaluated, but is likely to be enormous.

As one would expect, cardiovascular problems are more likely in patients starting long-term dialysis therapy who have pre-existent cardiovascular disease. This is true for many patients beginning renal replacement therapy; in the United States of America, for example, it was estimated that 41% of patients starting dialysis therapy had a prior history of ischemic heart disease; a similar percentage had experienced an episode of cardiac failure (USRDS, 1992). Preclinical cardiomyopathy was very common in our patient cohort when they started dialysis treatment: on baseline echocardiography left ventricular hypertrophy was present in 74%, left ventricular dilatation in 32%, and systolic dysfunction in 15% (Foley *et al.*, 1995*a*). Several other investigators reported that echocardiographic abnormalities are very common in ESRD patients (Hutting *et al.*, 1988*a*; Parfrey *et al.*, 1990; Morris *et al.*, 1993*a*; Greaves *et al.*, 1994*a*). The burden of peripheral vascular disease and cerebrovascular disease in patients starting dialysis therapy is not as well studied. At our institution 6% of patients starting maintenance dialysis therapy between 1980 and 1990 had either a gangrenous extremity, abdominal aortic surgery, or arterial bypass surgery in the previous 6 months (Foley *et al.*, 1994). It is likely that less severe manifestations of peripheral vascular disease are even more common. A recent non-invasive study using B-mode ultrasound suggested that the average dialysis patient has thicker carotid and femoral arteries, indirect evidence of more severe atherosclerosis than age- and sex-matched controls from the general population (Kawagishi *et al.*, 1995).

It is clear that the burden of cardiac disease in dialysis patients can only be partly explained by pre-existent disease. In our studies, over a mean follow-up of 41 months, 12% of patients developed new-onset ischemic heart disease (Parfrey *et al.*, 1996), while 24% went on to have a first episode of cardiac failure (Harnett *et al.*, 1995). Clinically defined cardiac failure was particularly deadly; almost two-thirds of all deaths in this study were preceded by admission for cardiac failure. A frequently raised issue is: is this true cardiac failure or simple fluid overload? This is often difficult to resolve with a routine clinical examination and a chest radiograph. It is likely that any clinical definition will include both types of patients. If one theorizes that patients with simple fluid overload are not at increased risk, one is left with the inescapable conclusion that true cardiac failure has an appalling prognosis, which is likely to have been underestimated in our studies.

Several recent studies confirm that each of the different clinical manifestations of cardiovascular disease is a strong and independent predictor of death in ESRD (USRDS, 1992; Foley *et al.*, 1995*a*; Harnett *et al.*, 1995; Parfrey *et al.*, 1996). The poor survival of patients with cardiac failure starting ESRD therapy is shown in Fig. 2.1 (Harnett *et al.*, 1995). Ischemic heart disease was also associated with reduced survival (Parfrey *et al.*, 1996*a*), but this effect was not independent of concomitant cardiac failure (Fig. 2.2) (Foley *et al.*, 1995*a*). Echocardiographic LV disorders—concentric LV hypertrophy, LV dilatation and systolic dysfunction—predispose to both ischemic heart disease (Parfrey *et al.*, 1996) and cardiac failure in dialysis patients (Fig. 2.3). Concentric LV hypertrophy and LV dilatation are associated with mortality after a lag phase of about 2 years, while systolic dysfunction is associated with increased mortality throughout follow-up (Fig. 2.4) (Foley *et al.*, 1995*b*).

In the remainder of this chapter, we review risk factors for cardiac disease in end-stage renal disease (Table 2.1) and discuss the appropriateness of different interventions. We believe that echocardiographic abnormalities are 'disease states', as opposed to 'risk factors'. This opinion is based on outcome: in our study it was clear that the following sequence of events took place: risk factor–echocardiographic abnormality–cardiac failure–death. The associations between echocardiographic abnormality and

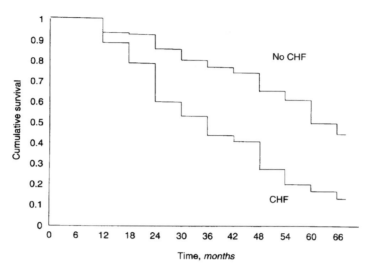

Fig. 2.1 The unadjusted survival of dialysis patients, who survived at least 6 months after starting ESRD therapy, comparing those with and without heart failure on starting dialysis. CHF, congestive heart failure. (Reproduced from Harnett *et al.*, 1995; with permission.)

subsequent ischemic heart disease and cardiac failure were strong. The baseline echocardiographic classification, based on left ventricular cavity volume and mass, was by far the greatest baseline predictor of death after 2 years on dialysis therapy (Foley *et al.*, 1995*b*). Other investigators have demonstrated an independent association between left ventricular mass and mortality in dialysis patients (Silberberg *et al.*, 1989).

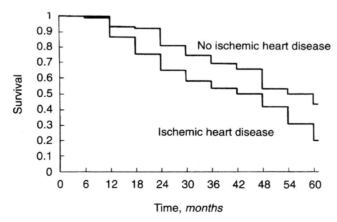

Fig. 2.2 The unadjusted survival of dialysis patients, who survived at least 6 months after starting ESRD treatment, comparing those with and without ischemic heart disease when starting dialysis. (Reproduced from Parfrey *et al.*, 1996*a*; with permission.)

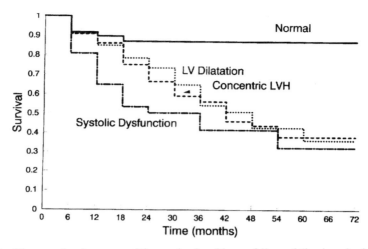

Fig. 2.3   Time to development of first episode of heart failure, following the initiation of dialysis therapy, in patients with normal echocardiogram (—), concentric LV hypertrophy (− − −), LV dilatation (. . .), and systolic dysfunction (− · −). (Reproduced from Parfrey *et al.*, 1996*b*, with persmission.)

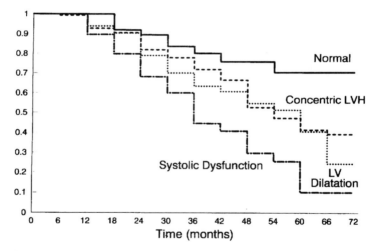

Fig. 2.4   Survival following the initiation of dialysis therapy of patients with normal echocardiogram, (—), concentric LV hypertrophy (− − −), LV dilatation (. . .), and systolic dysfunction (− · −). (Reproduced from Parfrey *et al.*, 1996*b*, with permission.)

Cardiovascular risk factors in long-term dialysis patients

Dialysis patients tend to be 'captive', by and large; they have regular clinical and laboratory tests; clinical events such as angina pectoris, myocardial infarction, cardiac failure, and death are very common. These features should make the clinical epidemiology of cardiac disease in ESRD attractive to study. In spite of these attractive features, the clinical epidemiology of cardiac disease in end-stage renal disease is in its infancy. Without ESRD-specific information, dialysis physicians have targeted general population-based risk factors, typified by those identified by the Framingham Study. In this section we will appraise the evidence that Framingham-type variables, like age, diabetes, hypertension, smoking, and dyslipidemias, are risk factors for cardiac disease in ESRD patients (Table 2.1 A); we will then examine the role of factors related to the uremic state, or its therapy (Table 2.1 B).

Table 2.1   Risk factors for cardiac disease in ESRD

A. *Framingham-type risk factors*
Age
Diabetes mellitus
Smoking
Hypertension
Dyslipidemia

B. *Uremic risk factors*
Anemia
Hyperparathyroidism
Uremia
Malnutrition
Mode of renal replacement therapy

Framingham-type risk factors

Age

Most epidemiological studies have implicated age as a predictor of mortality in ESRD patients. In our studies, age was independently associated with echocardiographic abnormalities, *de-novo* ischemic heart disease, *de-novo* cardiac failure, cardiac mortality, and overall mortality (Foley *et al.*, 1995*a, b*; Harnett *et al.*, 1995; Parfrey *et al.*, 1996). In the non-uremic general population, the effects of aging on the heart include increases in myocyte size, rates of degenerative change, fibrosis, loss of myoctyes, amyloidosis, and calcification (Yin, 1980; Wei, 1992). Older age increases the risk of coronary artery disease in the general public (Kannel *et al.*, 1960; Castelli and Anderson, 1986). The vascular changes associated with old age include atheroma deposition, increased intimal heterogeneity, and subendothelial hardening (Yin, 1980; Wei, 1992). Age has been associated with arteriographic coronary artery disease in the ESRD population as a whole (Rostand *et al.*, 1984) and in diabetic patients without symptomatic ischemic heart disease (Manske *et al.*, 1993).

Diabetes mellitus

In many countries diabetic nephropathy is the commonest cause of incident ESRD. It is widely recognized that this patient group is at a very high risk of cardiovascular disease. Many previous studies have excluded diabetics, based on the quite reasonable opinion that risk factors may be different in diabetics and non-diabetics. There is a glaring disparity in the amount of clinical research on diabetics with nephropathy before and after the start of renal replacement therapy. The natural history and risk factors of cardiovascular disease in diabetic dialysis patients need to be prioritized. In our study, diabetes was independently associated with concentric LV hypertrophy on baseline echocardiography (odds ratio 2.4) (Foley *et al.*, 1995*b*), the development of *de-novo* ischemic heart disease (relative risk 4.0) (Parfrey *et al.*, 1996), overall mortality (relative risk 2.0), and mortality after 2 years (relative risk 1.9) (Foley *et al.*, 1995*a*). These results suggest that much of the cardiac disease seen in diabetic ESRD patients is new and possibly preventable.

There is evidence for a specific diabetic cardiomyopathy in patients without ESRD, manifested by left ventricular diastolic dysfunction, which is believed to be caused by microvascular coronary disease (Schultz, 1876; Blumental *et al.*, 1960; Zoneraich and Silverman, 1978; Shapiro *et al.*, 1981*a*, *b*; Theusen *et al.*, 1988; Galderisi *et al.*, 1991; Grossmann *et al.*, 1992; van Hoeven and Factor, 1990). Left ventricular hypertrophy is found more frequently in hypertensive diabetics than hypertensive non-diabetics (Grossmann *et al.*, 1992). In an autopsy study, hypertensive diabetic hearts were heavier and more fibrotic than diabetic non-hypertensive and hypertensive non-diabetic hearts (van Hoeven and Factor, 1990). Greaves *et al.*, (1994*a*) have reported an independent association between the presence of diabetic nephropathy and left ventricular hypertrophy.

Diabetes mellitus is an independent risk factor for the development of coronary artery disease in the general population, quite apart from the large burden of other risk factors, such as hypertension and dyslipoproteinemia (Kannel and McGee, 1979; Valsania *et al.*, 1991). Our study defined ischemic heart disease on the basis of clinical symptoms; such an approach is highly likely to underestimate the degree of coronary artery disease because there is a very marked prevalence of silent ischemic heart disease in diabetic ESRD patients. It has been estimated that one-third of asymptomatic diabetic patients on dialysis therapy have 50% or more stenosis of at least one coronary artery (Weinrauch *et al.*, 1978; Braun *et al.*, 1984; Rostand *et al.*, 1984; Lorber *et al.*, 1987). This prevalence rises markedly with age. Manske *et al.* (1993) reported that 88% of asymptomatic diabetics undergoing pretransplant screening coronary angiography had coronary artery stenosis. In patients under 45 years of age, only those with each of the following characteristics—diabetes less than 5 years, normal ST segments on arteriography, and a smoking history of less than 5 pack-years—could be predicted not to have angiographic coronary artery disease with any degree of confidence (sensitivity 97% and negative predictive accuracy 96%). These latter studies are probably subject to unavoidable selection bias; it is also probable that the true prevalence of asymptomatic coronary artery disease is much higher when the diabetic-ESRD population is considered in its entirety. Several basic questions need to be answered:

1. Does uremia accelerate the vasculopathy of diabetics?
2. Can reversible risk factors, specific for uremic diabetics, be identified?
3. What are the differences in the risk factors and natural history of cardiovascular disease in non-insulin-dependent and insulin-dependent diabetes mellitus?

Smoking

Smoking is a powerful risk factor for coronary artery disease in the general population, approximately doubling the risk of cardiovascular disease (Kannel, 1981). In the
USRDS Special Study of Case Mix Severity smoking independently increased mortality by 26% in hemodialysis patients (USRDS, 1992). Smoking appears to be especially lethal in diabetics with ESRD, in whom it more than doubles mortality rates
(McMillan *et al.*, 1990). In the study of Kawagishi *et al.*, (1995), smoking was independently associated with greater intima-media thickness in both the femoral and
carotid arterial systems.

Hypertension

Hypertension is a well-established risk factor for left ventricular hypertrophy, coronary artery disease, stroke, and death in the general population (Kannel, 1975).
Hypertension is very common in ESRD populations (Weidmann and Beretta-Picoli,
1983; Paganini *et al.*, 1984; Ritz *et al.*, 1985). It has been widely held that hypertension is a
major cause of mortality in dialysis patients (Degoulet *et al.*, 1982; Neff *et al.*, 1983;
Charra *et al.*, 1992*a*; Fernandez *et al.*, 1992; Ritz and Koch, 1993). There is very little
controlled evidence that directly supports this contention: in fact two very large epidemiological studies have suggested that low (Lowrie and Lew, 1990; USRDS, 1992),
not high, blood pressure is independently associated with mortality in dialysis
patients. Another recent study suggested that the absence of hypertension predicted
more hospitalization days (Rocco *et al.*, 1996). Taken at face value, this inverse association between blood pressure and mortality and morbidity, suggests that we are
overtreating hypertension in our dialysis patients. In our patient cohort, mean arterial
blood pressure levels were 101 ± 11 mmHg. There was an inverse relationship between
blood pressure levels and mortality, with an (adjusted) increase in mortality of 22% for
each 10 mmHg in mean arterial blood pressure. However, within this blood pressure
range, rising blood pressure was independently associated with an increase in LV mass
index and cavity volume on follow-up echocardiography, *de-novo* ischemic heart disease, and *de-novo* cardiac failure (Table 2.2). These effects were apparent even within a
range of blood pressure considered to be 'normotensive'. It was apparent in this
patient cohort that the inverse association between blood pressure and mortality was
a statistical epiphenomenon, and was due to the large burden of cardiac failure, a very
lethal occurrence, in whom *low* blood pressure was the single greatest predictor of
subsequent death. These data strongly suggest that a lower blood pressure is highly
desirable in dialysis patients, principally because it decreases the likelihood of cardiac
failure (Foley *et al.*, 1996*a*).

The majority of ESRD patients receive antihypertensive medication. There are no
trials to guide our choice of agent(s) in ESRD patients. In our study ($n = 433$, followed
for a mean duration of 41 months), patients received an average of 1.2 different agents;
calcium channel blockers (3147 patient-months) were the most frequently used
agents, followed by beta-blockers (2707 patient-months), ACE-inhibitors (1546
patient-months), vasodilators (1457 patient-months), and centrally acting agents (520
patient-months). There was a large increase in calcium blocker use during the course

of this study, a trend which has been seen in the general public (Manolio *et al.*, 1995). The use of calcium channel blockers for the treatment of hypertension has come under public scrutiny, based on observational data that showed an excessive incidence of myocardial infarction and mortality compared with other antihypertensive agents (Furberg *et al.*, 1995; Psaty *et al.*, 1995). Clearly, randomized controlled trials are needed to determine:

1. What target blood pressures are appropriate in different subgroups of ESRD patients?
2. What agents, and groups of agents should be used?
3. How should we use them, given that both volume-related hypertension, which is only adequately treated by the achievement of euvolemia, and symptomatic hypotension are so common in dialysis patients?

Table 2.2   Association between blood pressure (the effect of a rise in mean arterial blood pressure level of 10 mmHg) and echocardiographic and clinical outcomes in the combined group of hemodialysis and peritoneal dialysis patients[a]

Outcome	Odds ratio (p)
Normal LV (reference category)	—
Concentric left ventricular hypertrophy	1.48 (0.020)
Left ventricular dilatation	1.48 (0.063)
Systolic dysfunction	No association
	β (p)
Change in left ventricular:	
Mass index (g/m^2)	5.4 (0.027)
Cavity volume (ml/m^2)	4.3 (0.048)
Fractional shortening (%)	No association
	Relative risk (p)
De-novo ischemic heart disease	1.39 (0.051)
De-novo cardiac failure	1.44 (0.007)
Death	0.82 (0.009)

[a]The covariates entered in each multivariate analysis were age, diabetes mellitus, ischemic heart disease (excluded for the outcomes *de-novo* and recurrent ischemic heart disease) as well as the average monthly mean arterial blood pressure, serum albumin, and hemoglobin level before the index event (From Foley *et al.*, 1996a).

Dyslipidemia

Elevated LDL, decreased high-density lipoprotein (HDL), an elevated ratio of total cholesterol to HDL cholesterol, and high lipoprotein(a) levels are associated with coronary artery disease in the general population (Kannel, 1983, 1985; Castelli *et al.*, 1986; Dahlen *et al.*, 1986). It is not clear whether high triglyceride levels are associated with coronary artery disease, although recent evidence suggests that hypertriglyceridemia may be an additional risk factor when it coexists with a high LDL to HDL cholesterol ratio (Assmann and Schulte, 1992).

Dialysis patients have both quantitative and qualitative lipid disturbances. High triglyceride levels and decreased HDL levels are seen in both hemodialysis and peritoneal dialysis patients, while peritoneal dialysis patients also tend to have high LDL levels (Shapiro, 1992; Toto *et al.*, 1993). Several studies have shown that ESRD patients have higher lipoprotein Lp(a) levels than the general population (Parra *et al.*, 1987; Murphy *et al.*, 1992; Auguet *et al.*, 1993; Hirata *et al.*, 1993; Okura *et al.*, 1993; Thillet *et al.*, 1993; Webb *et al.*, 1993). The qualitative abnormalities seen in ESRD patients include:

(1) a defect in postprandial lipid disposal, which exposes the vasculature to high chylomicron remnant concentrations;
(2) elevated intermediate density lipoprotein levels;
(3) increased heterogeneity of LDL and HDL apoproteins;
(4) abnormalities of size and composition of LDL and HDL particles;
(5) increased LDL susceptibility to oxidation; and
(6) altered cell surface LDL epitope recognition (Joven *et al.*, 1992; Weintraub *et al.*, 1992; Reade *et al.*, 1993; Maggi *et al.*, 1994).

In general, the design of studies relating outcome to lipid status in ESRD has been suboptimal. The situation is made more difficult by the observation that low serum cholesterol levels, which probably reflect malnutrition, may be associated with mortality in dialysis patients (Lowrie and Lew, 1990). Recent studies, however, have associated dyslipidemia with cardiac death in diabetic ESRD patients (Tschope *et al.*, 1993*a*, *b*), lipoprotein(a) levels with cardiovascular disease (Cressman *et al.*, 1992), and vascular access loss (Goldwasser *et al.*, 1993) in ESRD patients. It remains to be demonstrated whether aggressive therapy of dyslipidemia has an impact on cardiovascular outcomes in ESRD.

Anemia

Anemia is an independent contributor to the cardiac abnormalities seen in dialysis patients. In our study, which spanned the introduction of recombinant human erythropoietin (HEPO) mean ($\pm$ standard deviation) hemoglobin levels were 88 ± 15 g/l. Within this range a fall in hemoglobin level was independently associated with LV dilatation on follow-up echocardiography, the development of *de-novo* cardiac failure, and overall mortality (Table 2.3). This effect was greater in hemodialysis patients than peritoneal dialysis patients, possibly because the latter group had higher mean hemoglobin levels while on dialysis therapy (9.6 ± 1.5 *vs.* 8.4 ± 1.4 g/dl, $p < 0.0001$) (Foley *et al.*, 1996*b*). Other epidemiological studies have associated anemia and left ventricular dilatation and/or left ventricular hypertrophy on echocardiography (Hutting *et al.*, 1988*b*, 1990; Greaves *et al.*, 1994*b*). A number of other investigators have noted an independent association between anemia and mortality (Lowrie *et al.*, 1994; Yang *et al.*, 1996). In the study of Yang *et al.* (1996) each 1% fall in hematocrit was independently associated with a 14% increase in mortality within a hematocrit range of $26 \pm 5\%$. Lowrie *et al.* (1994), in a very large group of hemodialysis patients, also showed a stepwise increase in mortality as hematocrit levels fell progressively below 30%; on a cautionary note, however, mortality also increased as hematocrits climbed above 35%.

There have been several studies examining the effect of partial correction of anemia with rHEPO on echocardiographic abnormalities. Most of these have been before–

after surveys of small numbers of patients, without an untreated control group. In spite of these limitations, the studies have uniformly shown that partial correction of anemia decreases hypoxic vasodilatation, increases peripheral resistance, reduces cardiac output, and leads to a partial reversal of left ventricular dilatation and hypertrophy (London *et al.*, 1989; Low *et al.*, 1989; Canella *et al.*, 1990; Macdougall *et al.*, 1990; Silberberg *et al.*, 1990; Low-Friedrich *et al.*, 1991; Pascual *et al.*, 1991; Tagawa *et al.*, 1991; Goldberg *et al.*, 1992; Martinez-Vea *et al.*, 1992; Fellner *et al.*, 1993; Morris *et al.*, 1993*b*; Rogerson *et al.*, 1993). None of the published literature to date has had adequate power to test the hypothesis that improvement of echocardiographic parameters will reduce cardiac morbidity or mortality. Currently, there are several ongoing clinical trials to assess the risks and benefits of complete normalization of the hematocrit in ESRD patients. Whether complete correction of anemia leads to further regression of these abnormalities as well as the cost of such an approach—in terms of finances, hypertension (Winnearls *et al.*, 1986; Eschbach *et al.*, 1987), and vascular access loss (Winnearls *et al.*, 1986; Casati *et al.*, 1987; Eschbach *et al.*, 1987; Paganini *et al.*, 1989; Sundal and Kaeser, 1989; Canadian Erythropoietin Study Group, 1990; Churchill *et al.*, 1994)—are areas of major current interest.

Table 2.3   Association between anemia (the effect of a fall in mean hemoglobin level of 10 g/l) and echocardiographic and clinical outcomes in the combined group of hemodialysis and peritoneal dialysis patients[a]

Outcome	Odds ratio (*p*)
Normal LV (reference category)	—
Concentric left ventricular hypertrophy	No association
Left ventricular dilatation	1.42 (0.018)
Systolic dysfunction	No association
	Relative risk (*p*)
De-novo ischemic heart disease	No association
De-novo cardiac failure	1.28 (0.017)
Death	1.14 (0.024)

[a]The covariates entered in each multivariate analysis were age, diabetes mellitus, ischemic heart disease (excluded for the outcomes *de-novo* and recurrent ischemic heart disease) as well as the average monthly mean arterial blood pressure, serum albumin, and hemoglobin level before the index event. (From Foley *et al.*, 1996*b*.)

A randomized, controlled clinical trial of the normalization of hemoglobin with erythropoietin in hemodialysis patients who had symptomatic cardiac disease was prematurely stopped in the USA, because the intervention group had a higher mortality and vascular access loss when compared to a control group in whom anemia was partially corrected. This suggests that the target hemoglobin level for erythropoietin therapy in dialysis patients with symptomatic cardiac disease should be 100–110 g/litre. The target hemoglobin level for patients without symptomatic cardiac disease is unclear, particularly as this group of patients may develop anemia-induced cardiomyopathy, which may predispose to earlier death.

Abnormal calcium–phosphate homeostasis

In our patient cohort, hypocalcemia was strongly associated with ischemic heart disease, even after adjusting for age, diabetes, blood pressure, hemoglobin, and several other covariates. The effect was seen in both peritoneal dialysis and hemodialysis patients, and was only partly explained by the relationship between mean serum calcium and time spent on dialysis therapy (Foley *et al.*, 1996*c*). Another group has shown that low calcium levels are independently associated with mortality in a very large cross-section of dialysis patients (Lowrie and Lew, 1990). The interpretation of these data is difficult without information on parathyroid hormone levels. Hypocalcemia induces hyperparathyroidism, which leads to intracellular calcium overload (Massry and Smogorzweski, 1994), followed by profound disturbances of myocardial bioenergetics and myocardial ischemia in experimental models (Raine *et al.*, 1993), and possibly to LV hypertrophy (Stefenelli *et al.*, 1993). In the study of Kawagishi *et al.* (1995) high phosphorus and parathyroid hormone levels were independently associated with arterial thickening in hemodialysis patients. In rats, calcitriol and a synthetic analog inhibit smooth muscle cell growth and enhance the production of prostacyclin by the vasculature, effects that would be expected to protect against atherosclerosis (McCarthy *et al.*, 1989; Inoue *et al.*, 1992). Hypocalcemia and hyperparathyroidism have been associated with reduced activities of the lipoprotein-regulating enzymes HTGL and Lecithin–Cholestorol amino transferase (LCAT) (Shoji *et al.*, 1992). These preliminary data suggest that maintaining a normal calcium–phosphate balance may benefit the cardiovascular system as much as the skeletal system of dialysis patients.

Uremic risk factors

Uremia and malnutrition

Malnutrition and dialysis intensity have been shown by several authors to be perhaps the greatest predictors of outcome in ESRD patients (Acchiardo *et al.*, 1983; Gotch and Sargent, 1985; Held *et al.*, 1991; Charra *et al.*, 1992*b*; Iseki *et al.*, 1993; Owen *et al.*, 1993; Collins *et al.*, 1994; Kopple, 1994; Lowrie *et al.*, 1994; Parker *et al.*, 1994; Spiegel and Breyer, 1994; CANUSA, 1996; Yang *et al.*, 1996). In these studies the relationship between hypoalbuminemia and death was particularly strong; this observation, and the observation that cardiovascular disease far overshadows any other cause of death in ESRD, suggest that some of the adverse impacts of malnutrition might be mediated via cardiac disease. Low serum albumin levels are independently associated with coronary heart disease in the general population (Phillips *et al.*, 1989; Kuller *et al.*, 1991; Gillum and Makuc, 1992; Corti *et al.*, 1996). The mechanism for this effect is unknown. It has been suggested that vascular injury can lead to increased vascular permeability and then to hypoalbuminemia, suggesting that low albumin levels are a result of vascular injury and not vice versa (Fleck *et al.*, 1985). In our study mean serum albumin levels were 39 ± 4 g/l in hemodialysis patients, compared with 35 ± 5 g/l in peritoneal dialysis patients ($p < 0.0001$). Among hemodialysis patients, each 10 g/l fall in mean serum albumin was independently associated with the development of *de-novo* and recurrent cardiac failure, *de-novo* and recurrent ischemic heart disease, cardiac

mortality, and overall mortality. Among PD patients, hypoalbuminemia was associated with progressive LV dilatation, *de-novo* cardiac failure, and overall mortality
(Table 2.4; Foley *et al.*, 1996*d*).

Table 2.4   Association between mean serum albumin and clinical outcomes (expressed as the
effect of a 10 g/1 fall), analyzed separately in hemodialysis ($N = 261$) and peritoneal dialysis
($N = 171$) patients[a]

Outcome	Hemodialysis		Peritoneal dialysis	
	Relative risk	p	Relative risk	p
Ischemic heart disease:				
De-novo	5.29	0.001	No association	No association
Recurrent	4.24	0.005	No association	No association
Cardiac failure:				
De-novo	2.22	0.001	4.16	0.003
Recurrent	3.84	0.003	No association	No association
Mortality:				
All-cause	4.33	< 0.001	2.06	< 0.001
Cardiac	5.60	0.001	No association	No association
Non-cardiac	3.58	< 0.001	3.52	< 0.001

[a]The covariates entered in each multivariate analysis were age, diabetes mellitus, ischemic heart disease
(excluded for the outcomes *de-novo* and recurrent ischemic heart disease) as well as the average monthly
mean arterial blood pressure, serum albumin, and hemoglobin level before the index event (Foley *et al.*,
1996*d*).

It is not clear how malnutrition might cause cardiomyopathy in dialysis patients.
Malnutrition can have effects on cardiac structure and function in non-uremic individuals. For example, 'brown atrophy' of the heart was seen in autopsy studies of
individuals dying of starvation in the Warsaw ghetto during World War II (Follis, 1958).
Low cardiac output, cardiac fibrosis, fatty infiltration, myofibrillar atrophy, and frank
cardiac failure have been seen in individuals with kwashiorkor (Smythe *et al.*, 1962;
Wharton *et al.*, 1967, 1969). Both cardiac atrophy and hypertrophy (Piza *et al.*, 1971) are
seen in marasmus. The diets of many ESRD patients are like those that result in
kwashiorkor (inadequate protein intake, with adequate caloric intake) and marasmus
(inadequate intake of both protein and calories).

It is equally unclear how hypoalbuminemia could cause ischemic heart disease. In
elderly, non-uremic patients malnutrition is associated with heparin cofactor 2 and
antithrombin 3 deficiency, which limits the ability to inhibit thrombin generation
(Kario *et al.*, 1992). Low serum albumin levels were the single factor most predictive of
access thrombosis in the Canadian Hemodialysis Morbidity Study; the authors
speculated that the low oncotic pressure associated with hypoalbuminemia leads to a
hypercoagulable state, by mechanisms analogous to those seen in nephrotic syndrome and other protein-losing states (Churchill *et al.*, 1992). The association between
hypoalbuminemia and ischemic heart disease could be a surrogate marker for a more
severe uremic state, which is not adequately captured by current estimates of dialysis
adequacy, such as Kt/V_{Urea} or per cent urea-reduction. There is accumulating

evidence that inflammation is an important factor in atherogenesis (Alexander, 1994). It is well known that low serum albumin levels occur in response to any illness, especially if it is inflammatory, independent of protein intake. Whether this may explain the recently reported excessive mortality seen with proinflammatory, bio-incompatible hemodialysis membranes (Hakim *et al.*, 1994) is unknown. It is possible that low albumin levels are associated with other nutritional deficiencies that lead to ischemic heart disease. Recent evidence suggests that hyperhomocysteinemia is a risk factor for vascular disease in the general (Stampfer *et al.*, 1992) and ESRD populations (Chauveau *et al.*, 1992, 1993). Others have suggested that malnutrition in ESRD may lead to chronic vasodilatation (possibly because of excessive NO production) and an increase in oxidant stress (Ponka and Kuhlback, 1983; Cohen *et al.*, 1986; Foote *et al.*, 1987; Ono, 1989; Paul *et al.*, 1993; Ritz *et al.*, 1994; Roselaar *et al.*, 1995; Yokokawa *et al.*, 1995).

In experimental studies, uremia leads to the increased deposition of interstitial ground substance, collagen deposition, and a reduction in capillary surface density. These effects are largely independent of blood pressure (Mall *et al.*, 1988; Amann *et al.*, 1992). Uremic serum is a direct myodepressant (Scheuer and Stezoski, 1973; Penpargkul and Scheuer, 1978). The uremic toxins responsible for this effect have not been identified. Some authors believe that the depressant factors are water soluble and filterable, with a molecular weight between 10 000 and 30 000 daltons (Horl and Riegel, 1993). Experimental work suggests that uremia leads to chronic activation of the vascular endothelium (Gris *et al.*, 1994). There is indirect evidence that uremia is cardiotoxic in human ESRD. In the National Cooperative Dialysis Study there were more cardiac events in patients who received less intensive dialysis (Lowrie *et al.*, 1981). In chronic renal failure left ventricular echocardiographic abnormalities are commoner in dialysis patients than in predialysis patients (Greaves *et al.*, 1994a). Churchill *et al.*, (1993), in a randomized crossover trial, have reported that more intensive dialysis tended to partially correct cardiac abnormalities.

Renal transplantation is a natural experiment that allows one to assess the impact of uremia. In our study, a total of 102 patients had an echocardiogram less than 1 year prior to transplantation as well as a repeat investigation a year or more following transplantation. In this population, which was free of coronary artery disease, the left ventricular mass index fell from 175 g/m^2 to 148 g/m^2 ($p < 0.0001$); left ventricular cavity volume fell from 86 ml/m^2 to 77 ml/m^2 ($p = 0.003$); left ventricular fractional shortening rose from 35% to 37% ($p = 0.036$). The most dramatic changes were seen in the 12 patients with systolic dysfunction (fractional shortening less than 25%) immediately prior to transplantation. Systolic dysfunction reversed in all these patients, increasing from 22% to 34% ($p < 0.0001$) (Parfrey *et al.*, 1995). These data suggest a role for uremia in the pathogenesis of uremic cardiomyopathy. Whether intensifying dialysis therapy can have the same effect is currently under investigation.

Mode of renal replacement therapy

It has long been held that hemodialysis and peritoneal dialysis (PD) are similar in terms of patient outcome. It has recently been confirmed that a large burden of uremic toxicity and malnutrition are as detrimental to PD patients as they are to hemodialysis patients (CANUSA, 1996). It is already well known that conventional

PD is associated with a much lower uremic solute clearance and serum albumin levels than conventional PD. It is difficult to provide a rational explanation of how PD and HD could have similar survival characteristics when the odds are so heavily stacked against the former in terms of the 'big two' risk factors. There has been concern recently that hemodialysis may have a survival advantage over peritoneal dialysis (Bloembergen *et al.*, 1995*a*). In our study, peritoneal dialysis consisted of 8 liters of dialysis fluid per day for almost all patients. A biphasic mortality pattern was seen. Compared to hemodialysis patients, PD patients had an excessive mortality, which became apparent after 2 years, and could not be explained by differences in baseline age and comorbidity. This excess mortality was not due to progressive cardiomyopathy or new cardiac failure, which were less likely in PD patients (Foley *et al.*, 1998). It is noteworthy that in the CANUSA study (1996) the efficiency of peritoneal dialysis fell to levels associated with high mortality by 2 years, because of loss of residual renal function. We conjecture that the late mortality effect in PD patients in our study was due to uremia, that became more marked as residual renal function fell. Whether enhanced peritoneal dialysis prescription could negate this difference in treatment efficacy needs to be determined as a matter of urgency. It seems, from our study, that the path to death may differ in hemodialysis and peritoneal dialysis, although the causes of death are similar (Bloembergen *et al.*, 1995*b*; Foley *et al.*, 1998).

Cardiac risk factor intervention in long-term dialysis patients

Table 2.5 lists some recommendations regarding targets for various cardiac risk factors in dialysis patients and how to achieve these targets. There are no ESRD-specific randomized trials to support or refute any of the opinions presented here. As a consequence we are forced to use the next best levels of evidence, prospective epidemiological studies in dialysis patients and randomized interventions in non-dialysis populations.

Table 2.5 Intervening cardiac risk factors in long-term dialysis patients

Risk factor	Target level and R_x	RCT in general population?	Prospective evidence in ESRD population
Smoking	Stop	No	Yes
Blood pressure	< 140/90	No	Yes
Cholesterol	< 6.0 mmol/l	Yes	No
Uremia	URR > 70%	NA	Yes
Albumin	As high as possible	No	Yes
Calcium	> 2.2 mmol/l	NA	Yes
Phosphorus	< 2.0 mmol/l	NA	No
PTH	< 200	NA	No
Hemoglobin	100 g/l	No	Yes

R_x treatment; RCT, randomized controlled trial; URR, urea reduction ratio; PTH, parathyroid hormone; NA, not applicable.

These interventions are recommended with the 'average' dialysis patient in mind. The potential loss and gain in terms of longevity and quality of life need to be considered in each patient individually. It goes without saying that we should encourage all our patients to give up smoking. There is convincing evidence that aggressive treatment of hypercholesterolemia improves the prognosis in non-uremic patients with clinical manifestations of atherosclerosis. The average dialysis patient is likely to have cardiomyopathy and/or coronary disease. As such they have a high cardiac risk; this is underscored by the observation that the incidence of new ischemic heart disease in dialysis patients is probably greater than the rate of reinfarction among survivors of myocardial infarction in the general population. Cholesterol-lowering agents have shown to be of greatest benefit in preventing further cardiovascular events in the latter group (Scandinavian Simvastatin Survival Study Group, 1994). Based on these data, as well as the results of the primary prevention WOSCOPS trial (Shepherd *et al.*, 1996), it is probably reasonable to aim for cholesterol levels under 6.0 mmol/l, and possibly lower in the average dialysis patient. Patients with serum cholesterol levels greater than 5.5 mmol/l with angina or myocardial infarction were studied in the 4S trial, with a target level of 3.0–5.0 mmol/l. In this study mortality and the incidence of major cardiac events were reduced by a third (Scandinavian Simvastatin Survival Study Group, 1994). In the WOSCOPS study middle-aged men with a mean cholesterol of 7.0 mmol/l were randomized to placebo or pravastatin. A reduction in serum cholesterol of 20% and LDL of 26% in the intervention group translated into a 31% reduction in death or non-fatal myocardial infarction over 4.9 years of follow-up (Shepherd *et al.*, 1996). These data, though yet to be validated in dialysis patients, are striking, and difficult to discount. Diet, HMG–CoA inhibitors, and fibrates form the cornerstones of therapy at our institution. We believe that aggressive blood-pressure targets are warranted, at least in patients who have never had cardiac failure; a predialysis BP of 140/90 or better is a reasonable target. There is no compelling evidence that any type of agent is more efficacious in treating hypertensive dialysis patients.

In the most recent studies, there has been no threshold level of serum albumin level or dialysis intensity at which the prognosis death risk appears to accelerate. It is therefore difficult to suggest a dichotomous target level. This is especially true for serum albumin. How we can most effectively reverse malnutrition in dialysis patients remains to be determined. Chertow *et al.* (1994) have shown epidemiological evidence that intradialytic parenteral nutrition may be of benefit. It is possible that increasing dialysis intensity may be the single most efficacious intervention. Currently, we aim for a urea-reduction ratio of over 70% in hemodialysis patients. With regard to the treatment of anemia with erythropoietin, there is no evidence that full correction, as opposed to partial correction of anemia, benefits hemodialysis patients with symptomatic cardiac disease. The risk–benefit ratio of such an approach in dialysis patients without symptomatic cardiac disease is currently under investigation. Our current recommendation is a target hemoglobin level of 100 g/l, similar to that proposed in a recent consensus document (Muirhead *et al.*, 1995).

References

Acchiardo, S. R., Moore, L. W., and La Tour, P. A. (1983). Malnutrition as the main factor in the morbidity and mortality of hemodialysis patients. *Kidney International*, **24** (Suppl. 16), 199–203.

Agadoa, L. Y., and Eggers, P. W. (1955). Renal replacement therapy in the United States: data from the United States renal data system. *American Journal of Kidney Diseases*, **25**, 119–33.

Alexander, R. W. (1994). Inflammation and coronary artery disease. *New England Journal Medicine*, **331**, 468–9.

Amann, K., Wiest, G., Zimmer, G., *et al.* (1992). Reduced capillary density in the myocardium of uremic rats—a stereological study. *Kidney International*, **42**, 1079–85.

Assmann, G., and Schulte, H. (1992). Relation of high-density lipoprotein cholesterol and tri-glycerides to incidence of atherosclerotic coronary artery disease (the PROCAM experience). *American Journal of Cardiology*, **70**, 733–7.

Auguet, T., Senti, M., Rubies-Prat, J., *et al.* (1993). Serum lipoprotein(a) concentrations in patients with chronic renal failure receiving hemodialysis: influence of apolipoprotein(a) genetic polymorphism. *Nephrology, Dialysis, Transplantation*, **8**, 1099–103.

Bloembergen, W., Port, F. K., Mauger, E. A., and Wolfe, R. A. (1995*a*). A comparison of mortality between patients treated with hemodialysis and peritoneal dialysis. *Journal of the American Society of Nephrology*, **6**, 177–83.

Bloembergen, W., Port, F. K., Mauger, E. A., and Wolfe, R. A. (1995*b*). A comparison of cause of death between patients treated with hemodialysis and peritoneal dialysis. *Journal of the American Society of Nephrology*, **6**, 184–91.

Blumental, H. T., Alex, M., and Goldenberg, S. (1960). A study of lesions of the intramural coronary by branches in diabetes mellitus. *Archives of Pathology*, **70**, 27–42.

Braun, W. E., Phillips, D. F., Vidt, G. D., *et al.* (1984). Coronary artery disease in 100 diabetics with end-stage renal failure. *Transplantation Proceedings*, **16**, 603–7.

Brunner, F. P., Garland, H. J., Harlen, H., Scharer, K., and Parsons, F. M. (1972). Combined report on regular dialysis and transplantation in Europe. *Proceedings of the European Dialysis and Transplantation Association*, **9**, 3.

CANUSA (Canada–USA) Peritoneal Dialysis Study Group. (1996). Adequacy of dialysis and nutrition in continuous peritoneal dialysis: Association with clinical outcome. *Journal of the American Society of Nephrology*, **7**, 198–207.

Canadian Erythropoietin Study Group. (1990). Association between recombinant human erythropoietin and quality of life and exercise capacity of patients receiving haemodialysis. *British Medical Journal*, **300**, 573–8.

Canella, G., LaCanna, G., Sandrini, M., *et al.* (1990). Renormalization of high cardiac output and left ventricular size following long-term recombinant human erythropoietin treatment of anemia dialyzed uremic patients. *Clinical Nephrology*, **34**, 272–8.

Casati, S., Passerini, P., Campise, M. R., *et al.* (1987). Benefits and risks of protracted treatment with human recombinant erythropoietin in patients having hemodialysis. *British Medical Journal*, **295**, 1017–20.

Castelli, W. P., and Anderson, K. M. (1986). A population at risk. *American Journal of Cardiology*, **80** (Suppl. 2A), 23–32.

Castelli, W. P., Garrison, R. J., Nelson, N. P. F., *et al.* (1986). Incidence of coronary artery disease and lipoprotein cholesterol levels: the Framingham Study. *Journal of the American Medical Association*, **256**, 2835–8.

Charra, B., Calemard, E., Ruffet, M., *et al.* (1992*a*). Survival as an index of adequacy of dialysis. *Kidney International*, **41**, 1286–91.

Charra, B., Calemard, E., Ruffet, M., *et al.* (1992*b*). Survival as an index of adequacy of dialysis. *Kidney International*, **41**, 1286–91.

Chauveau, P., Chadefaux, B., Coude M., *et al.* (1992). Increased plasma homocysteine concentrations in patients with chronic renal failure. *Mineral and Electrolyte Metabolism*, **18**, 196.

Chauveau, P., Chadefaux, B., Coude, B., *et al.* (1993). Hyperhomocysteinemia, a risk factor for atherosclerosis in chronic uremic patients. *Kidney International*, **44**, 881–6.

Chertow, G. M., Ling, J., Lew, N. L., Lazarus, J. M., and Lowrie, E. G. (1994). The association between intradialytic parenteral nutrition administration with survival in hemodialysis patients. *American Journal of Kidney Diseases*, **24**, 912–20.

Churchill, D. N., Taylor, D. W., Cook, R. J, *et al.* (1992). Canadian Hemodialysis Morbidity Study. *American Journal of Kidney Diseases*, **19**, 214–34.

Churchill, D. N., Taylor, D. W., Tomlinson, C. W., *et al.* (1993). Effects of high flux hemodialysis on cardiac structure and function among patients with end-stage renal failure. *Nephron* **65**, 573–7.

Churchill, D. N., Muirhead, N., Goldstein, M., *et al.* (1994). Probability of thrombosis of vascular access among hemodialysis patients treated with recombinant human erythropoietin. *Journal of the American Society of Nephrology*, **4**, 1809–13.

Cohen, J. D., Viljoen, M., Clifford, D., De Oliveira, A. A., Veriava, Y., and Milne, F. J. (1986). Plasma vitamin E levels in a chronically hemolyzing group of dialysis patients. *Clinical Nephrology*, **25**, 42–7.

Collins, A. J., Ma, J. Z., Umen, A., and Keshaviah, P. (1994). Urea index and other predictors of hemodialysis patient survival. *American Journal of Kidney Diseases*, **23**, 272–82.

Corti, M.-C, Salive, E., and Guralnik, J. M. (1996). Serum albumin and physical function as predictors of coronary heart disease mortality and incidence in older persons. *Journal of Clinical Epidemiology*, **49**, 519–26.

Cressman, M. D., Heyka, R. J., Paganini, E. P., *et al.* (1992). Lipoprotein(a) is an independent risk factor for cardiovascular disease in hemodialysis patients. *Circulation*, **86**, 475–82.

Dahlen, G. H., Guyton, J. R., Arrar, M., *et al.* (1986). Association of lipoprotein Lp(a), plasma lipids and other lipoproteins with coronary artery disease documented by angiography. *Circulation*, **74**, 758–68.

Degoulet, P., Legrain, M., Reach, I., *et al.* (1982). Mortality factors in patients treated by chronic hemodialysis. *Nephron* **31**, 103–10.

Disney, A. P. S. (1995). Demography and survival of patients receiving treatment for chronic renal failure in Australia and New Zealand: report on dialysis and renal transplantation treatment from the Australia and New Zealand Dialysis and Transplant Registry. *American Journal of Kidney Diseases*, **25**, 165–75.

Drukker, W., Alberts, C., Ode, A., Roosendaal, K. J., and Wilmink, J. M. (1966). Report on regular dialysis treatment in Europe. *Proceedings of the European Dialysis and Transplantation Association*, **3**, 90.

Eschbach, J.W., Egrie, J. C., Downing, M. R., *et al.* (1987). Correction of the anemia of end-stage renal disease with recombinant human erythropoietin. *New England Journal of Medicine*, **316**, 73–8.

Fellner, S. K., Lang, R. M., Neumann, A., *et al.* (1993). Cardiovascular consequences of the correction of the anemia of renal failure with erythropoietin. *Kidney International* **44**, 1309–15.

Fenton, S., Desmeules, M., Copleston, P., *et al.*, (1995). Renal replacement therapy in Canada: a report from the Canadian organ replacement register. *American Journal of Kidney Diseases*, **25**, 134–50.

Fernandez, J. M., Carbonell, M. E., Mazzucchi, N., and Petrucelli, D. (1992). Simultaneous analysis of mortality and morbidity factors in chronic hemodialysis patient. *Kidney International*, **41**, 1029–34.

Fleck, A., Raines, G., Hawker, F., *et al.* (1985). Increased permeability: a major cause of hypoalbuminemia in disease and injury. *Lancet*, **i**, 781–4.

Foley, R. N., Parfrey, P. S., Hefferton, D., Singh, I., Simms, A., and Barrett, B. J. (1994). Advance prediction of early death in patients starting maintenance hemodialysis. *American Journal of Kidney Diseases*, **23**, 836–45.

Foley, R. N., Parfrey, P. S., Harnett, J. D., *et al.* (1995*a*). Clinical and echocardiographic disease in patients starting end-stage renal disease therapy. *Kidney International*, **47**, 186–92.

Foley, R. N., Parfrey, P. S., Harnett, J. D., Kent, G. M., Murray, D. C., and Barre, P. E. (1995*b*). The prognostic importance of left ventricular geometry in uremic cardiomyopathy. *Journal of the American Society of Nephrology*, **5**, 2024–31.

Foley, R. N., Parfrey, P. S., Harnett, J. D., Kent, G. M., Murray, D. C., and Barre, P. E. (1996*a*). Impact of hypertension on cardiomyopathy, morbidity and mortality in end-stage renal disease *Kidney International*, **49**, 1379–85.

Foley, R. N., Parfrey, P. S., Harnett, J. D., Kent, G. M., Murray, D. C., and Barre, P. E. (1996*b*). The impact of anemia on cardiomyopathy, morbidity and mortality in end-stage renal disease. *American Journal of Kidney Diseases*, **28**, 53–61.

Foley, R. N., Parfrey, P. S., Harnett, J. D., Kent, G. M., Murray, D. C., and Barre, P. E. (1996*c*). Hypoalbumiemia, cardiac morbidity and mortality in end-stage renal disease. *Journal of the American Society of Nephrology*, **7**, 728–36.

Foley, R. N., Parfrey, P. S., Harnett, J. D., *et al.* (1998). Mode of dialysis therapy, cardiac morbidity and mortality in end-stage renal disease. *Journal of the American Society of Nephrology*, **9**, 267–76.

Follis, R. H. (1958). *Deficiency disease: functional and structural changes in mammals, which result from exogenous or endogenous lack of one or more essential nutrients.* Charles C. Thomas, Springfield, I L.

Foote, J. W., Hinks, L. J., and Lloyd, B. (1987). Reduced plasma and white blood cell selenium levels in hemodialysis patients. *Clinica Chemica Acta*, **164**, 323–8.

Furberg, C. D., Psaty, B. M., and Meyer, J. V. (1995). Nifedipine. Dose-related increase in mortality in patients with coronary heart disease. *Circulation*, **92**, 1326–31.

Galderisi, M., Anderson, K. M., Wilson, P. W. F., *et al.* (1991). Echocardiographic evidence for a distinct diabetic cardiomyopathy (The Framingham Heart Study. *American Journal of Cardiology*, **68**, 85–9.

Gillum, R. F. and Makuc, D. M. (1992). Serum albumin, coronary heart disease and death. *American Heart Journal*, **123**, 507–13.

Goldberg, N., Lundin, A. P., Delano, B., *et al.* (1992). Changes in left ventricular size, wall thickness, and function in anemic patients treated with recombinant human erythropoietin. *American Heart Journal*, **124**, 424–7.

Goldwasser, P., Michel, M. A., Collier, M. A., *et al.* (1993). Prealbumin and lipoprotein(a) in hemodialysis: relationship with patients and vascular access survival. *American Journal of Kidney Diseases.* **22**, 215–25.

Gotch, F., and Sargent, J. (1985). A mechanistic analysis of the National Cooperative Dialysis Study. *Kidney International*, **28**, 526–34.

Greaves, S. C., Gamble, G. D., Collins J. F., *et al.* (1994*a*). Determinants of left ventricular hypertrophy and systolic dysfunction in chronic renal failure. *American Journal of Kidney Diseases*, **24**, 768–76.

Greaves, S. C., Gamble, G. D., Collins, J. F., *et al.* (1994*b*). Determinants of left ventricular hypertrophy and systolic dysfunction in chronic renal failure. *American Journal of Kidney Diseases.* **24**, 768–76.

Gris J-C, Branger B, Vecina F, Sabadini BA, Fourcade J, Schved J-F. (1994). Increased cardio-vascular risk factors and features of cardiovascular activation and dysfunction in dialyzed uremic patients. *Kidney International*, **46**, 807–13.

Grossmann, E., Shemesh, J., Shamiss, A., *et al.* (1992). Left ventricular mass in diabetes-hypertension. *Archives of Internal Medicine*, **152**, 1001–4.

Hakim, R. M., Stannard, D., Port, F., and Held P. (1994). The effect of the dialysis membrane on mortality of chronic hemodialysis patients in the U.S. *Journal of the American Society of Nephrology.* **5**, 451. (Abstract).

Harnett, J. D., Foley, R. N., Parfrey, P. S., Kent, G. M., Murray, D. C., and Barre, P. (1995). Congestive heart failure in dialysis patients: prevalence, associations and prognosis. *Kidney International*, **47**, 884–90.

Held, P. J., Levin, N. W., Bovbjerg, R. R., *et al.* (1991). Mortality and duration of hemodialysis treatment. *Journal of the American Medical Association*, **265**, 871–5.

Hirata, K., Kikuchi, S., Saku, K., *et al.* (1993). Apolipoprotein(a) phenotypes and serum lipoprotein(a) levels in hemodialysis patients with/without diabetes mellitus. *Kidney International*, **44**, 1062–70.

Horl, W. H., and Riegel, W. (1993). Cardiac depressant factors in renal disease. Circulation, **87** (Suppl. 5), IV77–82.

Hutting, J., Kramer, W., Schutterle, G., and Wizemann, V. (1988*a*). Analysis of left ventricular changes associated with chronic hemodialysis: a non-invasive follow-up study. *Nephron*, **49**, 284–90.

Hutting, J., Kramer, W., Schutterle, G., and Wizemann, V. (1986*b*). Analysis of left ventricular changes associated with chronic hemodialysis: a non-invasive follow-up study. Nephron, **49**, 284–90.

Hutting, J., Kramer, W., Reitinger, J., *et al.* (1990). Cardiac structure and function in continuous ambulatory dialysis: influence of blood purification and hypercirculation. *American Heart Journal*, **119**, 344–352.

Inoue, M., Wakasugi, M., Wakao, R., *et al.* (1992). A synthetic analogue of vitamin D_3 22-oxa-1,25-dihydroxyvitamin D_3, stimulates the production of prostacyclin by vascular tissues. *Life Sciences*, **51**, 1105–12.

Iseki, K., Kawazoe, N., and, Fukiyama, K. (1993). Serum albumin is a strong predictor of death in chronic dialysis patients. *Kidney International*, **44**, 115–19.

Jacobs, C., and Selwood, N. H. (1995). Renal replacement therapy in France: current status and evolutive trends over the last decade. *American Journal of Kidney Diseases*, **25**, 188–95.

Joven, J., Vilella, E., Ahmed, S., *et al.* (1992). Lipoprotein heterogeneity in end stage renal disease. *Kidney International*, **42**, 1247–52.

Kannel, W. B. (1975). Role of blood pressure in cardiovascular disease: The Framingham Study. Angiology **26**, 1–14.

Kannel, W. B., (1981). Update on the role of cigarette smoking in coronary artery disease. *American Heart Journal*, **101**, 319–25.

Kannel, W. B. (1983). Epidemiological profile and risks of coronary artery disease. *American Journal of Cardiology*, **52**, 9B–13B.

Kannel, W. B. (1985). Cholesterol and risk of coronary heart disease in men. *Clinical Chemistry*, **34**, 353–9.

Kannel, W. B., and McGee, D. L. (1979). Diabetes and cardiovascular disease: the Framingham Study. *Journal of the American Medical Association*, **241**, 2035–8.

Kannel, W. B., Dawber, T. R., Kagan, A., *et al.* (1960). Factors of risk in the development of coronary artery disease—six year follow-up experience: The Framingham Study. *Annals of Internal Medicine*, **55**, 33–50.

Kario, K., Matsuo, T., Kobaysahi, H. (1992). Heparin cofactor II deficiency in the elderly: comparison with antithrombin III *Thrombosis Research*, **66**, 489–98.

Kawagishi, T., Nishizawa, Y., Konishi, T., *et al.* (1995). High resolution B-mode ultrasonography in evaluation of atherosclerosis in uremia. *Kidney International*, **48**, 820–6.

Kopple, J. D. (1994). Effect of malnutrition on morbidity and mortality in maintenance dialysis patients. American Journal *of Kidney Diseases*, **24**, 1002–9.

Kuller, L. H., Eichner, J. E., and Orchard, T. J. (1991). The relationship between serum albumin levels and risk of coronary heart disease in Multiple Risk Factor Intervention Trial. *American Journal of Epidemiology*, **134**, 1266–77.

Lindner, A., Charra, A., Sherrard, D. J., and Scribner, B. H. (1974). Accelerated atherosclerosis in prolonged maintenance hemodialysis. *New England Journal of Medicine*, **290**, 697.

London, G. M., Zins, B., Pannier, B., *et al.* (1989). Vascular changes in hemodialysis patients in response to recombinant human erythropoietin. *Kidney International*, **36**, 878–82.

Lorber, M. L., Van Buren, C. T., Flechner, S. M., *et al.* (1987). Pre-transplant arteriography for diabetic renal transplant recipients. *Transplantation Proceedings*, **19**, 1539–41.

Low, I., Grutzmacher, P., Bergmann, M., *et al.* (1989). Echocardiogrpahic findings in patients on maintenance hemodialysis substituted with recombinant human erythropoietin. *Clinical Nephrology*, **31**, 26–30.

Low-Friedrich, I., Grutzmacher, P., Marz, W., *et al.* (1991). Therapy with recombinant human erythropoietin reduces cardiac size and improves cardiac size in chronic hemodialysis patients. *American Journal of Nephrology*, **11**, 54–60.

Lowrie, E. G., and Lew, N. L. (1990). Death risk in hemodialysis patients: the predictive value of commonly measured variables and an evaluation of death rate differences between facilities. *American Journal of Kidney Diseases*, **15**, 458–82.

Lowrie, E. G., Laird, N. M., Parker, T. F., *et al.* (1981). Effect of the hemodialysis prescription on patient morbidity. Report from the National Co-operative Dialysis Study. *New England Journal of Medicine*, **305**, 1176–81.

Lowrie, E. G., Huang, N. L., Lew, N. L., and Liu, Y. (1994). The relative contribution of measured variables to death risk among hemodialysis patients. In *Death on hemodialysis: preventable or inevitable?* (ed. E. A. Friedman), pp. 121–41. Kluwer Academic, Dordrecht.

McCarthy, E. P., Yamashita, W., Hsu, A., and Ooi, B. S. (1989). 1,25-dihydroxyvitamin D_3 and rat vascular smooth muscle cell growth. *Hypertension*, **13**, 954–9.

Macdougall, I. C., Lewis, N. P., Saunders, M. J., *et al.* (1990). Long-term cardiorespiratory effect of amelioration of renal anaemia by erythropoietin. *Lancet*, **335**, 489–93.

McMillan, M. A., Briggs, J. D., and Junor, B. J. (1990). Outcome of renal replacement therapy in patients with diabetes mellitus. *British Medical Journal*, **301**, 540–4.

Maggi, E., Bellazzi, R., Falaschi F., *et al.* (1994). Enhanced LDL oxidation in uremic patients. An additional mechanism for accelerated atherosclerosis? *Kidney International*, **45**, 876–83.

Mall, G., Rambausek, N., Neumeister, A., *et al.* (1988). Myocardial interstitial fibrosis in experimental uremia—implications for cardiac compliance. *Kidney International*, **33**, 804–11.

Mallick, N. P., Jones, E., and Selwood, N. (1995). The European (European Dialysis and Transplantation Association—European Renal Association) Registry. *American Journal of Kidney Diseases*, **25**, 176–87.

Manolio, T. A., Cutler, J. A., Furberg, C. D., Psaty, B. M., Whelton, P. K., and Applegate, W. B. (1995). Trends in pharmacologic management of hypertension in the United States. *Archives of Internal Medicine*, **155**, 829–37.

Manske, C. L., Thomas, W., Wang, Y., *et al.* (1993). Screening diabetic transplant candidates for coronary artery disease: identification of a low risk subgroup. *Kidney International* **44**, 617–21.

Martinez-Vea, A., Bardaji, A., Garcia, C., *et al.* (1992). Long-term myocardial effects of correction of anemia with recombinant human erythropoietin in aged patients on hemodialysis. *American Journal of Kidney Diseases*, **14**, 353–7.

Massry, S. G., Smogorzweski, M. (1994). Mechanisms through which parathyroid hormone mediates its deleterious effects on organ function in uremia. *Seminars in Nephrology*, **14**, 219–31.

Morris, K. P., Skinner, J. R., Wren, C., *et al.* (1993*a*). Cardiac abnormalities in end-stage renal failure and anemia. *Archives of Disease in Childhood*, **68**, 637–43.

Morris, K. P., Skinner, J. R., Hunter, S., *et al.* (1993*b*). Short term correction of anaemia with recombinant human erythropoietin and reduction of cardiac output in end-stage renal failure. *Archives of Disease in Childhood*, **68**, 644–8.

Muirhead, N., Bargman, J., Burgess, E., *et al.* (1995). Evidence-based recommendations for the clinical use of human erythropoietin. *American Journal of Kidney Diseases*, **26** (Suppl. 1), S1–S24.

Murphy, B. G., McNamee, P., Duly, E., *et al.* (1992). Increased serum apolipoprotein(a) in patients with chronic renal failure treated with continuous ambulatory peritoneal dialysis. *Atherosclerosis* **93**, 53–7.

Neff, M. S., Esier, A. R., Slifkin, R. F., *et al.* (1983). Patients surviving 10 years of dialysis. *American Journal of Medicine*, **74**, 996–1004.

Okura, Y., Saku, K., Hirata, K., *et al.* (1993). Serum lipoprotein(a) levels in maintenance hemodialysis patients. *Nephron*, **65**, 46–50.

Ono, K. (1989). The effect of vitamin C supplementation and withdrawal on the mortality and morbidity of regular hemodialysis patients. *Clinical Nephrology*, **31**, 31–4.

Owen, S. R., Lew, N. L., Yan Liu, S. M., Lowrie, E. G., and Lazarus J. M. (1993). The urea reduction ratio and serum albumin concentrations as predictors of mortality in patients undergoing hemodialysis. *New England Journal of Medicine*, **329**, 1001–6.

Paganini, E. P., Fouad, F. M., and Tarazi, R. C. (1984). Systemic hypertension in chronic renal failure. In *The heart and renal disease*, (ed. R. A. O'Rourke, B. M. Brenner, and J. H. Stein), pp. 127. Churchill Livingstone, New York.

Paganini, E. D., Lathaur, D., and Abdulhadi, M. (1989). Practical considerations of recombinant human erythropoietin therapy. *American Journal of Kidney Diseases*, **14**, 19–28.

Parfrey, P. S., Harnett, J. D., Griffiths, S. M., *et al.* (1990). The clinical course of left ventricular hypertrophy in dialysis patients. *Nephron*, **55**, 114–20.

Parfrey, P. S., Harnett, J. D., Foley, R. N., *et al.* (1995). Impact of renal transplantation on uremic cardiomyopathy. *Transplantation*, **60**, 908–14.

Parfrey, P. S., Foley, R. N., Harnett, J. D., Kent, G. M., Murray, D., and Barre, P. E. (1996*a*). Outcome and risk factors of ischemic heart disease in chronic uremia. *Kidney International*, **49**, 1428–34.

Parfrey, P. S., Foley, R. N., Harnett, J. D., *et al.* (1996*b*). Outcome and risk factors for left ventricular disorders in chronic uraemia. *Nephrology, Dialysis and Transplantation*, **11**, 1277–85.

Parker, T. F., Husni, L., Huang, W., *et al.* (1994). Survival of hemodialysis in the U.S. is improved with a greater quantity of dialysis. *American Journal of Kidney Diseases*, **23**, 670–80.

Parra, H. J., Mexdour, H., Cachera, C., *et al.* (1987). *Clinical Chemistry*, **33**, 721.

Pascual, J., Teruel, J. L., Moya, J. L., *et al.* (1991). Regression of left ventricular hypertrophy after partial correction of anaemia with erythropoietin in patients on hemodialysis: a prospective study. *Clinical Nephrology*, **35**, 280–7.

Paul, J. L., Sall, N. D., Soni, T., *et al.* (1993). Lipid peroxidation abnormalities in hemodialyzed patients. Nephron, **64**, 106–9.

Penpargkul, S. and Scheuer, J. (1978). Effect of uremia upon the performance of the rat heart. *Cardiovascular Research*, **6**, 702–8.

Phillips, A., Shaper, A. G., and Whincup, and P. H. (1989). Association between serum albumin and mortality from cardiovascular disease, cancer and other causes. *Lancet*, **i**, 1434–6.

Piza, J., Troper, L., Cespedes, R., *et al.* (1971). Myocardial lesions and heart failure in infantile malnutrition. *American Journal of Tropical Medicine and Hygiene*, **20**, 343–55.

Ponka, A., and Kuhlback, B. (1983). Serum ascorbic acid in patients undergoing chronic hemodialysis. *Acta Medica Scandinavica*, **213**, 305–7.

Psaty, B. M., Heckbert, S. R., Koepsell, T. D., *et al.* (1995). The risk of myocardial infarction associated with antihypertensive drug therapies. *Journal of the American Medical Association*, **274**, 620–5.

Raine, A. E. G., Seymour, A.-M. L., Roberts, A. F. C., Radda, G. K., and Ledingham, J. G. C. (1993). Impairment of cardiac function and energetics in experimental renal failure. *Journal of Clinical Investigation*, **92**, 2934–40.

Reade, V., Tailleaux, A., Reade, R., *et al.* (1993). Expression of apolipoprotein B epitopes in low density lipoproteins of hemodialyzed patients. *Kidney International*, **44**, 1360–65.

Ritz, E., and Koch, M. (1993). Morbidity and mortality due to hypertension in patients with renal failure. *American Journal of Kidney Diseases*, **21** (Suppl. 2), 113–18.

Ritz, E., Strumpf, C., Katz, F., *et al.* (1985). Hypertension and cardiovascular risk factors in hemodialyzed diabetic patients. *Hypertension*, **7** (Suppl. II), 118.

Ritz, E., Vallance, P., and Nowicki, M. (1994). The effect of malnutrition on cardiovascular mortality in dialysis patients: is L-arginine the answer? *Nephrology, Dialysis, Transplantation*, **9**, 129–30.

Rocco, M. V., Soucie, M. J., Reboussin, D. M., McClellan, W. M., and the Southeastern Kidney Council (Network 6). (1996). Risk factors for hospital utilization in chronic dialysis patients. *Journal of the American Society of Nephrology*, **7**, 889–96.

Rogerson, M. E., Kong, C. H., Leaker, B., *et al.* (1993). The effect of recombinant human erythropoietin on cardiovascular responses to postural stress in dialysis patients. *Clinical Autonomic Research*, **3**, 271–4.

Roselaar, S. E., Nazhat, N. B., Winyard, P. G., Jones, P., Cunningham, J., and Blake, D. R. (1995). Detection of oxidants in uremic plasma by electron spin resonance spectroscopy. *Kidney International*, **48**, 199–206.

Rostand, S. G., Kirk, K. A., and Rutsky, E. A. (1984). Dialysis-associated ischemic heart disease: insights from coronary angiography. *Kidney International*, **25**, 653–9.

Scandinavian Simvastatin Survival Study Group. (1994). Randomised trial of cholesterol lowering in 4444 patients with coronary heart disease and: the (4S). *Lancet*, **344**, 1383–9.

Scheuer, J., and Stezoski, S. N. (1973). Effect of uremic compounds on cardiac function and metabolism. Journal of Molecular and *Cellular Cardiology*, **4**, 287–300.

Schreiner, G. E., and Maher, J. F. (1961). *Uremia; biochemistry, pathogenesis and treatment*. Charles C. Thomas, Springfield.

Schultz, R. (1876). Advanced cardiac insufficiency, a frequent complication of diabetes mellitus, requiring attention, *Berliner Klinische Wochenschift*, **6**, 4–5.

Shapiro, J. (1992). Atherogenesis in chronic renal failure. In *Cardiac dysfunction in chronic uremia*, (ed. P. S. Parfrey and J. D. Harnett) pp. 187–204. Kluwer Academic, Boston.

Shapiro, L. M., Howatt, A. P., and Calter, M. M. (1981*a*). Left ventricular function in diabetes mellitus I. Methodology and prevalence and spectrum of abnormalities. *British Heart Journal*, **45**, 122–8.

Shapiro, L. M., Leatherdale, B. A., MacKinnon, J., *et al.* (1981*b*). Left ventricular function in diabetes mellitus II. Relation between clinical features and left ventricular function. *British Heart Journal*, **45**, 129–32.

Shepherd, J., Cobbe, S. M., Ford, I., *et al.* (1996). Prevention of coronary heart disease with pravastatin in men with hypercholesterolemia. *New England Journal of Medicine*, **333**, 1301–7.

Shoji, T., Nishizawa, Y., Nishitani, H., Yamakawa, M., and Morii, H. (1992). Impaired metabolism of high density lipoproteins in uremic patients. *Kidney International*, **41**, 1653–61.

Silberberg, J. S., Barre, P., Prichard, S., Sniderman, A. D. (1989). Left ventricular hypertrophy: an independent determinant of survival in end stage renal disease. *Kidney International*, **36**, 286–90.

Silberberg, J. S., Racine, N., Barre, P. E., *et al.* (1990). Regression of left ventricular hypertrophy in dialysis patients following correction of anemia with recombinant human erythropietin. *Canadian Journal of Cardiology*, **6**, 1–4.

Smythe, P. M., Swanepoel, A., and Campbell, J. A. H. (1962). The heart and kwashiorkor. *British Medical Journal*, **1**, 67–73.

Spiegel, D. M., and Breyer, J. A. (1994). Serum albumin: a predictor of long-term outcome in peritoneal dialysis patients. *American Journal of Kidney Diseases*, **23**, 283–5.

Stampfer, M. J., Malinow, M. R., Willett, W. C., *et al.* (1992). A prospective study of homo-cyst(e)ine and risk of myocardial infarction in U.S. physicians. *Journal of the American Medical Association*, **268**, 877.

Stefenelli, T., Mayr, H., Bergler-Klein, J., Globits, S., Wolszezuk, W., and Niederle, B. (1993). Primary hyperparathyroidism: incidence of cardiac abnormalities and partial parathyroidectomy. *American Journal of Medicine*, **95**, 197–202.

Sundal, E., and Kaeser, U. (1989). Correction of anemia of chronic renal failure with recombinant human erythropoietin: safety and efficacy of one year's treatment in a European Multi-centre Study of 150 hemodialysis-dependent patients. *Nephrology, Dialysis, Transplantation*, **4**, 979–87.

Tagawa, H., Nagano, M., Saito, H., *et al.* (1991). Echocardiogrpahic findings in hemodialysis patients treated with recombinant human erythropoietin: proposal for a hematocrit most beneficial to hemodynamics. *Clinical Nephrology*, **35**, 35–8.

Teraoka, S., Toma, H., Nihei, H., *et al.* (1995). Current status of renal replacement therapy in Japan. *American Journal of Kidney Diseases*, **25**, 151–64.

Theusen, L., Christiansen, J. S., Mogensen, C. E., *et al.* (1988). Echocardiogrpahic-determined left ventricular wall characteristics in insulin dependent diabetic patients. *Acta Medica Scandinavica*, **224**, 343–8.

Thillet, J., Faucher, C., Issad, B., *et al.* (1993). Lipoprotein(a) in patients treated by continuous ambulatory peritoneal dialysis. *American Journal of Kidney Diseases*, **22**, 226–32.

Toto, R. D., Lena Vega, G. L., and Grundy, S. M. (1993). Mechanisms and treatment of dyslipidemia of renal diseases. *Current Opinion in Nephrology and Hypertension*, **2**, 784–90.

Tschope, W., Koch, M., Thomas, B., and Ritz E. (1993*a*). Serum lipids predict cardiac death in diabetic patients on maintenance hemodialysis. Results of a prospective study. The German Study Group Diabetes and Uremia. *Nephron*, **64**, 354–8.

Tschope, W., Koch, M., Thomas, B., and Ritz, E. (1993*b*). Survival and predictors of death in dialysed diabetic patients. *Diabetologia*, **36**, 1113–17.

USRDS (1992). U.S. Renal Data System 1992 Annual Report. IV. Comorbid conditions and correlations with mortality risk among 3,399 incident hemodialysis patients. *American Journal of Kidney Diseases* (Suppl. 2), 32–8.

Valsania, S. W., Zarich, S. W., Kowalchuk, G. J., *et al.* (1991). Severity of coronary artery disease in young patients with insulin-dependent diabetes mellitus. *American Journal of Cardiology*, **68**, 85–9.

van Hoeven, K. H., and Factor, S. M. (1990). A comparison of the pathological spectrum of hypertensive, diabetic and hypertensive-diabetic heart disease. *Circulation*, **82**, 848–55.

Webb, A. T., Reaveley, D. A., O'Donnell, M., *et al.* (1993). Lipoprotein(a) in patients on maintenance hemodialysis and continuous ambulatory peritoneal dialysis. *Nephrology, Dialysis, Transplantation*, **8**, 609–13.

Wei, J. Y. (1992). Age and the cardiovascular system. *New England Journal of Medicine*, **327**, 1735–9.

Weidmann, P. and Beretta-Picoli, C. (1983). Chronic renal failure and hypertension. In *Handbook of hypertension*, Vol. 2, (ed. J. I. S. Robertson), pp. 80. Elsevier Amsterdam.

Weinrauch, L., D'Elia, E. A., Healy, R. W., *et al.* (1978). Asymptomatic coronary artery disease: an assessment of diabetics evaluated for renal transplantation. *Circulation*, **58**, 1184–90.

Weintraub, M., Burstein, A., Rassin, T., *et al.* (1992). Severe defect in clearing post prandial chylomicron remnants in dialysis patients. *Kidney International*, **42**, 1247–52.

Wharton, B. A., Howells, G. R., and McGance, R. A. (1967). Cardiac failure in kwashiorkor. *Lancet* **2**, 384–7.

Wharton, B. A., Balmer, S. E., Somers, K., *et al.* (1969). The myocardium in kwashiorkor. *Quarterly Journal of Medicine*, **38**, 107–16.

Winnearls, C. G., Oliver, D. O., Pippard, M. J., *et al.* (1986). Effect of human erythropoietin derived from recombinant DNA on the anaemia of patients maintained by chronic haemo-dialysis. *Lancet* **ii**, 1175–7.

Yang, C. S., Chen, S. W., Chiang, C. H., Wang, M., Peng, S. J., and Kan, Y. T. (1996). Effects of increasing dialysis dose on serum albumin and mortality in hemodialysis patients. *American Journal of Kidney Diseases*, **27**, 380–6.

Yin, F. C. P. (1980). The ageing vasculature and its effect on the heart. In *The ageing heart: its function in response to stress*. (ed. M. L. Weisfeldt), pp. 137–214. Raven Press, New York.

Yokokawa, K., Mankus, R., Sakleyen, M. G., *et al.* (1995). Increased nitric oxide production in patients with hypotension during hemodialysis. *Annals of Internal Medicine*, **123**, 35–7.

Zoneraich, S., and Silverman, G. (1981*a*). Myocardial small vessel disease in diabetic patients. In *Diabetes and the heart* (ed. S. Zoneraich), pp. 3–18. Charles C. Thomas, Springfield.

3

Complications of long-term dialysis: cellular immunity, infection, and neoplasia

Izhar H. Khan and Graeme R. D. Catto

Introduction

The treatment of end-stage renal disease (ESRD) with dialysis has evolved greatly since the pioneering days of Wilhelm Kolf's experiments with the artificial kidney during the Second World War. Then, and in the early days of renal replacement therapy, dialysis was a novel treatment which sustained life in patients who would otherwise have succumbed to uremia. During the 1970s in the United States of America, and in the past two decades in the United Kingdom and Europe, improvements in the technological aspects of dialysis and the ability to offer this treatment to patients with a variety of renal diseases, irrespective of age or of the presence of comorbidity, have resulted in a great increase in the number of patients receiving dialysis therapy. In the USA 200 patients per million of the population start dialysis each year (USRDS Report, 1991). However, in the UK around 80 patients per million of the population commence dialysis each year (Feest *et al.*, 1990), but this number is likely to rise as the incidence of ESRD is much higher than the number of patients treated (Khan *et al.*, 1994). A greater proportion of patients now also receives a renal transplant and many patients currently receiving renal replacement therapy in Western countries have a functioning renal graft. Nevertheless, a significant proportion of patients with ESRD are kept alive with dialysis. Some patients are less likely to receive a renal transplant because of increased preformed antibodies as a result of previous unsuccessful grafts or transfusions. Furthermore, in some countries ethical and religious objections to cadaveric transplants have led to a much higher proportion of ESRD patients on dialysis. An increasing number of older patients now starting dialysis are also not considered for transplantation. There are many patients who are likely to remain on dialysis for years and be at risk of long-term complications.

There is a general perception among nephrologists that patients on long-term dialysis are at an increased risk of developing infection and neoplasia compared to the general population. This perception is largely based on results of *in-vitro* studies of human and animal material showing evidence of impaired cellular and humoral immunity in the uremic state (reviewed in Khan and Catto, 1993). Although infections are a common cause of death and morbidity in patients receiving dialysis therapy, the incidence may be related primarily to a breach of mechanical barriers during vascular and peritoneal access for dialysis. Clinical studies undertaken almost a quarter of a century ago suggested that infection contributed to or caused 30% of deaths in patients receiving long-term dialysis. Current evidence, however, does not reveal serious infections as a major cause of morbidity or mortality; furthermore, rare fungal and parasitic infections associated with severe immunosuppression, as seen in transplant recipients and patients with AIDS, are not frequent in long-term dialysis patients.

Viral infections, however, remain a problem. Infection from hepatitis B and C virus is a concern in long-term dialysis patients. The routes of infection for hepatitis in dialysis patients are most probably contact with infected material within a renal unit. The spread of infection may be prevented by rigid adherence to preventive measures, disinfection, and the judicious use of vaccination where appropriate. Viral hepatitis will not be considered further in this chapter as it is covered by Pereira in Chapter 14.

There is also concern that neoplasms may occur more frequently in patients on long-term dialysis, probably as a consequence of impaired cellular defense mechanisms which impair tumor immune-surveillance. Evidence for a greater than expected incidence of malignant disease in dialysis patients is scarce and not as robust as for the well-established increased incidence of neoplasm in recipients of renal transplants. Studies which suggest an increase in incidence of neoplasia in long-term dialysis patients need to be carefully evaluated. First, the incidence of cancer increases with age even in the non-uremic population. Therefore it is important to determine relative risks adjusted for age. Second, patients who have previously received immunosuppressive agents following transplantation, and who return to dialysis therapy following a failed graft, may be at a higher risk of developing neoplasms than those who have received dialysis alone. It is also important to relate the incidence of cancer in dialysis patients to that observed in the native population; skin cancer, for example, may be common in dialysis patients in Australia where the incidence of such a cancer is also high in the general population. Finally, some cancers may be associated with the primary cause of renal failure such as tuberous sclerosis and von Hippel–Lindau disease which are associated with cystadenomas, and analgesic nephropathy which is associated with transitional cell carcinomas.

In this chapter we shall first review the evidence of impaired immune responses in dialysis. Then we will discuss the evidence for the increased incidence of infection and neoplasia in patients receiving long-term dialysis therapy.

The normal immune system

Central to understanding the clinical implications of impaired immune responses in uremia is an understanding of the mechanisms of the normal immune response. The human immune system comprises cellular and humoral components, both of which are intimately related and interact at various stages of the immune response.

Phagocytosis

Neutrophils and monocytes are mobilized from the circulation to the site of injury by migration towards the focus of injury (chemotaxis). Chemotactic factors such as the

C5a component of complement and bacterial products interact with neutrophils and macrophages through specific cell–surface receptors. Opsonization facilitates the process of phagocytosis of antigens. Following this the phagocytic neutrophil or macrophage releases lysosomal enzymes such as myeloperoxidase into the phagosome. A burst of oxygen consumption ensues in the cells which release highly toxic, oxygen free radicals from molecular oxygen. These toxic derivatives include superoxide, hydrogen peroxide, and singlet oxygen which are directly toxic to microorganisms.

Lymphocytes

Lymphocytes are an important cellular component of the immune system and comprise T (thymus–dependent) and B (bursa–equivalent) cells. The majority of circulating lymphocytes are T cells, accounting for around 70–80% of all cells. T cells are classified into T-helper, T-suppressor, and T-cytotoxic cells. The latter are involved in attacking cell membranes and releasing cytolytic substances which destroy antigens. T-helper cells, which carry the CD4 antigen are involved in facilitating antibody production by B cells and enhancing the cytotoxic activity of cytotoxic T cells, whereas T-suppressor cells, characterized by the CD8 antigen on their cell surface, inhibit these activities.

Antigen presentation and lymphocyte activation (Fig. 3.1)

Macrophages, which are activated monocytes, play an important role in the processing and presentation of antigens to lymphocytes, which in turn are activated and sensitized to the specific antigen. Antigen presentation to lymphocytes is carried out by cells which possess the class II molecules coded by the major histocompatibility complex (MHC) which is situated on Chromosome 6 in humans. These molecules are expressed constitutively by some cells which can be regarded as professional antigen-presenting cells. Other cells can be induced by suitable stimuli to express class II molecules and are regarded as facultative antigen-presenting cells. Apart from

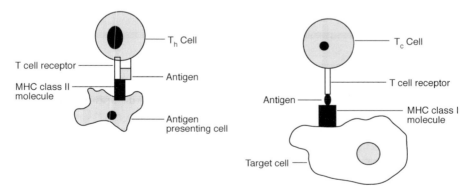

Fig. 3.1 T-helper (T_h) cell reception recognize processed antigen in association with MHC class II molecules. Cytotoxic T cells (T_c) may be MHC class I-restricted and recognize these molecules in association with antigen on target cells.

macrophage/monocyte cells, interdigitating dendritic cells and follicular dendritic cells are classical antigen-presenting cells of the lymphoid organs. Facultative antigen-presenting cells, such as macrophages and endothelial cells, require the presence of inducing signals such as interferon-gamma (IFN-γ) which is produced by activated T cells. Before antigens are presented to lymphocytes they undergo processing, during which large antigens are degraded into fragments which can be recognized by the lymphocytes. This processing takes place at the cell surface, or following ingestion by pinocytosis or phagocytosis in endosomes or phagolysosomes. The detailed mechanisms of antigen processing are the subject of intensive investigation and are not clear at present. When B lymphocytes are sensitized to a specific antigen they are transformed into plasma cells and produce immunoglobulins. T cells are able to recognize processed antigens presented by macrophages and dendritic cells through MHC class II restricted mechanisms. During the activation process, the surface of T cells alters and expresses receptors for interleukin-2 (IL-2) and HLA class II antigens.

Cell-mediated cytotoxicity

The term 'cell-mediated immunity' originally described immune responses mediated by lymphocytes and phagocytes rather than by antibody (humoral immunity). It is difficult, however, to consider cell-mediated and antibody-mediated processes entirely separately because the two are closely linked. T-helper lymphocytes are central to the development of immune responses. They help B cells to produce antibody and also modulate the actions of effector cells, including cytotoxic T cells, macrophages, natural killer (NK) cells, and antibody-dependent cytotoxic cells. Many of these effects are mediated by cytokines. Suppressor T cells also influence these processes. Cell-mediated cytotoxicity involves three main types of receptor–ligand interaction: MHC-restricted T-cell receptors (cytotoxic T cells), antibody Fc receptors (antibody-dependent, cell-mediated cytotoxicity), and determinants recognized by NK cells. Most cytotoxic cells express CD8 on their surface and recognize antigen in association with class I molecules. Cytotoxic cells which are required to destroy virally infected cells recognize antigen and class I molecules which are expressed on all nucleated cells. There are, however, cytotoxic cells which recognize antigen associated with class II molecules and which express CD4.

NK cells play an important role in cell-mediated immunity. These cells comprise 10–15% of the circulating lymphocytes. They are mostly derived from large granular lymphocytes (LGR) which are characterized by a high cytoplasmic/nuclear ratio compared with other lymphocytes. They are defined functionally by their ability to spontaneously lyse autologous and allogeneic target cells and are MHC-unrestricted. *In vivo* these cells are important in the destruction of autologous tumor cells and in resistance to viral infections.

Tumor immunology

The concept that tumor cells are antigenically distinct led to Burnet's hypothesis of tumor immunosurveillance, according to which the majority of potentially malignant cells are recognized and eliminated by the immune system before they can develop into clinically significant neoplasms. A consequence of such a mechanism may be the development of tumors in states of defective immunity. Such immunosuppression may arise as a result of drug therapy or irradiation, diseases affecting the immune system such as AIDS, and inherited deficiencies in immune responsiveness which lead to lymphoreticular neoplasms.

The immunosurveillance theory of tumor genesis is based on the concept that tumor cells express antigens that are not found on non-tumor cells of the body. Malignant transformation of cells may lead to phenotypic changes which include the loss of normally present antigens or the gain of neo-antigens. These neo-antigens may be capable of eliciting an immune response. A strong allogeneic immune response may lead to tumor removal, whereas little or no adaptive immune response may result in tumor expansion. In addition, it is possible that tumors may express neo-antigens which evoke no response at all or generate a response which is successfully evaded; a condition known as immunological escape.

If normal immune mechanisms prevent the emergence of clinically detectable tumors, then the development of tumors could arise from an alteration either in the efficiency of the immune response or in the immunogenicity of the tumor cells. There are a variety of possible mechanisms whereby tumor cells might 'escape' immuno-surveillance. The tumor cells may fail to elicit a response by alteration or loss of MHC class I antigens which would prevent recognition and lysis by cytotoxic T cells. The possible loss of non-antigen-specific adhesion molecules, such as LFA-1, on tumor cells may also contribute to escape from immunosurveillance. The host may be pre-disposed either genetically or as a result of acquired disease which may result in fail-ure of association of the MHC class II molecules with tumor antigens. A rapid growth rate of tumor cells may stimulate an immediate immune response but their rapid growth rate may favor net tumor proliferation. Antigen-shedding may be another mechanism whereby antibodies against tumor antigens are 'blocked'. Hence this may effectively abolish the action of antibody-dependent, cell-mediated cytotoxicity against the tumor cells. Tumor cell products other than antigens, such as anti-chemotactic and anti-inflammatory substances, may decrease the immune response in a non-specific manner.

The immune system in uremia

There is a considerable body of evidence in the literature of an impaired immune response in uremia based on both *in-vitro* and *in-vivo* studies. The earliest evidence of impaired immunity in uremia came from the observation that skin allograft survival was better in uremic subjects (Dammin, *et al.*, 1956). This was confirmed in other studies (Smiddy *et al.*, 1961). The observation that early renal allografts survived longer than other organs transplanted into non-uremic subjects (Hume *et al.*, 1955) provided further evidence of impaired immunity in uremia. Before the availability of immuno-suppressive agents used to prevent allograft rejection, some renal transplants from non-related donors survived for several months in their recipients with ESRD. Later studies provided evidence of anergy and sensitivity to viruses and mycobacteria

(Goldblum and Reed, 1980). It was observed that most patients on dialysis had lymphopenia, a suppressed delayed–hypersensitivity response to a number of stimuli (Casciani *et al.*, 1978), impaired proliferative responses to a number of mitogens (Kamata *et al.*, 1983), and decreased production of immunoglobulins by B lymphocytes (Weeke *et al.*, 1971). Since these early observations, numerous laboratory and research studies have shown impairment of all components of the immune system, such as chemotaxis, phagocytosis, neutrophil function, natural killer-cell activity, and cytokine production.

Chemotaxis

Neutrophil chemotaxis to a variety of stimuli, including *Escherichia coli*, C5a, and immune complexes, is impaired (Lewis and van, Epps 1987). The defects in chemotaxis have been reported in patients receiving both hemodialysis and peritoneal dialysis, although the significance of these observations with regard to any predisposition to infection remains speculative. In patients receiving hemodialysis, contact of blood with the dialyzer membrane causes activation of complement which may lead to saturation of receptors for the chemotactic factor C5a on monocytes and neutrophils, thus leaving receptor sites unavailable for C5a binding following further complement activation. The presence of a permanent catheter in the peritoneal cavity may similarly act as a source of complement activation in patients on peritoneal dialysis, leading to a similar deficiency of free C5a receptors on neutrophils and monocytes.

Phagocytosis

A number of studies have examined phagocytosis in patients receiving chronic dialysis, most, but not all, of which observed a reduction in the phagocytic function of neutrophils from dialysis patients (Goldblum and Reed, 1980; Lewis and van Epps, 1987). Oxidative metabolism is also reduced, resulting in a decrease in the generation of superoxide radicals during the oxidative burst following phagocytosis, which may impair the ability of macrophages to kill phagocytosed microorganisms. Macrophage Fc gamma receptors, which are important in clearing IgG-coated antigens and immune complexes, are shown to have marked functional abnormalities in uremia which may contribute to an increased susceptibility to infection (Ruiz *et al.*, 1990).

Neutrophil–membrane fluidity

Fluidity of the neutrophil membrane regulates receptor activity and has been shown to be reduced in uremic patients (Midory *et al.*, 1990). The reduced neutrophil–membrane fluidity was shown to be reversed with dialysis and has been attributed to uremic factors in blood. Alterations in this characteristic of neutrophil membranes may play a role in susceptibility to infection.

Lymphocytes

Dialysis patients generally tend to show moderate lymphopenia. In addition, a number of functional abnormalities have been observed which include suppressed delayed hypersensitivity to a number of antigenic stimuli such as vaccines (reviewed by Casciani *et al.*, 1978), impaired proliferative responses to stimulation by mitogens (Kamata *et al.*, 1983), and decreased immunoglobulin production by B cells (Weeke *et al.*, 1971).

Despite decreased absolute numbers of circulating B lymphocytes in uremic patients (which may be reversed with dialysis) the levels of circulating immunoglobulins, with the possible exception of IgE (Weeke *et al.*, 1971), are normal in patients on dialysis who are adequately nourished and do not suffer from plasma cell disorders. Investigations of the immunoglobulin response to specific antigen challenges have, however, produced interesting results. Injection of tetanus toxoid (Balch, 1955) and diphtheria toxoid (Stoloff *et al.*, 1958) to uremic patients produced a normal antitoxin response. However, diminished or subnormal antibody responses have been demonstrated following the administration to uremic patients of influenza vaccine (Jordan *et al.*, 1983), typhoid vaccine (Wilson *et al.*, 1965), and pneumococcal capsular-polysaccharide antigen (Simberkoff *et al.*, 1980).

Natural killer (NK) cells

There is also evidence of deficient cidal activity of killer cells in dialyzed patients, which may have a role in the surveillance of clones of cells which might undergo malignant transformation. Asaka *et al.* (1988) investigated the NK cell activity of peripheral blood mononuclear cells and the activity of the suppressor factor for NK cells in patients on maintenance hemodialysis. They found that NK cell activity was significantly lower in patients on hemodialysis than in healthy controls. Furthermore, they found no difference in NK cell activity between those treated with natural and synthetic dialysis membranes. NK cells from patients on hemodialysis showed a poor response to interleukin-2. Also, uremic sera significantly suppressed NK cell activity of normal peripheral blood mononuclear cells (Asaka *et al.*, 1988). Zaoui and Hakim (1993) reported a decrease in the ability of NK cells to lyse target cells derived from the K562 cell line, following 2 weeks' dialysis with the Cuprophan membrane, while their ability to lyse β2m/HLA-negative cells increased during the same period. The authors interpreted these findings as supporting *in-vitro* observations of the decrease in cytolytic activity of the NK cells when exposed to a Cuprophan membrane. The clinical importance of these observations and the finding of increased suppressor cell activity (Raskova *et al.*, 1984) is difficult to evaluate. It has been suggested that they may, in part, explain the possible increased incidence of malignant disease reported by Lindner and colleagues (Lindner *et al.*, 1981), as well as the abnormal host responses to antigenic stimuli.

Cytokine production is also abnormal in dialysis patients. Gamma-interferon, important for macrophage activation and interleukin-2, activates B lymphocytes and T-cell differentiation. The latter are both reduced, while interleukin-1, which stimulates T-cell activity and is released from activated monocytes, is increased (Gall *et al.*, 1981; Bingel *et al.*, 1986; and Chatenoud *et al.*, 1986).

Infections in long-term dialysis

Before the development of dialysis, infections were a major cause of death in patients with chronic renal failure (Montgomerie *et al.*, 1968). Renal replacement in the form of dialysis is, at best, a life-sustaining intervention with intermittent clearance of known and unknown uremic toxins. The state of uremia is therefore not completely reversed by dialysis. The patient who receives dialysis therapy is under the constant threat of infection from breach of the integument and exposure to the synthetic material used for vascular and peritoneal access. It is, therefore, not surprising that device-related and access-related infection are commonly encountered in patients with end-stage renal disease; indeed infections are second only to cardiovascular diseases as the major cause of death in patients on long-term dialysis (Kaslow and Zellner, 1972; Jacobs *et al.*, 1981; Gabriel, 1984; and Lewis, 1990; Lowrie *et al.*, 1973). Tuberculosis has been reported with increased frequency in dialysis patients, as have viral diseases such as hepatitis A, hepatitis B, and hepatitis C.

Most studies detailing infections encountered in dialysis patients were carried out more than a quarter of a century ago. Despite a considerable and often conflicting body of data on *in-vitro* defects in the immune system in uremia, it has not been definitely established whether patients receiving dialysis therapy are at greater risk of developing infectious complications other than those related to vascular access and to nosocomial spread of viral infections. The introduction of CAPD during the late 1970s and 1980s provided further evidence of the increased risk of infections associated with uremia. Recurrent episodes of peritonitis proved to be not only the most common complication (Gokal *et al.*, 1982, Heaton *et al.*, 1986) but a potent stimulus for further research into mechanisms of chronic immunosuppression.

Bacterial infections in patients receiving long-term dialysis

Evidence for an increased incidence of bacterial infection among patients receiving dialysis comes from three main sources. First, single case reports, or small case series, of patients from a single center detailed unusual infections or presentations in dialysis patients, such as rare causes of bacterial peritonitis. These anecdotal reports are sporadic and of limited interest to the practising nephrologist. The second source of information is that derived from registry reports on a national and international level, in which data from many centers are collated under standard conditions and are of a general nature. Finally, large, individual dialysis centers have reviewed their clinical experience and provided detailed analyses of infections occurring in their patient population over a period of time. These studies probably provide the most valuable and reliable information on infectious problems in dialysis. Data from nine studies which have described infections as a cause of mortality in dialysis patients are summarized in Table 3.1 (modified from Lewis, 1990).

Studies carried out before 1980 showed that infection was a frequent cause of morbidity and mortality in patients on long-term hemodialysis. Most episodes of infection, however, comprised those related to vascular access. Kaslow and Zellner (1972) reviewed all infectious episodes in 309 hemodialysis patients from five centers over a period of 12–45 months. Their observations covered 2943 patient-months during which a mean incidence of 6.5 infections per 100 patient-months was recorded, of which 3.5 infections per 100 patient-months were attributed to arteriovenous-shunt infections. Bacteremia accounted for 4–33% of the totals for the centers, urinary tract infections for 0–17%, with respiratory and other infections responsible for smaller proportions of the total number of infections observed. These authors unfortunately did not provide information about the number of deaths attributed to infectious causes.

Table 3.1 Percentage of deaths caused by infection in patients on long-term dialysis (modified from Lewis, 1990). (Reproduced with permission from Khan and Catto, 1993.)

Percentage of deaths	No of patients	Length of study (years)	References
19.8	45	3.5	Keane *et al.*, 1977
32.4[a]	445	3.5	Keane *et al.*, 1977
19.8	1014	11	Nsouli *et al.*, 1979
24	333	NR[b]	Berman *et al.*, 1979
35.7	24	14	Lundin *et al.*, 1980
13.1	1453	6	Degoulet *et al.*, 1982
14.9	373	15	Laurent *et al.*, 1983
15.7	83	10	Neff *et al.*, 1983
13	NR	NR	Nissenson *et al.*, 1986
31	NR	NR	Rubin *et al.*, 1983

[a] Includes infections contributing to death.　　NR, Not reported.

Keane *et al.*, (1977) report that infection was the primary or a contributory factor in more than 30% of deaths. Of the 445 patients studied for 42 months, 111 died, and infection either as a primary or contributory factor was responsible for 4.4 deaths/1000 treatment-months. Non-diabetics over 60 years of age had a higher incidence of death related to infection than younger patients (7.8 deaths vs. 1.4 deaths/1000 treatment-months). The incidence of deaths related to infection was similar in diabetic patients (6.6 deaths/1000 treatment-months) and non-diabetic patients (4.2/1000 treatment-months). Analysis of the various sources of infection indicated that vascular access site and respiratory infections were the most frequent problems, particularly in older patients. A total of 40 episodes of pneumonia were reported in 35 patients, giving an incidence of 4.9 episodes per 1000 patient-months. *Streptococcus pneumoniae* was isolated in 53% of patients, Gram-negative organisms from 33%, and *Staphylococcus aureus* from 13%. Almost two-thirds of the episodes occurred while the patients were already in hospital. They frequently followed such procedures as splenectomy and bilateral nephrectomy, at that time undertaken prior to renal transplantation.

Access-site infection was particularly common in this series, with an incidence of 72.3 episodes per 1000 treatment-months. The incidence of bacteremia was 15.3 per 1000 treatment-months. Cannulas were responsible for almost 80% of access-site related infections—an incidence of 5–7 times that observed with arteriovenous fistulas. The incidence of bacteremia secondary to access-site infection was significantly higher in diabetic than in non-diabetic patients (16.6 vs. 7.5 episodes per 1000 treatment-months). Access-site infections not only were associated with a 10% mortality rate but caused substantial morbidity, including septic pulmonary emboli, endo-carditis, and osteomyelitis. The authors concluded that infection was the major cause of morbidity and mortality in their patients on hemodialysis. The most common source was vascular access particularly when cannulas were used.

Higgins (1989) examined the incidence of infections in 211 hemodialysis and 99 peritoneal dialysis patients over a one-year period. Apart from infections related to vascular or peritoneal access, long-term dialysis patients developed few serious infections unless they had another disease causing immunosuppression. Out of 18 cases of septicemia, 16 were caused by Gram-positive organisms and were related to vascular access infection, but other infections were uncommon in patients on hemodialysis.

The hypothesis that patients receiving dialysis treatment are at risk of infections, primarily due to the processes involved in the dialysis procedure rather than to the defects in immune mechanisms observed in *in-vitro* studies, is supported by the observation that rare opportunistic infections seen in AIDS and with immunosup-pressive treatment are uncommon in dialysis patients. A recent study (Hoen *et al.*, 1995) reported the incidence of bacterial infection in over 600 patients receiving hemodialysis in 13 French dialysis units during a 6-month period. Patients had received dialysis for a mean duration of 4.7 years. They found that 118 patients (19%) developed at least one bacterial infection during this period. Patients who developed infection were comparable to those who were infection-free with respect to age, duration of dialysis, and cause of renal failure. Of the 30 episodes of bacteremia, 22 (73%) were due to *Staphylococcus aureus* infection and 17 of these were related to vascular access infection. In a multivariate analysis, three variables were found to be significant and independent risk factors for bacterial infection: previous history of bacterial infection, the presence of a dialysis catheter as opposed to a fistula, and an elevated serum ferritin concentration (>500 μmol/l). The study suggested that factors predisposing to bacterial infection in hemodialysis patients were those related to treatment. The authors point out that most of the patients studied had received multiple blood transfusions as the use of erythropoietin had not been common during the study period. Other studies have also suggested iron overload as a predis-posing factor for infections; iron overload impairs the chemotactic and phagocytic properties of neutrophils (Tielemans *et al.*, 1989), and iron is an essential element for bacterial growth. With the need for blood transfusions decreasing as more patients are treated with erythropoietin there may be a further reduction in the infectious com-plications of long-term dialysis therapy.

Tuberculosis

Patients receiving long-term dialysis therapy may be at increased risk of tuberculosis, although the evidence for such a risk is inconclusive. The diagnosis is often difficult to establish because the symptoms may mimic those of uremia and because intermediate-strength tuberculin tests may be negative (Pradham *et al.*, 1974; Lundin *et al.*, 1979; Andrew *et al.*, 1980). Pradham and colleagues (1974) reported a series of five patients with active tuberculosis among 136 hemodialysis patients over an average period of 1.4 years. Later Lundin *et al.* reported eight cases of tuberculosis in hemodialysis patients over a period of 10 years (Lundin *et al.*, 1979). Soon after this report was published, Andrew and colleagues reported tuberculosis in 10 out of 172 adult patients on hemodialysis (Andrew *et al.*, 1980). It is perhaps relevant that the vast majority of patients reported in these three papers were either black American or Chinese in origin, ethnic groups which have a high incidence of tuberculosis in the general population. Nevertheless, the incidence of tuberculosis was considered high even for these ethnic groups.

Prevention of infections in dialysis patients

It is apparent that the majority of infections encountered in patients receiving dialysis are related to vascular and peritoneal access, and to breach of the mechanical barriers to infection. Meticulous aseptic techniques during needling of fistulas, insertion of temporary central venous catheters, and exchange of peritoneal dialysis fluid remain the key preventive measures. The introduction of new peritoneal dialysis delivery systems such as the Y-set and flush-before-fill techniques have led to a reduction in the incidence of peritonitis. In patients with nasal carriage of Staphylococcus, the use of topical mupirocin ointment or a 5-day course of oral rifampicin (600 mg/day) may prevent recurrent peritonitis. This is particularly useful for the prevention of exit-site infections.

Malnutrition, an important cause of a suppressed immune system (Glassock, 1983), is not uncommon in uremic patients. Patients on dialysis often suffer from protein–calorie malnutrition (Lowrie and Lew, 1990). In a study involving two hemodialysis patients with protein–calorie malnutrition, protein and calorie supplementation for 3 months resulted in improved skin responses to four different antigens tested (Hak *et al.*, 1982). Of the many studies of the immunological changes in uremia and the clinical studies regarding infections in patients on maintenance dialysis, none has taken account of the nutritional status of their patients. Further studies to examine the role played by malnutrition in the susceptibility of dialysis patients to infection are required. It is possible that by improving the nutritional status of long-term dialysis patients the incidence of infection may be reduced. The increased availability and use of recombinant human erythropoietin for the treatment of anemia in dialysis patients should lead to a reduced need for blood transfusions, and this should decrease the risk of transmission of blood-borne infections. There is some evidence that the use of biocompatible membranes, as opposed to cellulose acetate and modified cellulose acetate membranes, in hemodialysis may be associated with a reduced risk of infection, although this needs to be assessed in large controlled trials (Himmelfarb and Hakim, 1994).

The use of vaccines in dialysis patients

In patients receiving dialysis for ESRD, the response to vaccination is usually suboptimal. There is evidence, however, that vaccinations against pneumococcus, hepatitis, and influenza are effective in most dialysis patients and should be undertaken. For hepatitis B, an increase in the dosage schedule to double that used for normal individuals is recommended and is likely to result in successful immunization. A course of three doses (40 μg per dose) of intramuscular hepatitis B vaccine is recommended at 0,1, and 6 months. There is some evidence that intradermal injection may be more effective than the intramuscular route. In dialysis patients without an antibody response after three doses of vaccine, a fourth dose is recommended which may be given 9–12 months after the initiation of vaccination (Kohler *et al.*, 1984). In patients who are non-responders, low dose interleukin-2 administration together with the vaccine may induce a response (Meuer *et al.*, 1989)—an observation that needs to be confirmed in larger controlled studies.

Although most renal units now immunize staff against hepatitis B, and vaccination against hepatitis B is recommended for hemodialysis patients in the UK (UK Health Departments, 1992), immunization against hepatitis B has not been adopted in most dialysis units. A postal survey of 73 UK renal units (Jibani *et al.*, 1994) revealed that only four (5%) routinely immunized their patients. Vaccination against pneumococcus and influenza are also recommended in patients receiving dialysis.

Malignant disease in long-term dialysis patients

The increased incidence of cancer in recipients of renal transplants has been recognized since 1972. Whether patients receiving long-term dialysis treatment are at an increased risk of developing cancer is less clear. Matas *et al.* (1975) first reported a higher than expected incidence of malignant disease in patients with chronic renal failure. In a study of 646 patients with renal failure (78 on dialysis) they showed a 7-fold increased incidence of malignant disease in patients with chronic renal failure (creatinine greater than 220 μmol/l) compared with the general population matched for age. Slifkin *et al.* (1977) studied the incidence of cancer in 712 dialysis patients, but did not find a higher incidence than was expected for age and sex, with the exception of renal cell carcinoma and reticulum cell sarcoma. A study of 1651 patients followed over a period of 10 years in six English dialysis units also did not show an increased incidence of cancer in dialysis patients, with the exception of non-Hodgkin's lymphoma (Kinlen *et al.*, 1980). The authors suggested that the small (not statistically significant) increase in non-lymphoid tumors might have resulted from better surveillance of dialysis patients. Another study showed a decreased incidence of cancer in patients with chronic renal failure (Bush and Gabriel, 1984). Kantor *et al.* excluded patients whose cancer was diagnosed during the first 3 months of dialysis, to reduce the possible confounding factor of patients whose tumors might be related to the cause of renal failure, and showed a reduced incidence of cancer in dialysis patients (Kantor *et al.*, 1987).

When considering whether long-term dialysis is associated with an increased risk of malignancy it should be borne in mind that a number of primary renal diseases are associated with an increased risk of renal cancer, such as polycystic kidneys and analgesic nephropathy. The former is associated with renal cell carcinoma and the latter with transitional carcinoma (Jacobs *et al.*, 1979; Kjellstrand, 1979). Thus in a study from North America 36 tumors were detected in 33 patients receiving dialysis; a tumor occurrence rate 20 times higher than expected in the general population. Most of the tumors were urogenital, and six of the seven bladder tumors were reported in patients with analgesic nephropathy (Pecqueux *et al.*, 1990).

Port *et al.* (1989) studied the incidence of cancer in those patients on dialysis using data from the Michigan Kidney Registry, and reported an increased relative risk of cancer in dialysis patients for renal cell cancer (X5), uterine cancer (X4), myeloma (X4), and prostatic cancer (X2). The authors attribute the high risk of renal cell cancer to underlying, acquired cystic kidney disease and polycystic disease.

Inamato and colleagues (1991) studied the incidence and risk of malignancy in a large population of patients undergoing dialysis. The authors performed a questionnaire study among 23,209 dialysis patients in 589 institutions. They excluded patients whose renal failure was secondary to malignant disease and those with a previous history of malignancy or of renal transplantation. The authors found an incidence of cancer 1.4 times the expected rates in the general population and a mortality rate 1.9 times the expected rate. The respective rates for cancer incidence and mortality were 1.9-fold and 2.6-fold higher for males than for females. The incidence was higher during the first 6 months of dialysis therapy than during later years. It was higher in younger dialysis patients relative to the general population in the same age group; over the age of 60 years the influence of age was greater than that of renal failure. The frequency of malignant diseases of the liver, colon, rectum, bladder, kidney, larynx, and skin were higher and that of pancreatic cancer was lower than in the general population. The risk of dying from cancer of the lungs, colon, rectum, bladder, kidney, and prostate was higher than in patients suffering from these cancers among the non-dialysis population. An interesting observation made in this study was the so-called detection bias; a high incidence rate was seen in university institutions where patients were more likely to undergo more intensive investigations and where autopsy rates were high.

Marple and MacDougall (1993) recently reviewed studies addressing the incidence of malignant disease in dialysis patients. They concluded that even studies indicating no overall increased risk of malignancy showed a higher risk of certain malignant diseases, such as non-Hodgkin's lymphoma, renal cell carcinoma, and some *in-situ* cancers. A summary of the relative risk of malignancy in different studies is shown in Table 3.2. These studies did not report the presence or absence of underlying, acquired cystic disease; the prevalence of renal cancer was more than 10 times that reported in the general population. Acquired cystic disease and its complications are more fully discussed elsewhere (Chapter 7).

A more recent study from the Lombardy Regional Dialysis and Transplant Registry reported the incidence of cancer in 44023 patient-years (25684 in men and 18339 in women). Patients with a history of cancer or those who developed cancer during the first year of dialysis were excluded. Only the first cancer was considered; 479 cases of cancer were recorded. The mean age of patients at diagnosis was 59.5 years and they had been on dialysis for a mean duration of 6.37 years. The relative risks of cancers in patients were calculated using data from the Varese Cancer Registry. There were significantly raised relative risks of primary liver cancer (2.41), renal cancer (2.82), thyroid cancer (2.22), lymphoma (2.19), and multiple myeloma (2.39). There were significantly decreased risks of cancers of the oral cavity and larynx (Buccianti *et al.*, 1996).

Table 3.2 Relative risk of malignancy in ESRD (modified from Marple and MacDougall 1993, with permission).

Increased Risk	Reference	Unchanged Risk	Reference
1.4	Inamoto *et al.*, 1991	0.9	Kantor *et al.*, 1987[a]
2.5	Lindner *et al.*, 1981	1.3	Kinlen *et al.*, 1980[b]
7.0	Matas *et al.*, 1975	1.0 (male)	Slifkin *et al.*, 1977
2.5	Sheil *et al.*, 1985	1.1 (female)	
22.6	Pecqueux *et al.*, 1990	0.45	Bush and Gabriel 1984
3.8	Herr *et al.*, 1979	1.1	Port *et al.*, 1989[c]
21.0	Miach *et al.*, 1976		
10.0	Sutherland *et al.*, 1977		
2.8	Robles *et al.*, 1990		
2.4	Jacobs *et al.*, 1981		

[a] Chronic GN-RR 2.6 for non-Hodgkin's lymphoma.
[b] Increased risk of non-Hodgkin's lymphoma (RR 26.6).
[c] Increased risk (5.0) for: renal cell carcinoma; (3.1) *in-situ* carcinoma; (4.3) uterine; and (1.8) prostatic carcinoma.

Taken together most studies addressing cancer incidence in dialysis patients seem to show an increased risk of cancer, especially for renal cancer and lymphoma. Longer and better patient survival, the availability of improved screening methods (such as magnetic resonance imaging and tumor markers), and improved clinical surveillance may contribute to an apparent rise in cancer in patients on long-term dialysis therapy in the future.

Screening for malignant disease in dialysis patients

There are no accepted guidelines for screening for malignant disease in dialysis patients, who are often seen in clinics by nursing and medical staff. This presents plenty of opportunities to examine patients and to undertake routine screening for the emergence of cancer. This is particularly important in patients with analgesic nephropathy who are at risk of developing transitional cell tumors of the urothelium, and those with acquired polycystic kidneys who are at an increased risk of renal cell carcinoma. The usefulness of urine cytology as a screening method for transitional cell carcinoma in dialysis patients with analgesic nephropathy was studied in 9 out of 138 patients with analgesic nephropathy. Urine cytology led to a suspicion of malignancy in three patients which was confirmed on further investigation (Veltman *et al.*, 1991).

The unexpected development of polycythemia or an unexplained lack of response or resistance to erythropoietin treatment should raise the suspicion of cancer as should flank pain and hematuria and dysfunctional uterine bleeding in women especially over the age of 40 years who have not menstruated for at least 1 year. It has been suggested (Pahl and Vaziri, 1994) that stools for occult blood and rectal examination in those patients over 40 years of age and cervical cytology in women should be performed annually. Women should be instructed in self-examination of the breast regularly. Older women (over 50 years) with a family history of breast cancer should probably have a yearly mammogram. In a study of mammography in 16 women on dialysis, however, a significant increase in vascular and parenchymal calcification was observed compared to age-matched controls. Ductal calcifications were no more prevalent in patients on dialysis and in no case did the calcification simulate malignancy (Evans *et al.*, 1992).

Tumor markers play an important role in the assessment of patients with some types of malignant tumors. Lye and colleagues (1994) studied the effects of dialysis and transplantation on the serum levels of five tumor markers; alpha-fetoprotein (AFP), carcinoembryonic antigen (CEA), cancer antigen-125 (CA-125), cancer antigen-19.9 (CA-19.9), and prostate-specific antigen (PSA). Serum tumor markers were measured in patients who had been on dialysis treatment or had had a renal transplant for at least 1 month. Serum AFP and PSA levels were within normal limits in the dialysis and transplant patients. CEA, CA-125, and CA-19.9 were raised in the hemodialysis and peritoneal dialysis patients compared with transplant patients and controls. Thus serum PSA and AFP may be useful markers for screening for prostatic and hepatic tumors in dialysis patients.

Conclusions

The morbidity and mortality rates associated with long-term dialysis treatment are well documented. The hypothesis that dialysis patients are at substantially greater risk of infection than control subjects has not—with two exceptions—been supported by good evidence in recent years. The exceptions are the infections associated with vascular and peritoneal access and viral hepatitis. With appropriate prophylaxis and treatment both are manageable, but remain significant threats to the health of dialysis patients. The evidence currently available suggests that patients on dialysis should be immunized against hepatitis B, pneumococcus, and influenza and thereafter reassessed.

The evidence for an increased risk of malignant disease remains controversial. At present there are few well-controlled studies showing a significantly greater risk of cancer in dialysis patients—despite the very great changes in immunological tests reproducibly detectable *in vitro*.

References

Andrew, O. T., Schonfeld, P. Y., Hopwell, P. C., and Humphreys, M. H. (1980). Tuberculosis in patients with end stage renal disease. *American Journal of Medicine*, **68**, 59–65.

Asaka, M., Iida, H., Izumino, K., and Sasayama, S. (1988). Depressed natural killer cell activity in uraemia: evidence for immunosuppressive factor in uraemic sera. *Nephron*, **49**, 291–5.

Balch, H. H. (1955). The effect of severe battle injury and post traumatic renal failure on resistance to infection. *Annals of Surgery*, **142**, 145–63.

Berman, S. J., Hess, J. R., Sugihara, J. G., Wong, E. G. C., Wong, L., and Semson, A. W. (1979). Morbidity of infection in chronic haemodialysis. *Dialysis and Transplantation*, **8**, 324–8.

Bingel, M., Lonnemann, G., Shaldon, S., Koch, K. M., and Dinarello, C. A. (1986). Human interleukin-1 production during haemodialysis. *Nephron*, **43**, 161–3.

Buccianti, G., Ravasi, B., Cresseri, D., Maisonneuve, P., Boyle, P., and Locatelli, F. (1996). Cancer in patients on renal replacement therapy in Lombardy, Italy. *Lancet*, **347**, 59–60 (letter).

Bush, A., and Gabriel, R. (1984). Cancer in uraemic patients. *Clinical Nephrology*, **22**, 77–81.

Caramelo, C., Navas, S., Alberola, M. L., Bermejillo, T., Reyero, A., and Carreno, V. (1994). Evidence against transmission of hepatitis C virus through hemodialysis ultrafiltrate and peritoneal fluid. *Nephron*, **66**, 470–3.

Casciani, C. U., Simone, C. D., Bonini, S., *et al.* (1978). Immunological aspects of chronic uraemia. *Kidney International*, **13** (Suppl. 8), S49–S54.

Chatenoud, L., Dugas, B., and Beaurain, G., *et al.* (1986). Presence of reactivated T cells in haemodialysed patients. Their possible role in altered immunity. *Proceedings of the National Academy of Sciences*, **83**, 7457–61.

Dammin, G. J., Couch, N. P., and Murray, J. E. (1956). Prolonged survival of skin homografts in uremic patients. *Annals of the NY Academy of Sciences*, **64**, 967–76.

Degoulet, P., Legrain, M., Reach, R., *et al.* (1982). Mortality risk factors in patients treated by chronic haemodialysis. *Nephrology*, **32**, 103–10.

Evans, A. J., Cohen, M. E., and Cohen, G. F. (1992). Patterns of breast calcification in patients on renal dialysis. *Clinical Radiology*, **45**, 343–4.

Feest, T. G., Mistry, C. D., Grimes, D. S., and Mallick, N. P. (1990). Incidence of advanced chronic renal failure and the need for end-stage renal replacement treatment. *British Medical Journal*, **301**, 897–900.

Gabriel, R. (1984). Morbidity and mortality of long term dialysis: a review. *Journal of the Royal Society of Medicine*, **77**, 595–601.

Gal, G., Toth, M., and Toth, S. (1981). Interferon production of leukocytes of dialysed chronic uraemic patients. *Proceedings of the European Transplantation Association*, **18**, 188–92.

Glassock, R. J. (1983). Nutrition, immunology and renal disease. *Kidney International*, **74**, S194–S198.

Gokal, R., Ramos, J. M., Francis, D. M. A., *et al.* (1982). Peritonitis in continuous ambulatory peritoneal dialysis. *Lancet*, **2**, 1388–91.

Goldblum, S. E., and Reed, W. P. (1980). Host defences and immunological associated with chronic haemodialysis. *Annals of Internal Medicine*, **93**, 597–613.

Hak, L. J., Lefell, M. S., Lamanna, R. W., Teasley, K. M., Bazzarre, L. H., and Mattern, W. D. (1982). Reversal of skin test anergy during maintenance haemodialysis by protein and calorie supplementation. *American Journal of Clinical Nutrition*, **36**, 1089–92.

Heaton, A., Rodger, R. S. C., Sellars, L., *et al.* (1986). Continuous ambulatory peritoneal dialysis after the honeymoon: review of experience in Newcastle. *British Medical Journal*, **293**, 938–41.

Herr, H. W., Engen, D. E., and Hostetler, J. (1979). Malignancy in uremia: dialysis versus transplantation. *Journal of Urology*, **121**, 584–6.

Higgins, R. M. (1989). Infections in a renal unit. *Quarterly Journal of Medicine*, **70**, 41–51.

Himmelfarb, J., and Hakim, R. M. (1994). Biocompatibility and risk of infection in haemodialysis patients. *Nephrology, Dialysis, Transplantation*, **9** (Suppl. 2), 138–44.

Hoen, B., Kessler, M., Hestin, D., and Mayeux, D. (1995). Risk factors for bacterial infections in chronic haemodialysis adult patients: a multicentre prospective study. *Nephrology, Dialysis, Transplantation*, **10**, 377–81.

Hume, D. M., Merrill, J. P., Miller, B. F., and Thorn, G. W. (1955). Experiences with renal transplantation in the human: report of nine cases. *Journal of Clinical Investigation*, **34**, 327–82.

Inamoto, H., Ryoko, O., Takako, M., Masatoshi, W., Takao, S., and Osawa, A. (1991). Incidence and mortality pattern of malignancy and factors affecting the risk of malignancy in dialysis patients. *Nephron*, **59**, 611–17.

Jacobs, C., Reach, I., and Degoulet, P. (1979). Cancer in patients on haemodialysis. *New England Journal of Medicine*, **300**, 1279–80.

Jacobs, C., Broyer, M., and Brunner, F. P., *et al.* (1981). Combined report on regular dialysis and transplantation in Europe XI 1980. *Proceedings of the European Dialysis and Transplantation Association*, **18**, 4–58.

Jibani, M. M., Heptonstall, J., Walker, A. M., Bloodworth, L. O., and Howard, A. J. (1994). Hepatitis B immunisation in UK renal units: failure to put policy into practice. *Nephrology, Dialysis, Transplantation*, **9**, 1765–8.

Jordan, M. C., Rousseau, W. E., Tegtmeier, G. E., Noble, G. R., Myth, R. G., and Chin, T. D. Y. (1973). Immunogenicity of inactivated influenza virus vaccine in chronic renal failure. *Annals of Internal Medicine*, **79**, 790–4.

Kamata, K., Okubo, M., and Sada, M. (1983). Immunosuppressive factors in uraemic sera are composed of both dialysable and non-dialysable components. *Clinical and Experimental Immunology*, **54**, 277–81.

Kantor, A. F., Hoover, R. N., Kinlen, L. J., McMullan, M. R., and Fraumeni, J. F. (1987). Cancer in patients receiving long-term dialysis treatment. *American Journal of Epidemiology*, **126**, 370–6.

Kaslow, R. A., and Zellner, S. R. (1972). Infections in patients on haemodialysis. *Lancet*, **2**, 117–18.

Keane, W. F., Shapiro, F. L., and Raij, L. (1977). Incidence and type of infections occurring in 445 chronic haemodialysis patients. *Transactions of the American Society of Artificial Internal Organs*, **23**, 41–6.

Khan, I. H., and Catto, G. R. D. (1993). Long-term complications of dialysis: infections. *Kidney International*, **41**, S143–148.

Khan, I. H., Catto, G. R. D., and Edward, N. (1994). Chronic renal failure: factors influencing nephrology referral. *Quarterly Journal of Medicine*, **87**, 559–64.

Kinlen, L. J., Eastwood, J. B., Kerr, D. N. S., *et al.* (1980). Cancer in patients receiving dialysis. *British Medical Journal*, **280**, 1401–3.

Kjellstrand, C. M. (1979). Are malignancies increased in uraemia? *Nephron*, **23**, 159–61.

Kohler, H., Arnold, W., Renschin, G., Dormeyer, H. H., and Meyer zum Buschenfelde, K. H. (1984). Active hepatitis B vaccination in dialysis patients and medical staff. *Kidney International*, **25**, 124–8.

Laurent, G., Calemard, E., and Charra, B. (1983). Long dialysis: a review of 15 years experience in one centre 1968–1983. *Proceedings of the European Dialysis and Transplantation Association*, **20**, 122–9.

Lewis, S. L. (1990). Alteration of host defence mechanisms in chronic dialysis patients. *Association of Nephrology Nurses of America Journal*, **17**, 170–80.

Lewis, S. L., and Van Epps, D. E. (1987). Neutrophil and monocyte alterations in chronic dialysis patients. *American Journal of Kidney Diseases*, **9**, 381–95.

Lindner, A., Farewell, V. J., and Sherrard, D. J. (1981). High incidence of neoplasia in uraemic patients receiving long-term dialysis. *Nephron*, **27**, 292–6.

Lowrie, E. G., and Lew, N. L. (1990). Death risks in haemodialysis patients: the predictive value of commonly measured variables and an evaluation of death rate differences between facilities. *American Journal of Kidney Diseases*, **15**, 458–82.

Lowrie, E. G., Lazarus, J. M., Mocelin, A. J., *et al.* (1973). Survival of patients undergoing chronic haemodialysis and renal transplantation. *New England Journal of Medicine*, **288**, 863–7.

Lundin, A. P., Adler, A. J., Berlyne, G. M., and Friedman, E. A. (1979). Tuberculosis in patients undergoing maintenance haemodialysis. *American Journal of Medicine*, **67**, 597–602.

Lundin, A. P., Adler, A. J., Feinroth, M. V., Berlyne, G. M., and Freedman, E. A. (1980). Maintenance haemodialysis: survival beyond the first decade. *Journal of the American Medical Association*, **244**, 38–40.

Lye, W. C., Tambyah, P., Leong, S. O., and Lee, E. J. (1994). Serum tumor markers in patients on dialysis and kidney transplantation. *Advances in Peritoneal Dialysis*, **10**, 109–11.

Marple, J. T., and MacDougall, M. (1993). Development of malignancy in the end-stage renal disease patient. *Seminars in Nephrology*, **13**, 306–14.

Matas, A. J., Simmons, R. L., Kjellstrand, C. M., Buselmeier, T. J., and Najarian, J. S. (1975). Increased incidence of malignancy during chronic renal failure. *Lancet*, **1**, 883–6.

Meuer, S. C., Dumman, H., Meyer zum Buschenfelde, K. H., and Kohler, H. (1989). Low-dose interleukin-2 induces systemic immune responses against HBsAg in immunodeficient non-responders to hepatitis B vaccination. *Lancet*, **1**, 15–18.

Miach, P., Dawborn, J., and Zipell, J. (1976). Neoplasia in patients with chronic renal failure on long-term dialysis. *Clinical Nephrology*, **5**, 101–4.

Midory, M., Komiyama, Y., Murakami, T., and Murata, K. (1990). Decrease of polymorphonuclear leucocyte membrane fluidity in uraemic patients on haemodialysis. *Nephron*, **54**, 36–41.

Montgomerie, J. Z., Kalmanson, G. M., and Guze, L. B. (1968). Renal failure and infection. *Medicine* (Baltimore), **47**, 1–32.

Neff, M. S., Eiser, A. R., Slifkin, R. F., *et al.* (1983). Patients surviving ten years of haemodialysis. *American Journal of Medicine*, **74**, 996–1004.

Nissenson, A. R., Gentile, D. E., and Soderblom, R. E. (1986). Morbidity and mortality of CAPD—regional experience and long-term prospects. *American Journal of Kidney Diseases*, **7**, 229–34.

Nsouli, K. A., Lazarus, J. M., Schoenbaum, S. C., Gottlieb, M., Laurie, E. G., and Shocair, M. (1979). Bacteremic infection in haemodialysis. *Archives of Internal Medicine*, **139**, 1255–9.

Pahl, M. V., and Vaziri, N. D. (1994). Cancer. In *Handbook of dialysis* (ed. J. T. Daugirdas and T. S. Ing), pp. 537–44. Little Brown and Co., Boston.

Pecqueux, J. C., Schwarz, A., Dieckmann, K. P., *et al.* (1990). Cancer incidence in patients on chronic dialysis and in renal transplant recipients. *Urology International*, **45**, 290–2.

Port, F. K., Ragheb, N. E., Schwartz, A. G., *et al.* (1989). Neoplasms in dialysis patients: a population based study. *American Journal of Kidney Diseases*, **14**, 119–23.

Pradham, R. P., Katz, L. A., Nidus, B. D., Malaton, R., and Eisinger, R. P. (1974). Tuberculosis in dialysed patients. *Journal of the American Medical Association*, **229**, 798–800.

Raskova, J., Ghobrial, I., Shea, S. M., Eisinger, R. P., and Raska, K. (1984). Suppressor cells in end stage renal disease. Functional assays and monoclonal antibody analysis. *American Journal of Medicine*, **76**, 847–53.

Robles, N. R., Calero, R., Rengel, M., *et al.* (1990). Hemodialysis and cancer. *Nephron*, **54**, 271–2.

Rubin, J., Barnes, T., and Bower, J. (1983). Morbidity and mortality in CAPD and home haemodialysis. *International Journal of Artificial Internal Organs*, **6**, 22–7.

Ruiz, P., Gomez, F., and Schreiber, A. D. (1990). Impaired function of macrophage Fc receptors in end-stage renal disease. *New England Journal of Medicine*, **322**, 717–22.

Sheil, A. G., Flavel, S., Disney, A. P., *et al.* (1985). Cancer in dialysis and transplant patients. *Transplantation Proceedings*, **17**, 195–8.

Simberkoff, M. S., Schiffman, G., Katz, L. A., Spicehandler, J. R., Moldover, N. H., and Rahal, J. J. (1980). Pneumococcal capsular polysaccharide vaccination in adult chronic haemodialysis patients. *Journal of Laborarory and Clinical Medicine*, **96**, 363–70.

Slifkin, R. F., Goldberg, J., Neff, M. S., Baez, A., Mattoo, N., and Gupta, S. (1977). Malignancy in end-stage renal disease. *Transactions of the American Society of Artificial Internal Organs*, **23**, 34–9.

Smiddy, F. G., Burwell, R. G., and Parsons, F. M. (1961). Influence of uraemia on the survival of skin homografts. *Nature*, **190**, 732.

Stolof, I. L., Stout, R., Myerson, R. M., and Havens, W. P. (1958). Production of antibody in patients with uraemia. *New England Journal of Medicine*, **259**, 320–3.

Sutherland, G., Glass, J., and Gabriel, R. (1977). Increased incidence of malignancy in chronic renal failure. *Nephron*, **18**, 182–4.

Tielemans, C. L., Lenclud, C. M., Wens, R., Collart, F. E., and Dratwa, M. (1989). Critical role of iron overload in haemodialysis patients to bacterial infections. Beneficial effects of desferrioxamine. *Nephrology, Dialysis, Transplantation*, **4**, 883–7.

UK Health Departments (1992). *Immunisation against infectious disease*. HMSO, London.

USRDS (1991). United States Renal Data System, Annual Data Report. *American Journal of Kidney Diseases*, **18**, 1–118.

Veltman, G. A., Bosch, F. H., van der Plas-Cats, M. B., and van Leusen, R. (1991). Urine cytology as a screening method for transitional cell carcinoma in dialysis patients with analgesic nephropathy. *Nephrology, Dialysis, Transplantation*, **6**, 346–8.

Weeke, B., Weeke E., and Bendixen, G. (1971). The variation in twenty one serum proteins before and after renal transplantation. I. General pattern. *Acta Medica Scandinavica*, **189**, 113–18.

Wilson, W. E. C., Kirkpatrick, C. H., and Talmage, D. W. (1965). Suppression of immunologic responsiveness in uraemic patients. *Annals of Internal Medicine*, **62**, 1–4.

Zaoui, P., and Hakim, R. M. (1993). Natural killer-cell function in haemodialysis patients: effect of the dialysis membrane. *Kidney International*, **43**, 1298–305.

4

Complications of long-term dialysis: bone disease

John Cunningham

General introduction

Normal role of the kidney in the maintenance of bone and mineral homeostasis

Divalent cation, phosphorus, and bone metabolism are critically dependent upon the fluxes of these mineral ions at the level of the kidney, the intestine, and bone itself. In the case of bone these fluxes are internal, and as such do not directly affect the overall balance of calcium, magnesium, or phosphorus whereas, in contrast, both the kidney and intestine are important sites of the regulation of their overall balance. Therefore, it is not surprising that disease of the kidney frequently leads to serious disturbances of mineral metabolism.

The integration of function between the kidney, the intestine and bone is achieved in a number of ways (Fig 4.1). Prominent amongst these are the roles exerted by the two major calcium regulating hormones, parathyroid hormone and 1,25-dihydroxyvitamin D (calcitriol), the latter being the hormonal form of vitamin D. In health, the kidney is by far the most important site for the synthesis of calcitriol, and the damaged kidney therefore has additional potential to perturb bone and mineral metabolism by failing to synthesize adequate amounts of calcitriol (Malluche and Faugere, 1990; Hruska and Teitelbaum, 1995).

The daily filtered load of calcium in health is approximately 230 mmol, of which a little over half is reabsorbed in the proximal tubule and the remainder in the thick ascending limb and more distal sites. In health, the reabsorption is almost complete, with only about 5 mmol of the daily filtered load of calcium appearing in the final urine. Parathyroid hormone (PTH) is an important controlling influence on urinary calcium—PTH serves to increase the tubular reabsorption of calcium, and its direct action on the kidney is therefore anticalciuric. Other important factors impacting on renal calcium handling are the sodium excretion rate and acid–base status. Both natriuresis and acidosis increase the level of calciuria. Predictably, increases in the filtered load of calcium, as occurs in the presence of hypercalcemia, also leads to increased calcium in the final urine.

The renal handling of phosphate is the major determinant of extracellular-fluid phosphate concentration. As with calcium, there is a huge filtered load, most of which is reabsorbed by tubular transport. Most phosphate reabsorption occurs proximally and the reabsorption can be adjusted over a wide range, mainly in response to changes in PTH or dietary phosphate intake. The list of hormones capable of modulating renal phosphate handling is long. Phosphaturia is promoted by PTH, PTH-related peptide, atrial natriuretic peptides, calcitonin, glucocorticoids, epidermal growth factor (EGF), and transforming growth factor-α (TGF-α). Antiphosphaturic actions emanate from insulin–like growth factor-1 (IGF-1), insulin, growth hormone, thyroid hormone, and calcitriol (Tenenhouse, 1997). Stanniocalcin (which has a clearly identi-fied role in fish) and phosphotonin have been identified recently—the latter is the principal mediator of phosphaturia in X-linked hypophosphatemic rickets and in its murine equivalent, the *hyp* mouse (Kumar, 1997).

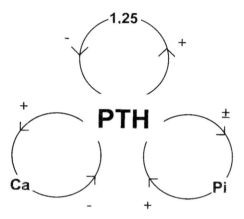

Fig. 4.1 Interrelationships between the parathyroid glands, calcium, inorganic phosphate, and calcitriol (1,25 dihydroxyvitamin D₃). + signs indicate stimulation and – signs inhibition. Each of the three modulators of PTH is itself influenced by PTH.

Calcitriol is synthesized in the mitochondria of the proximal tubular cells (Reichel, *et al.*, 1989). This is the site of the enzyme, 25-hydroxyvitamin D 1α-hydroxylase. The precursor for calcitriol, 25-hydroxyvitamin D, is itself the product of a hydroxylation carried out in the liver. Although 25-hydroxyvitamin D has vitamin D-like activity, it is at least three orders of magnitude less potent than calcitriol (Cunningham and Makin, 1997). In the context of mineral metabolism, the principal actions of calcitriol are to increase the intestinal absorption of calcium and phosphorus, to reduce the synthesis of PTH and the proliferation of parathyroid cells, and to enhance the release of calcium from bone (Reichel *et al.*, 1989; Hsu *et al.*, 1994; Cunningham and Makin, 1997). These actions are crucial to the normal regulation of mineral metabolism and, because calcitriol is so potent (the daily production rate is less than 0.5 μg) its synthe-sis has to be controlled very tightly. This takes place principally at the level of the kid-ney—the photolytic production of vitamin D₃ in the skin is not under metabolic con-trol, and the 25-hydroxylation of vitamin D in the liver is only regulated loosely. The activity of the 1α-hydroxylase is augmented by PTH and by reduction of the extracellular fluid (ECF) calcium or phosphate concentration, and is inhibited by calcitriol itself (feedback inhibition).

Consequences of renal failure

As renal function diminishes there is a progressive reduction in the excretory capacity for phosphorus and of the synthetic capacity for calcitriol. These are by far the most important consequences of renal damage so far as mineral metabolism is concerned. There is also a progressive reduction in the excretory capacity for calcium, culminating at end-stage renal disease (ESRD) with zero calcium excretion. However, because the parallel decrease in calcitriol availability leads to intestinal calcium malabsorption, excessive accumulation of calcium as a result of the failure of the kidneys to excrete is virtually never seen—most of these patients exhibit a substantial negative calcium balance at the level of the intestine unless treated with large doses of oral calcium or vitamin D metabolites (see below).

Phosphate retention

1. If there is an absolute increase in the ECF phosphate concentration, a reciprocal downward pressure is exerted on ECF calcium with resulting secondary hyperparathyroidism. In the past, reciprocity of phosphate and calcium was thought to be the major (and perhaps the only) drive to progressive hyperparathyroidism and this formed the basis of the 'trade-off' hypothesis as initially promulgated by Bricker and Slatopolsky (Bricker *et al.*, 1969; Reiss *et al.*, 1970). In practice, plasma phosphate is not invariably increased, especially in early and moderate renal insufficiency, and in some cases it may even be low. That hyperparathyroidism is often found in these early stages of renal insufficiency indicates that factors other than hyperphosphatemia must be implicated.
2. An increased ECF phosphate concentration has recently been shown to stimulate directly the synthesis of PTH (Kilav *et al.*, 1995; Almaden *et al.*, 1996; Denda *et al.*, 1996; Hernandez *et al.*, 1996). This partly explains why hyperphosphatemia is often associated with a poor therapeutic response to calcitriol.
3. Elevated ECF phosphate concentration, with a high Ca $\times$ Pi product, strongly predisposes to soft-tissue calcification.

Failure to synthesize calcitriol

1. Intestinal calcium malabsorption and a reduction in calcitriol-driven calcium efflux from the skeleton leads to downward pressure on ECF calcium concentration and resulting secondary hyperparathyroidism.
2. The normal inhibition of PTH synthesis in the parathyroid glands is reduced.
3. Parathyroid cell proliferative activity is increased.

Intestinal calcium malabsorption exacerbates secondary hyperparathyroidism, and the lack of a calcitriol effect on the parathyroids allows excessive PTH synthesis and excessive mitotic activity in the parathyroid cells with resulting hyperplasia (Silver and Naveh-Many, 1994). In some cases this hyperplasia may be complicated by the development of monoclonal proliferation within the parathyroids, a condition termed 'nodular hyperplasia'. The development of nodular hyperplasia is extremely important in pathophysiological and clinical terms because the nodules, while retaining all the normal PTH biosynthetic machinery, exhibit a relative lack of vitamin D receptors (Falchetti *et al.*, 1993; Fukada *et al.*, 1993). This results in the nodules being inappropriately autonomous and largely refractory to the suppressive role of calcitriol, whether this is synthesized endogenously or given as therapy. The prevention of the development of nodular hyperplasia has become a major therapeutic goal for nephrologists treating renal bone disease.

The discussion above would lead to the conclusion that renal failure, whether partial or complete, should normally be associated with a state of parathyroid overactivity, calcitriol insufficiency, and skeletal lesions consistent with hyperparathyroidism. Indeed, this is often the case, but by no means invariably so. Studies documenting the histological changes in bone in patients on dialysis have revealed a spectrum of bone disease which can best be classified according to the rate of bone turnover in relation to normality (Malluche and Faugere, 1990; Hruska and Teitelbaum, 1995). These issues will be discussed in more detail later in the chapter, but it is important to realize that the spectrum of renal osteodystrophy encompasses both abnormally high and abnormally low bone turnover. Thus, although many factors that would be expected to drive bone turnover to an abnormal degree have been clearly identified, such factors do not always dominate: by implication, the uremic state also appears to be associated with factors that act to diminish bone turnover. The nature of these remains to be determined.

Pathogenesis of renal osteodystrophy

Uremic hyperparathyroidism

At least six components of the uremic state with demonstrable stimulatory influence on the parathyroids have been identified: reduction of extracellular fluid calcium concentration, loss of normal PTH suppressability by calcium, reduced calcitriol synthesis and action, phosphate retention, metabolic acidosis, and target resistance to PTH.

Reduction of extracellular-fluid calcium concentration

Although the plasma calcium concentration is within the normal range in most uremic patients, this is so only because PTH is increased and supports plasma calcium in the face of downward pressure exerted by phosphate retention and calcitriol deficiency (Bricker *et al.*, 1969; Reiss *et al.*, 1970). Frank hypocalcemia exists in a proportion of patients, but it is important to realize that such is the sensitivity of the parathyroids to the plasma calcium concentration that, particularly when sustained, calcium decrements as small as 0.03 mmol/l are associated with marked increases in PTH secretion. The contribution of phosphate retention to this set of circumstances comprises the trade-off hypothesis already mentioned (Bricker *et al.*, 1969). At one time 'trade-off' was thought to explain adequately most, if not all, the observed increase in PTH in chronic renal failure, the postulated basis being that hyperphosphatemia leads to a reciprocal reduction of plasma calcium concentration. Subsequent observations have cast considerable doubt on this, not least because during the development of progressive renal insufficiency, PTH often rises well before there is any perceptible increment in plasma phosphate (Adler and Berlyne, 1986). The trade-off hypothesis therefore accounts, at most, for only a part of the stimulatory package that is faced by the parathyroids in uremia.

However, a sustained change in the calcium concentration may also have structural consequences for the parathyroids. A number of studies have shown convincingly that PTH mRNA per cell is substantially increased by a low calcium concentration (Silver and Naveh-Many, 1994). Of note is that the converse is probably *not* true—chronic exposure to an abnormally high calcium does not appear to suppress PTH mRNA below the normal ambient level (Silver and Naveh-Many, 1994). Teleologically, these findings are plausible, and suggest that the parathyroid cells have adaptive capability that is very well suited to chronic calcium deficiency but less so to the much rarer environmental insult of chronic calcium excess.

Aberrant parathyroid gland response to the extracellular fluid calcium concentration—loss of normal suppressibility by calcium

Much evidence suggests that uremia is associated with a variable loss of the normal suppressive influence of calcium on the parathyroids. Studies using human or animal parathyroid cells *in vitro* have shown that cells taken from pathologically overactive glands (primary hyperparathyroidism or secondary hyperparathyroidism in uremia) exhibited reduced suppressibility by calcium compared with cells from normal glands. The explanation remains uncertain and not all studies support this view (Cunningham, 1996; Goodman and Salusky, 1996; Goodman *et al.*, 1996). Much attention has focused on the possibility that the membrane-located calcium sensor is perturbed in uremia in a fashion that reduces its sensitivity to calcium (Brown *et al.*, 1995). No convincing evidence to this effect has been advanced, although if true the hypothesis would explain the experimental and clinical observations satisfactorily.

Similar results have been obtained by acutely perturbing extracellular fluid calcium concentration *in vivo*, both using normal subjects and those with clinical uremia being treated by dialysis. These studies have generally induced acute hypocalcemia either by means of an ethylenediaminetetraacetic acid (EDTA) infusion or by hemodialysis using a low- or zero-calcium dialysate, with hypercalcemia induced acutely by calcium infusion or by dialysis using a supraphysiological dialysate calcium concentration. Many, although not all, of these studies have suggested that the parathyroids have less calcium suppressibility in uremia and that this defect may be repaired partially or completely by the administration of calcitriol (Dunlay *et al.*, 1989; Kwan *et al.*, 1992).

Attempts have been made to quantify the calcium sensitivity of the parathyroids by the calculation of a parathyroid 'set point' for calcium. This is a derived calcium concentration, usually defined as: 'that calcium concentration at which PTH is 50% of the maximum PTH achieved during acute hypocalcemia'. Although of some use, the concept is of dubious biological relevance, as are a number of the other parameters that can be derived from the generation of sigmoidal curves relating PTH to calcium where the latter is perturbed acutely. This area has been extensively reviewed (Cunningham, 1996; Goodman and Salusky, 1996).

Reduced calcitriol synthesis and action

The development of significant renal insufficiency is associated with an increasingly severe impairment of calcitriol synthesis. Many studies have shown that a progressive reduction of the glomerular filtration rate (GFR) correlates with an increase in PTH and a decrease in calcitriol concentrations. However, the changes to calcitriol are subtle in early and moderate renal insufficiency, with the result that many patients manifest plasma calcitriol concentrations that remain within the arbitrarily defined 'normal range' until the GFR has fallen to 30% of normal or less (Cheung *et al.*, 1983). Nevertheless, it is clear that, although technically normal, the calcitriol concentration is inappropriately low given the accompanying drive to calcitriol synthesis provided by increased circulating PTH. Further evidence in support of this view comes from dynamic studies that have looked at the reserve synthetic capacity for calcitriol in patients with very mild chronic renal insufficiency. Even when the GFR was reduced by only 20–25% of normal, the administration of large doses of exogenous parathyroid hormone, which in normal subjects is associated with a prompt increase in calcitriol concentration, was essentially without effect, even though these patients had a normal, unstimulated, baseline calcitriol concentration (Ritz *et al.*, 1991). This suggests that the PTH–calcitriol endocrine system was already compensated maximally at this early stage of progressive renal insufficiency.

Parathyroid cells possess specific high-affinity receptors for calcitriol, in common with the other major sites for calcitriol action such as the intestine and bone (Reichel *et al.*, 1989). Radiolabeled calcitriol localizes in the nuclei of parathyroid cells, and physiological concentrations of calcitriol markedly reduce the cellular PTH mRNA content *in vitro* (Silver *et al.*, 1985). These changes are the result of a decrease in gene transcription and are therefore not instantaneous, but are first manifest approximately 5 hours after exposure and are maximal at 48 hours (Silver *et al.*, 1985). Even more rapid responses have been reported, although they are not wholly convincing. If present, these effects could not be the result of a genomic action of calcitriol, but may instead be mediated via the membrane-located calcium sensor itself.

In a number of tissues, including the parathyroids, calcitriol has been shown to up-regulate its own receptor, and in so doing calcitriol amplifies its actions. Conversely, calcitriol lack, as occurs in uremia, is associated with vitamin D receptor (VDR) down-regulation and target organ resistance (Reichel *et al.*, 1989; Naveh-Many, 1990).

The development of nodular hyperplasia in enlarged parathyroid glands has been recognized to have an important association with severe hyperparathyroidism, and is associated with a high degree of autonomy and relative lack of suppressibility by calcium and/or calcitriol (Fukayawa *et al.*, 1995). Together these disturbances constitute what has often been described as 'tertiary hyperparathyroidism', and recently the pathophysiological basis for this has become better understood. Areas of nodular hyperplasia in enlarged parathyroid glands bear the usual biosynthetic machinery for PTH but they exhibit a profound lack of vitamin D receptors, with the result that they are resistant to the normal suppressive influence of calcitriol (Fukayawa *et al.*, 1995). Thus even when calcitriol is given in supraphysiological amounts, the glands may fail to suppress adequately and the clinical problem can only be resolved by physical reduction of parathyroid mass by surgery or chemical ablation.

Phosphate retention

Phosphate retention is of importance for three principal reasons. First, overt elevation of the extracellular-fluid phosphate concentration is associated with a reciprocal downward pressure on ECF calcium, which in turn is rapidly sensed by the parathyroids with resulting secondary hyperparathyroidism—the trade-off hypothesis (Bricker *et al.*, 1969; Reiss *et al.*, 1970). Second, in early renal insufficiency, when calcitriol synthesis by the kidney is still significant, a tendency to retain phosphate would be expected to reduce the activity of the 1α-hydroxylase enzyme (Fraser, 1980). Both experimental and some clinical studies have provided support for this view, with dietary phosphate restriction being associated with an increase in calcitriol and a decrease in PTH concentrations (Portale *et al.*, 1984; Tessitore *et al.*, 1987; Lopez-Hilker *et al.*, 1990). Third, it has become clear that phosphate directly modulates PTH synthesis. It does this independent of either calcitriol or ECF calcium concentration. Several groups have shown that in animals with experimental renal insufficiency, dietary phosphate is an important regulator of PTH secretion and also that ambient phosphate concentration is a determinant of preproPTH mRNA content and parathyroid hyperplasia (Kilav *et al.*, 1995; Almaden *et al.*, 1996; Denda *et al.*, 1996; Hernandez *et al.*, 1996). Phosphate restriction in clinical uremia has recently been shown to shift the relationship between PTH and calcium in a manner that suggests increased parathyroid suppressibility by calcium during periods of dietary phosphate restriction (Combe and Aparicio, 1994).

Metabolic acidosis

Severe skeletal derangements may arise as a result of metabolic acidosis, particularly if it is sustained and severe (Cunningham *et al.*, 1982). In addition, several studies have pointed to a role of metabolic acidosis in the genesis of hyperparathyroidism in uremia. Very careful correction of uremic acidosis in these patients appears to alter the relationship between calcium and PTH in much the same way as does dietary phosphate restriction (Lefebvre *et al.*, 1989; Graham *et al.*, 1997). Of great interest, but not yet clear, is the possibility that acidosis is also involved in the genesis of parathyroid cell proliferation. If so, it is likely that uremic acidosis will have to be treated much more rigorously than has been the case hitherto.

Target resistance to parathyroid hormone

Much evidence has been accumulated to indicate the resistance of target tissues to PTH in uremia. The most obvious example is the kidney itself which, as disease progresses, becomes increasingly incapable of mounting an appropriate phosphaturic response to increased PTH levels. In parallel with this is a progressive reduction of the kidney's ability to synthesize calcitriol in response to stimulation by PTH and other factors (Ritz *et al.*, 1991). Elsewhere it is clear that the skeleton is significantly resistant to PTH in uremia, with the result that PTH rises still further (Somerville and Kaye, 1979; Rodriguez *et al.*, 1991 *a*, *b*). There are two important components of the uremic state that appear to underlie the skeletal resistance to PTH, i.e. deficiency of calcitriol and hyperphosphatemia (Somerville and Kaye, 1979; Rodriguez *et al.*, 1991 *a*, *b*). Replacement of deficient calcitriol largely repairs the defective skeletal responsiveness to PTH, and elegant experiments performed by Somerville and Kaye, in which phosphate was removed in acutely uremic animals that were reinfused with their own urine, led to restoration of the normal calcemic response to PTH (Somerville and Kaye, 1979).

Hypoparathyroidism in uremia

With the exception of patients who have coexisting idiopathic hypoparathyroidism (exceedingly rare), or postsurgical hypoparathyroidism, inappropriate underactivity of the parathyroids is not thought to be a primary event. Rather, it can be seen that in those patients in whom parathyroid activity is abnormally low the PTH suppression is demonstrably the result of elevation of the ECF calcium concentration as a result of adynamic bone disease (see below), or the ingestion of calcium salts and/or vitamin D metabolites. In such patients the withdrawal of the calcemic therapy is usually followed by a progressive increase in parathyroid activity to normal and eventually supranormal levels. In patients with underlying adynamic bone disease PTH is usually low, but it rises if the patients are rendered hypocalcemic acutely (EDTA infusion or low-calcium dialysis), or chronically by the continued use of a reduced calcium dialysate. The acute PTH response to induced hypocalcemia in these patients may be blunted (Sanchez *et al.*, 1995), almost certainly a reflection of the lack of significant parathyroid hyperplasia. Thus in the uremic patient with low parathyroid activity, parathyroid behavior is usually appropriate to the calcium/vitamin D status of the patient.

A possible exception to the above is seen in patients severely intoxicated with aluminum. At the level of bone, aluminum intoxication is associated with a profound reduction of osteoblastic activity with very low synthetic rates of bone matrix, severely impaired mineralization, and a coupled decrease in resorptive activity (Malluche and Faugere, 1990; Hruska and Teitelbaum, 1995). These effects reflect a direct toxic action of aluminum on bone. In addition, there is some evidence pointing to the direct suppressive actions of aluminum on the parathyroids (Morrisey *et al.*, 1983). High concentrations of aluminum suppressed PTH production by parathyroid tissue *in vitro*, but at a concentration higher than those encountered in clinical practice, even in cases of severe aluminum intoxication. The evidence that this form of direct aluminum action on the parathyroids is significantly operative in clinical practice is weak.

Skeletal consequences of uremia—histological features of renal osteodystrophy

Examination of specimens of bone taken from patients with uremia nearly always reveals clear-cut abnormalities which are often florid. Bone turnover rates may be low, normal, or high and is determined by a combination of static and dynamic parameters (Table 4.1). Specific histological abnormalities such as osteitis fibrosa, osteomalacia, or woven bone are still useful, but are now viewed in relation to their position on the spectrum of bone turnover (Malluche and Faugere, 1990; Hruska and Teitelbaum, 1995).

Table 4.1   Histological classification of uremic osteodystrophy

High turnover
—osteitis fibrosa
—hyperparathyroid bone disease
—mixed uremic bone disease
Low turnover
—adynamic/aplastic bone disease
      aluminum +ve
      aluminum −ve
—osteomalacia
      aluminum +ve
      aluminum −ve
Mild disease
Incidental aluminum

It is important to recognize that quantitative histomorphometry does not allow the direct measurement of bone turnover, although it does allow certain inferences to be drawn. Proper measurements relating to bone turnover can only be done following double-tetracycline labeling, whereby the transiently administered tetracycline is taken up at sites of active mineralization and demonstrated by fluorescence micro-scopy (Malluche and Faugere, 1990).

High-turnover bone disease

This lesion is the skeletal correlate of PTH excess and is characterized histologically by osteitis fibrosa. Evidence of accelerated bone resorption is abundant with increased osteoclast numbers and resorption bays (Malluche and Faugere, 1990; Hruska and Teitelbaum, 1995). In parallel, osteoblastic activity is also much increased, thereby accounting for the high bone turnover and remodeling rate that characterizes patients with PTH excess. Osteoblasts are increased in number and also assume a characteristic 'plump' morphology. Bone formation rate may be increased to five or more times the upper limit of normal. The rapid synthesis of osteoid covering the trabecular bone surface often runs ahead of mineralization, such that an excess of osteoid is evident; it is important to appreciate that this 'hyperosteoidosis' is not indicative of osteomalacia, in which bone turnover is low and the mineralization of osteoid is severely retarded. In some areas, osteoid seams may become disordered and acquire a woven appearance similar to that seen in other high-turnover conditions such as Paget's disease. Peritrabecular marrow fibrosis (hence the term 'osteitis fibrosa') is seen in severe cases. Patients with high-turnover bone disease usually manifest PTH concentrations at least four times the upper limit of normal, and sometimes much higher.

Low-turnover bone disease

This takes the form of osteomalacia or adynamic/aplastic bone disease. In both, the dynamic parameters assessed from tetracycline labeling are strikingly depressed (Malluche and Monier-Faugere, 1994). Bone formation is extremely low and mineralization appears virtually absent in many cases. Tetracycline uptake at the trabecular bone surface is minimal. The amount of osteoid helps to distinguish osteomalacia from adynamic/aplastic bone disease. Osteomalacia is associated with an excess of osteoid which, in contrast to the hyperosteoidosis of high-turnover bone disease, reflects a failure to mineralize osteoid rather than an overexuberant osteoid production. Osteoblasts are morphologically flat and inactive, and bone resorption indices are depressed in parallel—osteoclast numbers are low and resorption bays few.

In contrast, patients with adynamic/aplastic bone disease have reduced or occasionally normal amounts of osteoid. Osteoblasts and osteoclasts are reduced in number and the bone formation rate is low and often unmeasurable.

Aluminum has been important in the genesis of these low-turnover bone lesions. In patients in whom aluminum exposure has been substantial, linear aluminum can be identified using various stains and is seen to co-locate with areas of mineralization defect, as judged by poor tetracycline labeling (Malluche and Monier-Faugere, 1994; Hruska and Teitelbaum, 1995). Important aluminum deposition of this kind is now much less frequent as a result of the reduced aluminum exposure faced by the current cohort of ESRD patients.

For reasons that are not fully understood, low-turnover bone lesions have become relatively more common and high-turnover ones less common over the past decade Fig. 4.2. This change is not explicable in terms of aluminum exposure—only a minority of patients manifesting adynamic/aplastic bone disease have important aluminum deposition in bone—and a number of other factors have been identified that are clearly associated with the development of adynamic bone disease, even though a

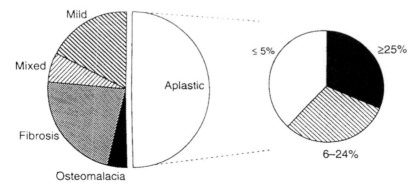

Fig. 4.2 Distribution of bone lesions in a large unselected dialysis population. Low-turnover lesions (aplastic plus osteomalacia) predominate over high-turnover lesions (mild, mixed, fibrosis). The aplastic lesions are further sub divided on the basis of surface aluminum staining which is heavy (> 25%), moderate (6–24%), or low (< 5%). (From Hercz *et al.*, 1993; with permission.)

causal link is often speculative (Pei *et al.*, 1995). Prominent factors include diabetes, corticosteroid therapy, early use of calcium-containing phosphate binders and/or vitamin D metabolites, and, finally, advanced age. As a group, these patients manifest surprisingly low circulating PTH concentrations (just above normal, normal, or even subnormal in some cases), together with a tendency to develop hypercalcemia and resulting intolerance of calcemic therapies such as calcium carbonate or vitamin D sterols (Merie *et al.*, 1990; Hercz *et al.*, 1993).

Other lesions—mixed osteodystrophy and mild lesions

Mixed osteodystrophy is a term implying the presence of both osteitis fibrosa and osteomalacia. Nearly all these patients have secondary hyperparathyroidism with a concomitant impairment of bone formation, as may be found in early aluminum toxicity or persisting hypocalcemia, leading to impaired mineralization. There is some evidence to suggest that patients who have low circulating levels of the calcitriol precursor, 25-hydroxyvitamin D, are more likely to develop this type of lesion (Cunningham and Makin, 1997).

Mild lesions are seen in patients who have very limited elevation of PTH levels, in whom static and dynamic skeletal parameters point to modest increases of bone turnover only.

Replacement of renal function by dialysis—consequences for osteodystrophy

Dialysis provides a very imperfect substitute for normal kidney function. In the case of mineral metabolism and renal osteodystrophy this is reflected by both inadequate function (for example, hemodialysis and CAPD remove phosphate much less well than does the kidney) and also by the failure to correct biosynthetic deficits such as that of calcitriol. Further, dialysis has essentially no modulatory capacity—a crucial deficiency given the kidneys' dynamic role in the adjustment of mineral and skeletal homeostasis. It is therefore not at all surprising that the disturbances that develop as renal insufficiency becomes more severe tend to be perpetuated rather than corrected by extended dialysis. This limitation applies to both hemodialysis and CAPD, although some differences between the modalities are apparent (Coburn, 1993; Armstrong and Cunningham, 1994). On the other hand, successful kidney transplantation rapidly restores most of the crucial functions of normal native kidneys and, although skeletal outcomes after transplantation may be compromised by pre-existing bone disease and by long-term drug therapies, there is no doubt that in many respects transplantation can be regarded as the best treatment for renal osteodystrophy.

Diagnosis of renal osteodystrophy

Abnormalities of mineral ions, calcium regulating hormones, and markers of bone metabolism can be identified in virtually all patients with significant renal insufficiency. The magnitude and pattern of these abnormalities depends much on the duration and severity of the renal failure. Table 4.2 illustrates 'snapshot' profiles of the important biochemical parameters in patients at various levels of chronic renal failure (CRF).

Table 4.2 Minerals and hormones in various stages of uremia—metabolic snapshot

	Mild	Moderate	Severe/ESRD
Ca	$\rightarrow$	$\rightarrow$ or $\downarrow$	$\rightarrow$ or $\downarrow$
P_i	$\rightarrow$	$\rightarrow$ or $\uparrow$	$\uparrow$
PTH	$\uparrow$	$\uparrow$ $\uparrow$	$\uparrow$ $\uparrow$
Calcitriol	$\rightarrow$	$\rightarrow$ or $\downarrow$	$\downarrow$ $\downarrow$

Calcium and phosphate

In the untreated patient on dialysis, calcium is usually low or low normal and phosphate is invariably elevated. Dialysis treatment, during which phosphate is removed and calcium enters the patient, is usually sufficient to ameliorate but not to correct fully these abnormalities. Both the raised phosphate and low calcium levels independently drive parathyroid overactivity which manifests itself by the increased secretion of PTH, hyperplastic changes in the glands, and finally the development of nodular hyperplasia with increasing gland autonomy (Silver and Naveh–Many, 1994; Cunningham, 1996). The standard treatment package for renal osteodystrophy comprises measures to reduce hyperphosphatemia (adequate dialysis, dietary restriction, and oral phosphate binders) together with measures to increase the serum calcium concentration (calcium salts plus vitamin D metabolites). In most patients these treatments serve to reduce the drive to parathyroid overactivity but may also lead to hypercalcemia—by far the most common cause of hypercalcemia in dialysis patients is the excessive use of calcium-containing phosphate binders and/or vitamin D metabolites. Patients with underlying aplastic bone disease are likely to manifest serum calcium levels in the upper normal or supranormal range, probably because the inert skeleton incorporates calcium poorly (Merie *et al.*, 1990; Hercz *et al.*, 1993).

Patients with severe parathyroid hyperplasia are often hypercalcemic, in this case in a PTH-dependent manner. These patients will usually have substantially enlarged parathyroid glands with areas of nodular hyperplasia and an abnormal degree of parathyroid autonomy. These glands are not adequately suppressed by high calcium levels or by vitamin D metabolites. Other less frequent causes are the same as those of hypercalcemia in non-renal patients, for example malignancy, granulomatous disorders with the extrarenal production of calcitriol, or immobilization in Paget's disease.

Parathyroid hormone

Parathyroid hormone (PTH) is elevated to at least a moderate extent in most patients. Exceptions are those who have adynamic bone disease or who have been rendered hypercalcemic by overtreatment with calcium salts or vitamin D metabolites. Currently,

PTH is usually measured using assays to detect the intact 84 amino-acid peptide. This is important because normal ranges between such assays are fairly comparable. Earlier assays measured different fragments of the PTH molecule with a very wide inter-assay variation as a result. In particular, the accumulation of C-terminal fragments in renal failure led to extremely high levels of C-PTH compared with those in normal subjects, or even patients with primary hyperparathyroidism (Slatopolsky *et al.*, 1980). PTH appears to have as good a specificity and sensitivity as do the biochemical bone remodeling markers (Alvarez-Ude *et al.*, 1978; Hruska *et al.*, 1978; Hutchison *et al.*, 1993; Joffe *et al.*, 1994; Salusky *et al.*, 1994; Torres *et al.*, 1995; Urena *et al.*, 1995). As can be seen from Table 4.3, both low PTH concentrations (less than 120 pg/ml) and high PTH concentrations (above 400 pg/ml) predict, respectively, low-turnover or high-turnover bone disease with a good positive predictive value (Hutchison *et al.*, 1993; Torres *et al.*, 1995). Because PTH measurements are frequently conducted in routine clinical practise, and are now relatively inexpensive, it can be argued that little further useful information can be obtained from the biochemical markers of bone re-modeling (at least those currently available). A number of studies have shown that bone turnover rates are most likely to be normal when PTH is in the region of 100–200 pg/ml (two to four times the upper limit of normal) (Torres *et al.*, 1995).

Table 4.3 PTH as a predictor of bone histology

	PTH	Sensitivity	Specificity	PPV[a]
Low turnover	< 120 pg/ml	0.59	0.94	0.9
High turnover	< 400 pg/ml	0.50	1	1

[a] PPV, positive predictive value. Data taken from Torres *et al.*, 1995.

Bone markers

Much attention has focused on the use of various markers of bone metabolism to pre-dict bone histology. Bone biopsy remains the benchmark in this respect, but it is an invasive test and also an expensive and technically exacting one (Malluche and Monier-Faugere, 1994). The biochemical markers of bone remodeling most used to probe bone formation are alkaline phosphatase and osteocalcin, both synthesized and released by active osteoblasts (Joffe *et al.*, 1994). Bone-specific alkaline phosphat-ase is more useful than total alkaline phosphatase, but the assays suffer from substantial cross-reactivity between bone and liver isoenzymes which reduces their utility, especially when bone alkaline phosphatase is low. Markers of bone resorption measure products of type I collagen breakdown. Of these, pyridinoline appears promising (Urena *et al.*, 1995), and cross-linked type I carboxy-terminal telopeptide (ICTP) and type I carboxy-terminal extension peptide (PICP) somewhat less so (Urena *et al.*, 1995).

Aluminum

Serum aluminum is found to be elevated in almost all patients with end–stage renal disease: this is largely a reflection of the loss of normal renal excretory capacity for aluminum (Altmann *et al.*, 1987). Serious disease resulted from aluminum accumulation in the past, although now it is unusual following the appreciation of the dangers and the near-universal use of highly purified hemodialysates, aluminum-free peritoneal dialysates, and the reduction of oral aluminum ingestion. Aluminum loading to the point of detectable clinical sequelae is now exceedingly rare, although concern remains that more subtle toxicity to the central nervous system and/or the skeleton may exist with aluminum burden at levels widely thought to be safe. For a full discussion of aluminum loading and its consequences in uremia see Chapter 5.

Radiology in renal osteodystrophy

The role of radiology as a diagnostic and monitoring tool in dialysis patients has decreased as the sophistication of biochemical monitoring has increased. Some centers have almost abandoned regular radiographic monitoring, preferring instead to obtain a radiographic database for each patient at entry to the dialysis program followed by subsequent studies as and when dictated by clinical events.

Subperiostial bone resorption is one of the most frequently encountered radiographic abnormalities in patients with secondary hyperparathyroidism. Both the likelihood of this abnormality being seen and its extent correspond broadly with the serum levels of both PTH and alkaline phosphatase (Hruska *et al.*, 1978). Subperiostial erosions are best seen affecting the surfaces of the distal and middle phalanges of hands and feet. In more severe cases, erosion of the distal ends of the clavicles may be seen, together with erosion at the metaphyseal–diaphyseal junction of the long bones. In some patients, areas of osteosclerosis also develop in association with hyperparathyroid bone disease. These are particularly likely to be seen in the spine and lead to the characteristic 'rugger jersey' appearance seen on lateral radiographs of the dorsal spine. These changes are all associated with marked hyperparathyroidism, and would generally be seen in combination with elevation of alkaline phosphatase and PTH, elevation of bone formation and resorption markers, and be associated with an increased prevalence of clinical sequelae such as bone pain and fracture.

In low–turnover bone disease the radiographic features are less pronounced and less specific. Osteopenia is common but not invariable, and is often absent on standard radiographs which have poor precision and sensitivity in the diagnosis of osteopenia. Pathological fractures may be evident and pseudofractures are seen occasionally in adult patients with osteomalacia (Alvarez-Ude *et al.*, 1978).

Periarticular cystic lesions are often seen, particularly in patients who have received hemodialysis for extended periods. These are usually indicative of β_2-microglobulin amyloid deposition. They are most likely to be seen near sites of soft-tissue insertion and are usually multiple. Solitary bone cysts are more likely to be 'brown tumors' and are seen particularly in the jaw, pelvis, or ribs. They are associated with severe hyperparathyroidism.

Isotopic bone scanning using [^{99}Tc]methylene diphosphonate has limited utility in this setting. Skeletal uptake of the radiopharmaceutical is usually enhanced— partly as a result of accelerated bone turnover, but also as a result of prolonged whole-body retention of the isotope in these patients who have no renal excretory capacity. Patients with low-turnover bone lesions (aplastic or osteomalacic bone disease) generally have a less striking skeletal uptake of the isotope, but the changes are not sensitive or specific enough to be of significant clinical utility.

Bone histology

Transiliac bone biopsy, whereby a cortex-to-cortex core of iliac bone is obtained by trephine or a drill technique, has been used widely in clinical research, although less so in routine clinical practice (Malluche and Monier-Faugere, 1994). The reasons for this are the invasive nature of the tests and the technically exacting processing and interpretation that is needed. While clearly providing the benchmark against which all other markers of bone metabolism should be judged, biopsy findings rarely dictate important clinical management decisions, especially when PTH and bone markers suggest that bone turnover is high. In contrast, low bone-turnover states are less likely to be diagnosed non-invasively and bone biopsy is more likely to be useful, especially if aluminum toxicity is suspected (Malluche and Faugere, 1990; Malluche and Monier-Faugese, 1994).

A bone biopsy is performed after two, spaced, orally administered tetracycline labels have been given approximately 14 and 4 days prior to the procedure. This enables key dynamic parameters (mineralizing surface, mineral appositional rate, bone formation rate) to be evaluated, as well as static ones (trabecular bone volume, osteoid volume, osteoid surface, osteoblastic surface, osteoclast surface, osteoclast numbers, and, finally, aluminum surface) (Malluche and Faugere, 1990).

Who gets renal osteodystrophy?

In a study of 243 patients who underwent bone biopsy and metabolic assessment within 6 months of starting regular hemodialysis treatment, four risk factors were identified, each of them conferring at least a twofold increase of relative risk of developing histological bone disease compared with the remainder of the study population. These factors were youth (less than 21 years of age), female sex, prolonged duration of uremia prior to dialysis, and tubulointerstitial disease (Cundy *et al.*, 1995). Similar results come from a different approach in another study of 422 patients with end-stage renal disease in whom risk factors for radiographic hyperparathyroidism were sought. Factors identified were similar—female sex, age less than 20 years, and duration of chronic renal insufficiency (Pazianas *et al.*, 1992).

These findings underlie the importance of early identification of renal osteodystrophy and the institution of appropriate prophylactic and treatment measures, particularly in the at-risk subgroups identified above.

Management of renal osteodystrophy in ESRD

It is important to appreciate that the patient with severe hyperparathyroid bone dis-ease, or with adynamic/aplastic bone disease, has arrived at an extreme of the spec-trum of osteodystrophy from which it may be difficult to escape. As such, patients at these extremes can be regarded as management failures, thereby indicating a major role for prophylaxis which should be implemented as early in the natural history of renal osteodystrophy as possible. The objectives of therapy are as follows:

(1) to ensure that the calcium and phosphorus concentrations in blood and extracel-lular fluid remain within the physiological range;
(2) to ensure that bone metabolism is as near to normal as possible, both in regard to bone cell activity and bone turnover and also to structural bone integrity;
(3) to ensure that the circulating concentration of PTH is appropriate to the above objectives and that it does not rise to concentrations that might be associated with PTH toxicity; and
(4) to prevent the development of parathyroid hyperplasia.

In the majority of patients the realization of the above objectives requires a combin-ation of dietary phosphate restriction, the regular administration of oral phosphate binders, and the regular use of active metabolites of vitamin D, all coupled with an adequate dialysis prescription. Reaching the target of normal bone turnover is often difficult or impossible.

Dietary phosphorus restriction

The normal dietary intake of phosphorus exceeds quite substantially the average daily phosphate removal by dialysis (whether hemodialysis or CAPD). Typically, an unre-stricted dietary phosphorus intake is in the region of 30 mmol per day, which may be decreased by sterner dietary measures to approximately 20 mmol per day. Unfor-tunately, dialysis removes only about 10 mmol daily and, to prevent the inevitable ac-cumulation of phosphorus and development of hyperphosphatemia, dietary phosphate binders are required in the vast majority of patients (Delmez and Slato-polsky, 1992).

Phosphate binders

In the early days of hemodialysis, and in the era before calcitriol and other 1-hydro-xylated metabolites of vitamin D had been identified, calcium carbonate was given in large quantities in an attempt to establish a positive calcium balance. It was noted by investigators at that time that large doses of calcium carbonate, as well as raising the plasma calcium concentration, also reduced plasma phosphorus—and in many patients also reduced the Ca×Pi product (Clarkson *et al.*, 1966). In the 1970s it became apparent that aluminum salts were much better phosphate binders than calcium salts, and both aluminum hydroxide and aluminum carbonate became standard ther-apy for the control of hyperphosphatemia in dialysis patients. The identification of aluminum as a cause of neurological and skeletal toxicity did not initially give rise to concern in regard to the use of aluminum-containing phosphate binders—the initial presumption was that aluminum burden was derived almost entirely from contaminated hemodialysis fluid (Ward *et al.*, 1978) and that the bioavailability of orally ingested aluminum was so low that the agent could be ingested with impunity. Subsequently it became apparent that although many of the most extreme examples of aluminum toxicity were indeed the result of dialysate contamination, others could only be explained in terms of oral aluminum ingestion. In particular, it was found that some patients in the predialysis phase of chronic renal insufficiency developed significant aluminum toxicity with high serum aluminum concentrations, a situation that could only have developed as a result of oral aluminum ingestion (Andreoli *et al.*, 1983). These discoveries heralded a swing away from aluminum as a phosphate binder and back to calcium salts, with calcium carbonate initially being the favored agent. A number of studies subsequently attested to the efficacy of calcium carbonate as a phosphate binder, but increasingly it became apparent that a substantial number of patients so treated developed hypercalcemia, sometimes severely so (Sawyer *et al.*, 1989). Further, many of these patients experienced an increase in the $Ca \times Pi$ product with resulting concern about accelerated vascular and other soft-tissue calcification. Measures to counter this problem included the reduction of the dialysate calcium concentration used in both hemodialysis and CAPD. Both therapies had generally used a supraphysiological calcium concentration, typically at 1.65–1.75 mmol/l. These concentrations were high enough to ensure that the dialysis procedure itself was associated with significant calcium entry, which was an intended and useful aspect of therapy in the era before calcitriol was available. However, the influx of calcium via the dialysis process ensures that, if oral calcium entry is sufficiently high to make the overall calcium balance at the level of the intestine positive, hypercalcemia is inevitable in the ESRD patient in whom no other point of calcium egress exists. It subsequently became clear that the judicious reduction of the dialysate calcium to concentrations in the region of 1.25 mmol/l substantially reduced the likelihood of hypercalcemia in calcium-carbonate treated patients, although a minority still remained surprisingly intolerant of calcium (Sawyer *et al.*, 1989; Cunningham *et al.*, 1992; Hutchison *et al.*, 1992). For these patients a further reduction of dialysate calcium has been evaluated, particularly in CAPD patients, with concentrations as low as 0.6 mmol/l being used (Armstrong *et al.*, 1997).

Very careful studies by Sheikh *et al.* (1989) suggested that calcium acetate should be a superior phosphate binder to calcium carbonate, exhibiting a somewhat lower calcium bioavailability and higher phosphate binding potency. Calcium acetate has been widely used, particularly in North America, and comparative studies have in the main indicated a comparable or slightly superior efficacy of the acetate salt with regard to the control of calcium and phosphorus, but a somewhat poorer tolerability with an unpleasant taste in the mouth and/or diarrhea being frequently encountered (Mai *et al.*, 1989; Hamida *et al.*, 1993; Ring *et al.*, 1993). Calcium citrate has also been advanced as a possible phosphate binder, but its use cannot be recommended. Although able to reduce plasma phosphate, the citrate salt leads to striking increases in the intestinal absorption of aluminum (reviewed in Delmez and Slatopolsky, 1992). Calcium citrate has no clear advantage over either calcium carbonate or calcium acetate and should therefore be avoided. Magnesium salts (carbonate or hydroxide) have been used, generally in combination with a magnesium-free dialysate. Diarrhea has been troublesome, but this approach may have potential when combined with calcium carbonate (Shah *et al.*, 1987; Delmez and Slatopolsky, 1992; Parsons *et al.*, 1993).

New phosphate binding agents that do not contain either aluminum or calcium are currently the focus of great interest and several are at various stages of development, with results from the first clinical trials now beginning to appear (Ritz and Herzesell, 1996; Chertow *et al.*, 1997). It is not yet clear whether any of these will materially alter our approach to the management of hyperphosphatemia.

All phosphate binding therapies suffer from the disadvantage of requiring a relatively large dose to be taken at strictly controlled times in relation to food ingestion. These therapies, at least from the patients' standpoint, are quite demanding and are often associated with poor compliance and poor therapeutic outcomes. Calcium salts, in particular, need to be taken accurately, and it is quite clear that the ingestion of calcium carbonate or calcium acetate without food leads to excessive calcium absorption from the phosphate binding salt and also reduces phosphate binding efficacy. These salts should be taken with food and in a dose that approximately matches the phosphorus content of the accompanying meal. By balancing the therapy in this fashion it is possible to minimize unwanted calcium absorption and maximize phosphate binding.

Overall it is clear that the control of phosphate represents the weak link in the therapeutic approach to uremic osteodystrophy—we badly need a safe, potent, and effective agent that is simple to use and easy to take, preferably on a once-daily basis to improve compliance. Until this is realized, phosphate control is likely to remain suboptimal in large numbers of dialysis patients.

Vitamin D therapies

Chronic renal insufficiency is one of the classical forms of vitamin D resistance. This resistance to therapy exists in regard to the parent vitamin D and also to the hepatic metabolite, 25-hydroxyvitamin D. Only when 1 α-hydroxylated (or equivalent) metabolites are given is vitamin D resistance lost, such that, with therapy using calcitriol or alfacalcidol, therapeutic dosing in dialysis patients is at a level quite similar to that required to treat simple dietary vitamin D deficiency (Brickman *et al.*, 1972; Chalmers *et al.*, 1973). The principal actions of all the therapeutic agents currently available are to increase the intestinal absorption of calcium and phosphorus, increase calcium mobilization from bone, and finally to reduce the synthesis of parathyroid hormone precursors and the rate of mitosis in the parathyroid glands. The balance between the above actions varies according to the metabolite used, and those having a relatively potent action to suppress the parathyroids with a low propensity to induce hypercalcemia via the intestine and/or bone should be particularly useful (Brown *et al.*, 1989; Dusso *et al.*, 1991). Other more enigmatic hormonal and paracrine actions of these metabolites have been identified; some, but not all, of them are associated with bone and mineral metabolism (Reichel *et al.*, 1989). These will not be discussed further here.

Much debate revolves around the optimum choice of the vitamin D metabolite and of the dosing regimen. Before developing these issues further, it is important to emphasize that the similarities between the available vitamin D metabolites, and the various dose regimens that have been evaluated, are much more striking than the differences. The convention in the past has been to use daily regimens of alfacalcidol or calcitriol (the choice between these two being governed largely by issues of habit and economics rather than by any scientifically established differences). Typical doses for calcitriol would be 0.125–0.5 μg daily, and for alfacalcidol approximately 0.25–1 μg daily. These therapies have proved very effective in the prevention and amelioration of hyperparathyroid bone disease and run-away hyperparathyroidism, at least in the short and medium terms. However, accumulating experience has clearly indicated that the treatments are by no means perfect. Substantial numbers of patients 'break through' with progressive parathyroid hyperplasia, PTH-dependent hypercalcemia, and eventually require parathyroid ablation (Sharman *et al.*, 1982).

These treatment failures have driven a search to find better vitamin D therapies. Pulsed calcitriol regimens have been used extensively, both orally and intravenously. There is an abundance of anecdotal evidence that they are more efficacious than conventional daily dosing, but unfortunately more robust data from properly controlled comparative studies are less convincing. It seems likely that such advantages of intravenous or oral, pulsed-calcitriol regimens that do exist are relatively minor and/or confined to as yet poorly defined subgroups of patients. This issue has been reviewed by Coburn and Frazao (1996).

Several new 'non-calcemic' vitamin D analogs are at various stages of development—at least three are currently undergoing clinical evaluation. In early experimental studies, 22-oxacalcitriol appeared to have little or no calcemic activity in rats and dogs, while suppressing PTH with a potency equal to that of calcitriol—in many ways an ideal profile (Brown et al., 1989). However, the signs from early clinical studies suggest a significant amount of hypercalcemia complicating treatment (Akizawa *et al.*, 1996). Another new vitamin D_2 analog, 1α-hydroxyvitamin D_2 (1α(OH)D_2), is also under evaluation. In vitamin-D deficient rodents 1α(OH)D_2 was less calcemic and less toxic than 1α(OH)D_3. The first clinical reports of 1α(OH)D_2 are encouraging, although it is too early to know whether this vitamin D metabolite represents a clinically useful advance (Tan *et al.*, 1997).

A consistent picture emerging from many treatment studies of vitamin D metabolites is the crucial importance of phosphate control—the failure to control phosphate adequately is a strong predictor of poor response or intolerance to vitamin D metabolites (Coburn and Frazao, 1996).

Targeting the membrane calcium sensor—calcimimetic agents

Calcimimetic agents bind to the extracellular calcium sensor, mimic the effect of extracellular calcium, and thereby fool the parathyroid cells into thinking that the ECF calcium concentration is higher than it really is. PTH falls even when the ECF calcium level is low. One of these agents, norcalcin, has recently been evaluated in hemodialysis patients and, at least in the short-term, it lowered calcium and PTH and simultaneously increased calcitonin (Atonsen *et al.*, 1996). This approach has great promise, and because in effect it increases the suppressibility of the parathyroid cells by calcium, it serves to restore the aberrant response to calcium of uremic parathyroid glands to normal.

The effects of dialysis modality on renal osteodystrophy— hemodialysis vs. CAPD

As therapies for end-stage renal disease, hemodialysis and CAPD have the following features in common:

(1) an inadequate clearance of inorganic phosphate;
(2) no impact on the endocrine functions of the kidney, e.g. calcitriol synthesis; and
(3) an incomplete correction of the uremic milieu.

Therefore, it is not surprising that the disordered bone and mineral metabolism of uremia is affected in a broadly similar fashion by both hemodialysis and CAPD treatment (Coburn, 1993; Armstrong and Cunningham, 1994).

Some distortion of the literature has resulted from the evolution of dialysis therapies. The early literature was heavily biased towards hemodialysis and, at least so far as bone disease was concerned, an assumption was made that extrapolation from hemodialysis to CAPD was generally valid. This is partially true, but the position is complicated by differing patient demographics between CAPD and hemodialysis programs with a tendency for older patients, and often those with metabolic or multi-system diseases, being selected preferentially for CAPD programs.

Both modalities have evolved over the past decade with an increasing emphasis placed on the adequacy of the dialysis prescription and nutritional support. Alternative osmotic agents have been evaluated and are increasingly used in CAPD and, as mentioned earlier in this chapter, there have been profound changes in our approach to phosphate binding therapy. Finally, there has been increasing emphasis placed on the notion that early intervention in the predialysis setting is of benefit; with the result that the substrate upon which both hemodialysis and CAPD operate has changed, with a progressively higher proportion of patients entering programs when already established on phosphate binding and/or vitamin D therapy. Nevertheless, certain aspects of the therapies differ significantly, and it is now becoming clear that the spectrum of bone disease seen amongst CAPD patients is not the same as that in hemodialysis (Coburn, 1993; Armstrong and Cunningham, 1994) (Fig. 4.3).

Phosphate control should, in theory, be better in CAPD-treated patients. Although the total clearance of phosphate by CAPD is similar to that by hemodialysis, its continuous nature should allow smoother control of serum phosphate with less parathyroid stimulation as a result. Plasma phosphate decreases during the course of a hemodialysis session but recovers rapidly to levels close to those prior to dialysis, therefore it is almost impossible for this intermittent therapy to achieve normophosphatemia without interspersed periods of hypophosphatemia.

CAPD allows continuous rather than discontinuous fluxes of calcium, the direction of which can be set by making appropriate adjustments to the CAPD dialysate calcium concentration. Historically, CAPD dialysate calcium has been set at 1.75 mmol/l which is supraphysiological and is associated with continuous calcium entry into the patient via the peritoneum. In combination with other calcemic therapies, such as calcium carbonate and/or vitamin D metabolites, this leads to an upward pressure on calcium in many patients with the result that PTH is more likely to be suppressed during CAPD than during hemodialysis (Fig. 4.3). This may be one of the explanations for the greater propensity of CAPD patients to manifest low-turnover bone lesions (Hercz *et al.*, 1993; Pei *et al.*, 1995). Now that increasing numbers of CAPD patients are dialyzed using a 'low calcium' dialysate (actually a misnomer in that at 1.25 mmol/l the 'low calcium' solutions are more physiological) there may be a tendency for PTH and bone turnover to increase in CAPD-treated patients.

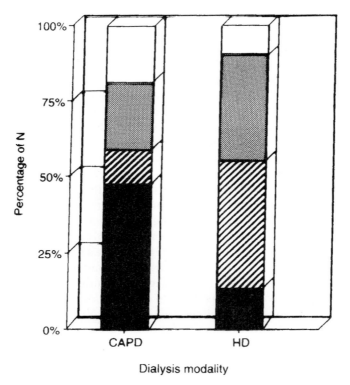

Fig. 4.3 Prevalence of bone lesions by dialysis modality. ■, aplastic bone disease (aluminum-negative). ▨, osteitis fibrosa; ▨, aluminum bone disease, □, mild lesions. Aluminum bone disease included aplastic and osteomalacic lesions with > 25% bone surface aluminum. (With permission from the *International Proceedings Journal*.)

Most CAPD solutions use lactate as a buffer, and recently solutions have appeared in which the lactate concentration has been raised to 40 mmol/l. This is likely to be associated with a more effective correction of uremic acidosis with potentially beneficial effects on the skeleton, although these have yet to be documented convincingly. Although it is possible to modify the hemodialysis prescription in such a way as to improve or to refine the control of acidosis, efficacy is likely to be limited by the intermittent nature of the treatment.

There is no evidence that CAPD patients are more prone to accumulate aluminum than are hemodialysis patients, except in so far that adynamic bone disease probably predisposes to aluminum accumulation and is also commoner in CAPD-treated patients. Aluminum is clearly much less important in the genesis of low-turnover bone disease than used to be the case, although large studies published in the early 1990s still showed that a significant minority of patients had substantial aluminum deposition (Hercz *et al.*, 1993), with the proportion being slightly higher in hemodialysis than in CAPD.

When should parathyroidectomy be performed?

This is an area of ongoing controversy. There is little doubt that PTH excess carries substantial skeletal and non-skeletal morbidity (Slatopolsky *et al.*, 1980), and less convincing evidence also points to an increased mortality. The need for parathyroidectomy is usually dictated by a failure of hyperplastic, overactive parathyroid glands to suppress adequately in response to optimal medical therapy. This assumes that the medical therapy prescribed is the best available, and also that the patient is able or willing to take it. Practicing nephrologists know to their chagrin that this is not always the case.

Optimal medical therapy in this setting can be defined as: the setting of plasma calcium at, or just above, the upper limit of normal; good phosphate control with serum phosphorus below 1.5 mmol/l; and continued administration of alfacalcidol or calcitriol given at the highest tolerated doses—at least 0.5 μg by mouth daily or 1 μg intravenously thrice weekly for calcitriol (alfacalcidol equivalents would be approximately double these). In practice, a substantial proportion of patients with severe hyperparathyroidism will be unable to tolerate these doses of vitamin D metabolites without developing unacceptable hypercalcemia and/or hyperphosphatemia.

The justification for parathyroidectomy depends on the clear demonstration of parathyroid-dependent hypercalcemia unresponsive to the non-surgical measures described above. It cannot be emphasized too strongly that an elevated PTH level *per se* is not an indication for parathyroidectomy—rather it is the elevation of the PTH concentration with concomitant hypercalcemia that provides the major indication. If calcium is low or normal, elevated PTH is indicative of secondary hyperparathyroidism and as such requires treatment with vitamin D metabolites and phosphate control. Implicit in the above comments is the notion that the patient must have a demonstrable PTH excess while hypercalcemic, and also must not have other causes of hypercalcemia such as low-turnover bone disease, granulomatous disease, malignancy, or the overzealous use of calcemic therapies. Inappropriate parathyroidectomy in this setting carries potentially deleterious consequences for the skeleton, almost certainly with an increased risk of aplastic bone disease (Felsenfield *et al.*, 1982). This may prove intractable.

Parathyroid ablation may be achieved surgically or by direct injection of ethanol into hyperplastic glands. The surgical approach is by far the most widely practiced and takes the form of: (a) subtotal parathyroidectomy (removal of obviously adenomatous tissue with the aim of about a seven-eighths reduction of total parathyroid tissue); (b) total parathyroidectomy with autotransplantation of a small amount of parathyroid tissue into the forearm; or (c) total parathyroidectomy with subsequent maintenance of the hypoparathyroid state using pharmacological doses of vitamin D metabolites. Few authorities now recommend total parathyroidectomy with vitamin D substitution. To render the uremic patient profoundly hypoparathyroid substantially increases the likelihood of the development of aplastic bone disease with its unknown long-term sequelae (Felsenfield *et al.*, 1982; Torres *et al.*, 1995). These concerns apply even though it is quite easy to maintain serum calcium levels within the normal range using sufficient doses of calcitriol—in the absence of one of its major stimulators, the osteoblasts will be insufficiently driven in the uremic environment with resulting aplastic bone disease.

Conversely, subtotal parathyroidectomy carries with it the risk of inadequate ablation or, in some cases, overablation. To some extent this problem can be circumvented by the technique of total parathyroidectomy with autotransplantation into the forearm, the hope being that a continued PTH excess from the grafted tissue can be dealt with more easily as a result of its greater surgical accessibility. This appealing idea is not always borne out in practice, with well-described instances of recurrent refractory hyperparathyroidism resulting from autografted tissue—as well as of unintended hypoparathyroidism such that, in one recent study, only a third of the patients avoided either hypoparathyroidism or hyperparathyroidism in the long-term after parathyroidectomy (Gagne *et al.*, 1992).

Ethanol injection into the parathyroids has been practised with considerable success by a limited number of groups (Giangrande *et al.*, 1994; Kitaoka *et al.*, 1994). The technique is highly operator-dependent, but in good hands appears to carry an acceptable success rate and also a low complication rate, the main concern being damage to the recurrent laryngeal nerve. Various strategies have been employed to minimize the risk of the extravasation of ethanol with subsequent damage to adjacent structures, and it is likely that with further refinement over the next few years this technique will find wider acceptance.

Defining the patients in need of parathyroidectomy, on the basis of advanced hyperparathyroidism with hyperparathyroid-dependent calcemia which is refractory to medical therapy, is fairly straightforward. Much less certain is the earlier identification of patients in whom the indications described above do not necessarily apply, but in whom progression of the disease is inevitable. That such patients exist is clear. Many of them would benefit from early parathyroidectomy, obviating the need for continued futile attempts at medical therapy and also minimizing the period of skeletal and other attrition from continuing uncontrolled hyperparathyroidism. The identification of nodular hyperplasia as an important part of the pathogenesis of progressive hyperparathyroidism should be a useful predictor. The approach to this problem has been discussed further by Gallieni and Brancaccio (1994). As a group, patients with nodular hyperplasia have been found to have larger glands which are less suppressible by calcium and in particular by vitamin D metabolites (Fukayawa *et al.*, 1995). These functional characteristics are almost certainly the result of a relative lack of vitamin D receptors in the nodules with resulting autonomy. Because the nodules bear chromosomal abnormalities (Falchetti *et al.*, 1993), it is conceivable that a fine-needle aspiration of suspicious glands could lead to the identification of monoclonal proliferation and to early surgery.

Effect of transplantation on renal osteodystrophy

Patients who undergo renal transplantation invariably do so on a background of previously disordered bone and mineral metabolism. Furthermore, these patients manifest a spectrum of bone disease with varying pathologies and bone turnover status. In addition, some may have comorbidity that bears on skeletal integrity, in particular type I diabetes mellitus which is associated with osteopenia and low-turnover bone disease, even in the absence of renal insufficiency. The substrate upon which transplantation works is therefore variable.

Metabolic and skeletal consequences of renal transplantation

Many of the components of the uremic syndrome are dramatically corrected by successful transplantation. Phosphate excretory capacity is returned to normal, eliminating the direct phosphate-mediated drive to secondary hyperparathyroidism. In addition, the transplanted kidney synthesizes calcitriol promptly after engraftment. This, together with the correction of hyperphosphatemia, leads to a rapid reduction in PTH concentration. Parathyroid hormone often, however, does not fall to unequivocally normal levels—even in patients with excellent graft function PTH is slightly higher than in comparable patients with native kidneys and lacking a previous history of uremia (Mitlak *et al.*, 1991; Pietschmann *et al.*, 1991). It is likely that the failure to suppress completely is the result of increased parathyroid gland mass, possibly complicated by the presence of autonomous areas of nodular hyperplasia.

Vitamin D receptor status is likely to improve as a result of kidney transplantation, although this has not been tested directly. The restoration of normal calcitriol synthesis would be expected to up-regulate the vitamin D receptor such that, not only is the hormone once again sufficient, but also the state of target organ resistance to vitamin D that characterizes uremia is corrected (Reichel *et al.*, 1989; Nareh-Many *et al.*, 1990).

Although uremic acidosis is usually corrected by successful transplantation, a minority of patients experience persisting type 4 renal tubular acidosis. This is particularly likely in cyclosporin-treated patients, and has potentially adverse consequences for the skeleton in the long term (Cunningham *et al.*, 1982; Lefebrre *et al.*, 1989).

Immune suppressive therapy

As indicated above, successful engraftment dramatically improves the disordered mineral metabolism of uremia. Unfortunately, the benefits to the skeleton are seriously compromised by the therapies that are usually given to transplant patients.

Glucocorticoids and cyclosporin in particular both have a range of skeletal consequences, some clearly established and some less so (Epstein, 1996).

Glucocorticoids

At the doses used in renal transplantation glucocorticoids have substantial skeletal toxicity (Lukert, 1996). This comment applies regardless of the indication for the glucocorticoid treatment, but is particularly relevant in patients in whom the skeleton is already compromised by pre-existing renal osteodystrophy. Prednisolone reduces intestinal calcium absorption (leading to a degree of secondary hyperparathyroidism) and also inhibits a number of osteoblast synthetic functions. The result of this is accelerated bone loss affecting principally the trabecular bone of the axial skeleton. Various treatment strategies have been evaluated in non-transplanted patients receiving glucocorticoids for other reasons. These include the administration of pharmacological doses of vitamin D (25-hydroxyvitamin D or calcitriol) and antiresorptive therapy with calcitonin or bisphosphonates (Reid *et al.*, 1988; Lukert, 1996).

Cyclosporin

Cyclosporin has dramatic effects on bone cells *in vitro* and in rodents *in vivo*. These effects are not consistent with one another in that while *in-vitro* cyclosporin exhibits inhibitory actions on bone cell activity, *in-vivo* studies in rats reveal high-turnover osteopenia in cyclosporin-treated animals (Epstein, 1996) Surprisingly, there is little direct evidence that cyclosporin-treated patients suffer more or different bone diseases in clinical practice.

Azathioprine and other immunosuppressive agents

Azathioprine and other cytotoxic agents are surprisingly devoid of important skeletal toxicity. The same appears to apply to mycophenolate mofetil, although data with regard to the latter are scarce at this stage. Tacrolimus (FK-506) appears to have some similarities to cyclosporin in experimental studies—no clear picture has yet emerged from clinical studies (Epstein, 1996).

Observational studies in transplant recipients

A number of reports have documented substantial and rapid bone loss, particularly early after transplantation (Julian *et al.*, 1991; Almond *et al.*, 1994; Horber *et al.*, 1994) Most point to a subsequent slowing of the loss rate, possibly with some recovery. Julian *et al.*, found an average bone loss of 6.8% in the first 6 months following transplantation of patients in the predialysis phase of chronic renal insufficiency. This slowed to 2.8% over the ensuing 12 months and the changes were largely confined to the axial skeleton—no significant changes were seen at the radial shaft (Julian *et al.*, 1991). Our own studies have also demonstrated a very high bone-loss rate, in this case during the first 3 months after transplantation, when the loss rate was equivalent to 15% per annum at both the lumbar spine and femoral neck. To put this in perspective, normal postmenopausal women typically lose bone at the rate of approximately 1.7% per annum. We also found that there are potentially important gender differences—women lost bone mainly from the axial skeleton and the loss was greatest in those with the highest pretransplant PTH concentration, whereas men lost bone mainly from the femoral neck and the major loss was seen in those with the lowest pretransplant PTH concentration (Almond *et al.*, 1994).

Prevention and treatment

Any strategy should focus initially on the reduction of the many skeletal insults described above (Horber *et al.*, 1994). Most important amongst these is glucocorticoid therapy, and this provides another strong indication for minimizing and, if possible, avoiding steroid therapy in transplant recipients. Persisting hyperparathyroidism should be sought and treated with vitamin D sterols, unless prohibited by hypercalcemia or hypercalciuria, in which case parathyroidectomy should be considered. Despite the animal data, clinical studies do not provide a justification for modifying our attitude to cyclosporin therapy. Azathioprine and other immunosuppressive agents appear to be relatively innocent.

Specific intervention should aim to decrease bone resorption, increase bone formation, or possibly both. The results of observational studies to date suggest that this intervention would best be applied early in the post-transplant phase when bone loss is as its most rapid.

We have recently completed a study looking at the effects of the second generation bisphosphonate, pamidronate, given after transplantation. The rationale behind this was that pamidronate and other bisphosphonates have been shown convincingly to ameliorate bone loss in patients receiving steroid treatment for non-renal conditions (Reid *et al.*, 1988; Lukert, 1996). The results showed that early bone loss was substantial and that this could be prevented during the first year by pamidronate (Fan *et al.*, 1996).

Other studies have looked at vitamin D metabolites, calcitonin, and estrogens following transplantation. Results are mixed, although estrogen therapy certainly merits further evaluation. Sodium fluoride is also being examined—it is a potent anabolic agent for osteoblasts and has proven efficacy when used to increase bone density in postmenopausal women. Preliminary data suggest that benefits may also be seen in transplant recipients.

Conclusions

It is clear that renal osteodystrophy is an almost inevitable consequence of long-standing renal insufficiency. The development of the hormonal, metabolic, and skeletal components of renal osteodystrophy begins early in the natural history of uremia with detectable abnormalities evident when the GFR is still above 50% of the predicted normal. There is a strong argument for instituting prophylactic measures at this stage in the hope of improving the substrate upon which dialysis therapy operates when the patients reach ESRD.

Unfortunately, dialysis has serious deficiencies in regard to the pathogenesis and treatment of renal osteodystrophy. Phosphate removal by all forms of dialysis is well short of that required to maintain appropriate phosphorus metabolism, thus imposing the need for various therapeutically inadequate phosphate binders which are often not taken reliably by patients. Further, dialysis in no way modifies the diseased kidneys' failure to synthesize calcitriol, which needs to be supplied exogenously. Although the combination of effective phosphate control and adequate calcitriol replacement undoubtedly greatly improves many of the components of renal osteodystrophy, this is not always the case and there is a difficult balance to be struck between, on the one hand, achieving normal bone turnover and, on the other, avoiding runaway hyperparathyroidism. It is clear that other components of the uremic state impact adversely on bone cell metabolism—these have not been clearly identified and until they are then no logical therapeutic strategy for dealing with the broader components of the uremic state will be forthcoming.

Prospects for the future center around the development of effective phosphate binders that do not contain calcium or aluminum, the identification of new vitamin D metabolites with a better therapeutic profile than exhibited by calcitriol itself, and finally the further evaluation of the calcimimetic agents in the treatment of hyperparathyroidism. Successful kidney transplantation overcomes many of the shortcomings of dialysis in regard to renal osteodystrophy, but transplanted patients are exposed to new and different threats to the skeleton.

References

Adler, A. J., and Berlyne, G. M. (1986). Phosphate retention and the genesis of secondary hyperparathyroidism. *American Journal of Nephrology*, 6, 417–21.

Akizawa, T., Kurakawa, K., Suzuki, M., *et al.* (1996). Suppressive effect of 22-oxacalcitriol (OCT) in secondary hyperparathyroidism (II HPT) of haemodialysis (HD) patients—a double blind comparison among four doses. *Journal of the American Society of Nephrology*, 71, 1810 (Abstract).

Almaden, Y., Canalejo, A., Hernandez, A., Ballesteros, E., Garcia-Navarro, S., and Torres, A. (1996). Direct effect of phosphorus on PTH secretion from whole rat parathyroid glands *in vitro*. *Journal of Bone and Mineral Research*, 11, 970–6.

Almond, M. K., Kwan, J. T., Evans, K., and Cunningham, J. (1994). Loss of regional bone mineral density in the first 12 months following renal transplantation. *Nephron*, 66, 52–7.

Altmann, P. A., Butter, K. C., Plowman, D., Chaput de Saintonge, D. M., Cunningham, J., and Marsh, F. P. (1987). Residual renal function in hemodialysis patients may protect against hyperaluminemia. *Kidney International*, 32, 710–13.

Alvarez-Ude, F., Feest, T. J., Ward, M. K., *et al.* (1978). Haemodialysis bone disease—correlation between clinical, histologic and other findings. *Kidney International*, 14, 68–73.

Andreoli, S. P., Bergstein, J. M., and Sherrard, D. J. (1983). Aluminum intoxication from aluminum containing phosphate binders in children with azotemia not undergoing dialysis. *New England Journal of Medicine*, 310, 1079–84.

Armstrong, A., and Cunningham, J. (1994). The treatment of metabolic bone disease in patients on peritoneal dialysis. *Kidney International*, 46 (Suppl. 48), 51–7.

Armstrong, A., Beer, J., Noonan, K., and Cunningham, J. (1997). Reduced calcium dialysate in CAPD patients: efficacy and limitations. *Nephrology Dialysis, Transplantation* (In press).

Atonsen, J. E., Brady, E., Sherrard, D. J., and Andress, D. L. (1996). A calcium receptor agonist acutely suppresses parathyroid hormone (PTH) in dialysis patients. *Journal of the American Society of Nephrology*, **71**, 1810 (Abstract).

Bricker, N. S., Slatopolsky, E., Reiss, E., and Avioli, L. V. (1969). Calcium, phosphorus, and bone in renal disease and transplantation. *Archives of Internal Medicine*, **123**, 543–53.

Brickman, A. S., Coburn, J. W., and Norman, A. W. (1972). Action of 1,25-dihydroxycholecalciferol, a potent, kidney-produced metabolite of vitamin D in uremic man. *New England Journal of Medicine*, **287**, 891–5.

Brown, A. J., Ritter, C. R., Finch, J. L., Morrissey, J., Martin, K. J., and Murayama, E. (1989). The noncalcemic analogue of vitamin D, 22-oxacalcitriol, suppresses parathyroid hormone synthesis and secretion. *Journal of Clinical Investigation*, **84**, 728–32.

Brown, E. M., Pollack, M., Seidman, C. E., *et al.* (1995). Calcium sensing cell surface receptors. *New England Journal of Medicine*, **333**, 234–40.

Chalmers, T. M., Davie, M. W., Hunter, J. O., and Szaz, K. F. (1973). 1-alpha-hydroxycholecalciferol as a substitute for the kidney hormone 1,25-dihydroxycholecalciferol in chronic renal failure. *Lancet*, **2**, 696–9.

Chertow, G. M., Burke, S. K., Lazarus, J. M., *et al.* (1997). Poly[allylamine hydrochloride] (RenaGel): a noncalcaemic phosphate binder for the treatment of hyperphosphatemia in chronic renal failure. *American Journal of Kidney Diseases*, **29**, 66–71.

Cheung, A. K., Manalagos, S. C., Cotterwood, B. D., *et al.* (1983). Determinants of serum 1,25 $(OH)_2D$ levels in renal disease. *Kidney International*, **24**, 104–9.

Clarkson, E. M., McDonald, S. J., and de Wardener, H. E. (1966). The effect of a high intake of calcium carbonate in normal subjects and patients with chronic renal failure. *Clinical Science*, **30**, 425–38.

Coburn, J. W., (1993). Mineral metabolism and renal bone disease: effects of CAPD versus hemodialysis. *Kidney International*, **43** (Suppl. 40), 92–100.

Coburn, J. W., and Frazao, J. (1996). Calcitriol in the management of renal osteodystrophy. *Seminars in Dialysis*, **9**, 316–26.

Combe, C., and Aparicio, M. (1994). Phosphorus and protein restriction and parathyroid function in chronic renal failure. *Kidney International*, **46**, 1381–6.

Cundy, T., Hand, D. J., Oliver, D. O., Wood, C. G., Wright, F. W., and Kanis, J. A. (1995). Who gets renal bone disease before beginning dialysis? *British Medical Journal*, **290**, 271–5.

Cunningham, J. (1996). Parathyroid pathophysiology in uraemia. *Nephrology, Dialysis, Transplantation*, **11** (Suppl. 3), 106–10.

Cunningham, J., and Makin, H. (1997). How important is vitamin D deficiency in uraemia? *Nephrology, Dialysis, Transplantation*, **12**, 16–18.

Cunningham, J., Fraher, L. J., Clemens, T. L., Revell, P. A., and Papapoulos, S. E. (1982). Chronic acidosis with metabolic bone disease. *American Journal of Medicine*, **73**, 199–204.

Cunningham, J., Beer, J., Coldwell, R. D., Noonan, K., Sawyer, N., and Makin, H. L. J. (1992). Dialysate calcium reduction in CAPD patients treated with calcium carbonate and alfacalcidol. *Nephrology, Dialysis, Transplantation*, **7**, 63–8.

Delmez, J. A., and Slatopolsky, E. (1992). Hyperphosphatemia: its consequences and treatment in patients with chronic renal disease. *American Journal of Kidney Diseases*, **XIX**, 303–17.

Denda, M., Finch, J., and Slatopolsky, E. (1996). Phosphorus accelerates the development of parathyroid hyperplasia and secondary hyperparathyroidism in rats with renal failure. *American Journal of Kidney Diseases*, **28**, 596–602.

Dunlay, R., Rodriguez, M., Felzenfeld, A. J., and Llach, F. (1989). Direct inhibitory effect of calcitriol on parathyroid function (sigmoidal curve) in dialysis. *Kidney International*, **36**, 1093–8.

Dusso, A. S., Negrea, L., Sunawardhana, S., Lopez-Hilker, S., Finch, J., and Mori, T. (1991). On the mechanism for the selective action of vitamin D analogs. *Endocrinology*, **128**, 1687–92.

Epstein, S. (1996). Post-transplantation bone disease: the role of immunosuppressive agents on the skeleton. *Journal of Bone and Mineral Research*, **11**, 127.

Falchetti, A., Bale, A. E., Amorosi, A., *et al.* (1993). Progression of uremic hyperparathyroidism involves allelic loss on chromosome 11. *Journal of Clinical Endocrinology and Metabolism*, **76**, 139–44.

Fan, S., Almond, M. K., Ball, E., Evans, K., and Cunningham, J. (1996). Randomised prospective study demonstrating prevention of bone loss by pamidronate during the first year after renal transplantation. *Journal of the American Society of Nephrology*, **7**, 1789 (Abstract).

Felsenfield, A. J., Harrelson, J. M., Gutman, R. A., Wells, S. A., and Drezner, M. K. (1982). Osteomalacia after parathyroidectomy in patients with uremia. *Annals of Internal Medicine*, **96**, 34–9.

Fraser, D. R., (1980). Regulation of the metabolism of vitamin D. *Physiological Reviews*, **40**, 551–613.

Fukayawa, M., Fukada, N., Ye, H., and Kurakawa, K. (1995). Resistance of parathyroid cell to calcitriol as a cause of parathyroid hyperfunction in chronic renal failure. *Nephrology, Dialysis, Transplantation*, **10**, 316–19.

Fukada, N., Tanaka, H., Toninayo, Y., Fukayawa, M., Kurakawa, K., and Seino, Y. (1993). Decreased 1,25-dihydroxyvitamin D_3 receptor density is associated with a more severe form of parathyroid hyperplasia in chronic uremic patients. *Journal of Clinical Investigation*, **92**, 1436–43.

Gagne, E. R., Urena, P., Leite-Silva, S., *et al.* (1992). Short and long-term efficacy of total parathyroidectomy with immediate autografting compared with subtotal parathyroidectomy in hemodialysis patients. *Journal of the American Society of Nephrology*, **3**, 1008–17.

Gallieni, M., and Brancaccio, D. (1994). Which is the preferred treatment of advanced hyperparathyroidism in a renal patient? 1. Medical intervention is the primary option in the treatment of advanced hyperparathyroidism in chronic renal failure. *Nephrology, Dialysis, Transplantation*, **9**, 1816–21.

Giangrande, A., Castiglioni, A., Solibiati, L., Ballarati, E., and Caligrara, F. (1994). Chemical parathyroidectomy for recurrence of secondary hyperparathyroidism. *American Journal of Kidney Diseases*, **24**, 421–6.

Goodman, W. G., and Salusky, I. B. (1996). Parathyroid gland function and the set point for PTH release: understanding the available data. *Nephrology, Dialysis, Transplantation*.

Goodman, W. G., Belin, T. R., and Salusky, I. S. (1996). *In vivo* assessments of calcium regulated parathyroid hormone release in secondary hyperparathyroidism. *Kidney International*, **50**, 1834–44.

Graham, K. A., Hoenich, N. A., Tarbit, M., Ward, M. K., and Goodship, T. H. J. (1997). Correction of acidosis in haemodialysis patients increases the sensitivity of the parathyroid glands to calcium. *Journal of the American Society of Nephrology*, **8**, 627–31.

Hamida, F. B., El Esper, I., Compagnon, M., Moriniere, Ph., and Fournier, A. (1993). Long-term (6 months) cross-over comparison of calcium acetate with calcium carbonate as phosphate binder. *Nephron*, **63**, 258–62.

Hercz, G., Pei, Y., Greenwood, C., *et al.* (1993). Aplastic osteodystrophy without aluminum: the role of 'suppressed' parathyroid function. *Kidney International*, **44**, 860–6.

Hernandez, A., Concepcion, M. T., Rodriguez, M., Salido, E., and Torres, A. (1996). High phosphorus diet increases preproPTH mRNA independent of calcium and calcitriol in normal rats. *Kidney International*, **50**, 1872–8.

Horber, F. F., Casez, J. P., Steiger, U., Czerniak, A., Montandon, A., and Jaeger, P. (1994). Changes in bone mass early after kidney transplantation. *Journal of Bone and Mineral Research*, **9**, 1–9.

Hruska, K. A., and Teitelbaum, S. L. (1995). Renal osteodystrophy. *New England Journal of Medicine*, July 20, 166–74.

Hruska, K. A., Teitelbaum, S. L., Kopelman, R., *et al.* (1978). The predictibility of the histological features of uraemic bone disease by non invasive techniques. *Metabolic Bone Disease and Related Research*, **1**, 39–44.

Hsu, C. S., Patel, S. R., Young, E. W., and Vanholder, R. (1994). The biological actions of calcitriol in uremia. *Kidney International*, **46**, 605–12.

Hutchison, A. J., Freemont, A. J., Boulton, H. F., and Gokal, R. (1992). Low–calcium dialysis fluid and oral calcium carbonate in CAPD. A method of controlling hyperphosphataemia whilst minimizing aluminium exposure and hypercalcaemia. *Nephrology, Dialysis, Transplantation*, **7**, 1219–25.

Hutchison, A. J., Whitehouse, R. W., Boulton, H. F., *et al.* (1993). Correlation of bone histology with parathyroid hormone, vitamin D_3, and radiology in end–stage renal disease. *Kidney International*, **44**, 1071–7.

Joffe, P., Heaf, J. G., and Hyldstrup, L. (1994). Osteocalcin: a non-invasive index of metabolic bone disease in patients treated by CAPD. *Kidney International*, **46**, 838–46.

Julian, B. A., Laskow, D. A., Dubovsky, J., Dubovsky, E. V., Curtis, J. J., and Quarles, L. D. (1991). Rapid loss of vertebral mineral density after renal transplantation. *New England Journal of Medicine*, **325**, 544–50.

Kilav, R., Silver, J., and Naveh-Many, T. (1995). Parathyroid hormone gene expression in hyperphosphatemic rats. *Journal of Clinical Investigation*, **96**, 327–33.

Kitaoka, M., Fukagawa, M., Ogata, E., and Kurokawa, K. (1994). Reduction of functioning parathyroid cell mass by ethanol injection in chronic dialysis patients. *Kidney International*, **46**, 1100–17.

Kumar, R. (1997). Phosphatonin—a new phosphaturic hormone? (Lessons from tumourinduced osteomalacia and X-linked hypophosphataemia). *Nephrology, Dialysis, Transplantation*, **12**, 11–13.

Kwan, J. T. C., Almond M. K., Beer, J. C., Noonan, K., Evans, S. J. W., and Cunningham, J. (1992). 'Pulse' oral calcitriol in uraemic patients: rapid modification of parathyroid response to calcium. *Nephrology, Dialysis, Transplantation*, **7**, 829–34.

Lefebvre, A., De Vernejoul, M. C., Gueris, J., Goldfarb, B., Graulet, A. M., and Morieux, C. (1989). Optimal correction of acidosis changes progression of dialysis osteodystrophy. *Kidney International*, **36**, 1112–18.

Lopez-Hilker, S., Dusso, A. S., Rapp, N. S., Martin, K. J., and Slatopolsky, E. (1990). Phosphate restriction reverses hyperparathyroidism in uremia independent of changes in calcium and calcitriol. *American Journal of Physiology*, **259** (Renal fluid electrolyte physiology 28) F432–F437.

Lukert, B. P. (1996). Glucocorticoid and drug induced osteoporosis. In *Primer on the metabolic bone diseases and disorders of mineral Metabolism*, (3rd edn) (ed. M. J. Favus), pp. 278–82. Lippincott–Raven.

Mai, M. L., Emmett, M., Sheikh, M. S., Santa Ana, C. A., Schiller, L., and Fordtran, J. S. (1989). Calcium acetate, an effective phosphorus binder in patients with renal failure. *Kidney International*, **36**, 690–5.

Malluche, H., and Faugere, M.-C. (1990). Renal bone disease: an unmet challenge for the nephrologist. *Kidney International*, **38**, 193–211.

Malluche, H. H., and Monier-Faugere, M. C. (1994). The role of bone biopsy in the management of patients with renal osteodystrophy. *Journal of the American Society of Nephrology*, **4**, 1631–42.

Merie, F., Yap, P., and Bia, M. J. (1990). Etiology of hypercalcemia in hemodialysis patients on calcium carbonate therapy. *American Journal of Kidney Diseases*, **16**, 459–64.

Mitlak, B. H., Alpert, M., Lo, C., Delmonico, F., and Neer, R. M. (1991). Parathyroid function in normocalcemic renal transplant recipients: evaluation by calcium infusion. *Journal of Clinical Endocrinology and Metabolism*, **72**, 350–5.

Morrisey, J., Rothestein, M., Mayer, G., and Slatopolsky, E. (1983). Suppression of parathyroid hormone secretion by aluminum. *Kidney International*, **23**, 699–704.

Naveh-Many, T., Marcz, R., Keshet, E., and Pike, J. W. (1990). Regulation of 1,25 dihydroxyvitamin D_3 receptor gene expression by 1,25 dihydroxyvitamin D in the parathyroid *in vivo*. *Journal of Clinical Investigation*, **86**, 1968–75.

Parsons, V., Baldwin, D., Moniz, C., Marsden, J., Ball, E., and Rifkin, I. (1993). Successful control of hyperparathyroidism in patients on Continuous Ambulatory Peritoneal Dialysis using magnesium carbonate and calcium carbonate as phosphate binders. *Nephron*, **63**, 379–83.

Pazianas, M., Phillips, M. E., MacRae, K. D., and Eastwood, J. B. (1992). Identification of risk factors for radiographic hyperparathyroidism in 422 patients with end-stage renal disease: development of a clinical predictive index. *Nephrology, Dialysis, Transplantation*, **7**, 1098–105.

Pei, Y., Hercz, G., Greenwood, C., *et al.* (1995). Risk factors for renal osteodystrophy: a multi-variant analysis. *Journal of Bone and Mineral Research*, **10**, 149–56.

Pietschmann P., Vychytyc, A., Woloszczuk, W., and Kovarik, J. (1991). Bone metabolism in patients with functioning kidney grafts: increases serum levels of osteocalcin and parathyroid hormone despite normalisation of kidney function. *Nephron*, **59**, 533–6.

Portale, A. A., Booth, B. E., Halloran, B. P., and Morris, R. C. Jr (1984). Effect of dietary phosphorus on circulating concentrations of 1,25-dihydroxyvitamin D and immunoreactive parathyroid hormone in children with moderate renal insufficiency. *Journal of Clinical Investigation*, **73**, 1580–9.

Reichel, H., Koeffer, H. P., and Norman, A. W. (1989). The role of the vitamin D endocrine system in health and disease. *New England Journal of Medicine*, **320**, 980–91.

Reid, I. R., King, A. R., Alexander, C. J., and Ibbertson, H. K. (1988). Prevention of steroid-induced osteoporosis with (3-amino-1-hydroxypropylidene)-1, 1-bisphosphonate (APD). *Lancet*, **23**, 143.

Reiss, E., Canterbury, J. M., Bercovitz, A. M., and Kaplan, E. L. (1970). The role of phosphate in the secretion of parathyroid hormone in man. *Journal of Clinical Investigation*, **49**, 2146–9.

Ring, T., Nielsen, C., Paulin Anderson, S., Behrens, J. K., Sodemann, B., and Kornerup, H. J. (1993). Calcium acetate versus calcium carbonate as phosphorus binders in patients on chronic haemodialysis: a controlled study. *Nephrology, Dialysis, Transplantation*, **8**, 341–6.

Ritz, E., and Herzesell, O. (1996). Oral phosphate binders without aluminium and calcium—a pipe dream? *Nephrology, Dialysis, Transplantation*, **11**, 766–8.

Ritz, E., Seidel, A., Ramisch, H., Szabo, A., and Bouillon, R. (1991). Attenuated rise of 1,25 $(OH)_2$ vitamin D_3 in response to parathyroid hormone in patients with incipient renal failure. *Nephron*, **57**, 314–18.

Rodriguez, M., Martin Malo, A., Martinez, M. E., Torres, A., Felsenfeld, A., and Llach, F. (1991*a*). Calcemic response to parathyroid hormone in renal failure: role of phosphate and its effect on calcitriol. *Kidney International*, **40**, 1055–62.

Rodriguez, M., Felsenfield, A., and Llach, F. (1991*b*). Calcemic response to PTH in renal failure: role of calcitriol and the effect of parathyroidectomy. *Kidney International*, **40**, 1063–8.

Salusky, I. B., Ramirez, J. A., Oppenheim, W., Gales, B., Segre, G. V., and Goodman, W. G. (1994). Biochemical markers of renal osteodystrophy in pediatric patients undergoing CAPD–CCPD. *Kidney International*, **45**, 253–8.

Sanchez, C. P., Goodman, W. G., Ramirez, J. A., *et al.* (1995). Calcium regulated parathyroid hormone secretion in adynamic renal osteodystrophy. *Kidney International*, **48**, 838–43.

Sawyer, N., Noonan, K., Altmann, P., Marsh, F., and Cunningham, J. (1989). High-dose calcium carbonate with stepwise reduction in dialysate calcium concentration: effective phosphate control and aluminium avoidance in haemodialysis patients. *Nephrology, Dialysis, Transplantation*, **4**, 105–9.

Shah, G. M., Winer, R. L., Culter, R. E., *et al.* (1987). Effects of a magnesium-free dialysate on magnesium metabolism during continuous ambulatory peritoneal dialysis. *American Journal of Kidney Diseases*, **X**, 268– .

Sharman, W. V., Brownjohn, A. M., Goodwin, F. J., *et al.* (1982). Long-term experience of alfacalcidol in renal osteodystrophy. *Quarterly Journal of Medicine (New Series)* **51**, 203, 271–87.

Sheikh, M. S., Maguire, J. A., Emmett, M., *et al.* (1989). Reduction of dietary phosphorus absorption by phosphorus binders. A theoretical, *in vitro*, and *in vivo* study. *Journal of Clinical Investigation*, **83**, 66–73.

Silver, J., and Naveh-Many, T. (1994). Regulation of parathyroid hormone synthesis and secretion. *Seminars in Nephrology*, **14**, 175–94.

Silver, J., Russell, J., and Sherwood, L. M. (1985). Regulation by vitamin D metabolites of messenger ribonucleic acid for preproparathyroid hormone in isolated bovine parathyroid cell. *Proceedings of the National Academy of Sciences, USA*, **82**, 4270–3.

Slatopolsky, E., Martin, K., and Hruska, K. (1980). Parathyroid hormone metabolism and its potential as a uremic toxin. *American Journal of Physiology*, **239** (Renal fluid electrolyte physiology 8), F1–F12.

Somerville, P. J., and Kaye, M. (1979). Evidence that resistance to the calcemic action of parathyroid hormone in rats with acute uraemia is caused by phosphate retention. *Kidney International*, **16**, 552–60.

Tan, A. V., Levine, B. S., Mazess, R. M., *et al.* (1997). Effective suppression of parathyroid hormone by 1α-hydroxyvitamin D_2 in hemodialysis patients with moderate to severe secondary hyperparathyroidism. *Kidney International*, **51**, 317–23.

Tenenhouse, H. S. (1997). Cellular and molecular mechanisms of renal phosphate control. *Journal of Bone and Mineral and Research*, **12**, 159–64.

Tessitore, N., Venturi, A., Adami, S., *et al.* (1987). Relationship between serum vitamin D metabolites and dietary intake of phosphate in patients with early renal failure. *Mineral and Electrolyte Metabolism*, **13**, 38–44.

Torres, A., Lorenzo, V., Hernandez, D., *et al.* (1995). Bone disease in predialysis, hemodialysis, and CAPD patients: evidence of a better bone response to PTH. *Kidney International*, **47**, 1434–42.

Urena, P., Ferreira, A., Kung, V. T., *et al.* (1995). Serum pyridinoline as a specific marker of collagen breakdown and bone metabolism in hemodialysis patients. *Journal of Bone and Mineral Research*, **10**, 932–9.

Ward, M. K., Feest, T. G., Ellis, H. A., *et al.* (1978). Osteomalacic dialysis osteodystrophy: evidence for a waterborn aetiological agent, probably aluminium. *Lancet*, **1**, 841–5.

5

Aluminum, silicon, and strontium accumulation/ intoxication as a complication of long-term dialysis

Patrick C. D'Haese and Marc E. De Broe

Introduction

A number of considerations indicate that trace elements may accumulate in dialysis patients. This is due to:

(1) the patients' uremic state;
(2) the dialysis treatment during which these constituents may be transferred to the patient;
(3) the diet; and
(4) the administration of pharmaceutical preparations which may contain high concentrations of a number of trace metals (Alfrey, 1989; Salusky *et al.*, 1991; D'Haese *et al.*, 1990*a*).

Aluminum accumulation is a well-known complication of long-term dialysis, and both acute and chronic intoxications have repeatedly been reported in the literature during the last two decades (Andress *et al.*, 1986; Simoes *et al.*, 1994; Burwen *et al.*, 1995). Aluminum overload in dialysis patients has been implicated in the pathogenesis of several clinical disorders of the musculoskeletal, central nervous, and hematological systems (De Broe and Coburn, 1990) and more subtle disorders at the level of parathyroid function and bone turnover, resistance to erythropoietin therapy, and anemia (De Broe *et al.*, 1993).

Recently increased *silicon* levels have also been reported in the serum of dialysis patients which significantly differed from center to center and from country to country (D'Haese *et al.*, 1995*a*). The clinical relevance of silicon accumulation is not yet clearly established, however, it is worthwhile considering in view of the element's suggested involvement in bone metabolism (Carlisle, 1972) and its potential effect on the absorption of aluminum (Edwardson *et al.*, 1993).

Data on increased *strontium* levels in dialysis patients is scarce, but it might become of particular interest in view of the reported association between increased concentrations of strontium in the bones of dialysis patients with osteomalacia (D'Haese *et al.*, 1995*b*). Although there is at present no clear-cut evidence regarding the causative role of strontium in the development of this potential new disease entity within the dialysis population, efforts should be undertaken to elucidate further the observed relationship and to search for factors underlying the accumulation of this element.

Aluminum

Aluminum (mol. wt, 27 Da) is the third most common element in the earth's crust, and is the most abundant metal. Although widely used by the food, cosmetic, and pharmaceutical industries, increased tissue aluminum was rarely considered to be a hazard until more accurate methods for measuring aluminum concentrations became available in the late 1970s, when the potential dangers of aluminum contamination of the water used for dialysis and the use of aluminum-containing phosphate binders were recognized.

Metabolism and aluminum-related disorders in dialysis

The protective mechanisms against aluminum accumulation (renal excretion and the gastrointestinal barrier) are either absent in dialysis patients or are highly challenged by the intake of pharmacological doses of aluminum salts for enteral phosphorous binding (Van de Vyver *et al.*, 1990). In serum, aluminum circulates 80–90% bound to transferrin (Van Landeghem *et al.*, 1994). The most important target organs for accumulation of the element are bone and liver. However, there is no clear-cut relationship between the concentration of aluminum in a given tissue and the toxicity the element exerts at that site. Thus, small concentrations of aluminum in brain have been associated with high toxicity expressed by either dialysis encephalopathy (Alfrey *et al.*, 1976), or Alzheimer's disease (Candy *et al.*, 1986), whereas high concentrations in the liver do not seem to induce any toxic effect. These data suggest that the toxicity of aluminum is related to the ultrastructural localization of the element; i.e. the accumulation of the element at critical metabolic sites, e.g. the osteoid calcified-bone boundary where mineralization takes place (Verbueken *et al.*, 1984).

The clinical consequences of aluminum overload in dialysis patients include a neurological syndrome, i.e. dialysis encephalopathy, disorders of the hematological system, and the development of the so-called aluminum-related bone disease (Tomson and Ward, 1989). The use of deionizers and reverse-osmosis filters for water purification and the replacement of $Al(OH)_3$ by calcium-containing phosphate-binding agents have markedly reduced the incidence and severity of the aluminum-related diseases. However, despite the availability of modern dialysis treatment modalities, acute, even fatal, intoxications cannot be excluded (Simoes *et al.*, 1994; D'Haese and De Broe, 1996*a*). Also, with the introduction of erythropoietin for the treatment of anemia, a new subgroup of subjects with relative iron deficiency has emerged within the current dialysis population. Interestingly, these patients appear to have higher serum aluminum levels (Vanuytsel *et al.*, 1992; Cannata *et al.*, 1993); this is most probably due to the higher affinity of transferrin (aluminum's transport protein in plasma) for aluminum at low iron–transferrin saturations (Van Landeghem *et al.*, 1997). In these patients, the aluminum–transferrin complex is supposed to preferentially accumulate at sites expressing transferrin receptors, where, at relatively low concentrations, it may be responsible for the development of rather subtle disorders involving, e.g. the parathyroid gland, erythropoiesis, the hepatocyte, or the osteoblast (Mladenovic, 1988; Abreo *et al.*, 1991; Smans *et al.*, 1996). On the other hand, in patients with transfusional iron overload or in those presenting with oversaturated transferrin secondary to the use of intravenous iron supplements (Zanen *et al.*, 1996), low serum-aluminum levels may be accompanied by distinct bone aluminum accumulation (Van Landeghem *et al.*, 1998), a site where the element is supposed to be deposited in its inorganic form; most probably as the citrate compound.

Aluminum-related bone disease (ARBD)

The most common types of ARBD are the so-called 'pure *osteomalacia*' and '*adynamic bone disease*'. Distinct features of aluminum-induced osteomalacia include extensive accumulation of the element at the mineralization front, a decreased number of osteoblasts and osteoclasts, increased osteoid volume, and a marked decrease of double-tetracycline-labeled surfaces. Sometimes increased osteoid is not seen, which is consistent with a picture of 'adynamic bone disease'. In some biopsies the *mixed lesion* is present with both features of hyperparathyroid bone disease and osteomalacia.

Although only limited information is available regarding the actions of aluminum as a direct inhibitor of mineralization, interference with calcium deposition and alterations in crystal seeding, structure, and growth of hydroxyapatite are the most likely explanation for the element's deleterious effect on bone mineralization (Blumenthal and Posner, 1984). However, the precise mechanisms by which aluminum alters calcification is not yet fully understood. Furthermore, mechanisms other than physicochemical interactions may contribute to the adverse interactions of aluminum on mineralization. Disturbances in osteoblast metabolism characterized by changes in cell enzyme activity and cell membrane function may represent another important mechanism by which aluminum could alter the process of calcification (Goodman, 1990); these cell-mediated actions of aluminum on the process of bone mineralization, however, have yet to be firmly established.

Apart from the element's effects on bone mineralization, interferences of aluminum with bone collagen synthesis may result in diminished bone formation (an important hallmark in the development of adynamic bone disease). Here, a transferrin-mediated effect of aluminum on osteoblast proliferation (Kasai *et al.*, 1991) has been suggested. The extent to which aluminum also alters osteoblast function is much less clear (Goodman, 1990). Furthermore, aluminum may indirectly influence bone remodeling by interfering with the actions of the parathyroid hormone (PTH). Indeed, in dialysis patients with ARBD serum PTH is often only moderately elevated or may be within the normal range for non-uremic subjects; findings that are distinctly uncommon in patients with advanced renal failure. Although a direct effect of aluminum on the PTH secretion (not synthesis) has been established (Morrissey *et al.*, 1983) it should be noted that many patients with ARBD have persistent elevations in serum calcium concentrations, which elicited the suggestion that the aluminum-related hypercalcemia mediates (at least in part) the decrease in serum PTH levels (Cannata *et al.*, 1983).

Clinically, ARBD is manifested by severe and diffuse bone pain, muscle weakness, and spontaneous fractures. Laboratory findings include slightly elevated serum calcium levels, which may rise dramatically after vitamin D administration and are persistent after parathyroidectomy. Furthermore, serum alkaline phosphatase levels are expected to be normal (D'Haese and De Broe, 1994). Although, in general, serum aluminum levels will be increased, patients with iron overload may present with ARBD in the presence of a low serum aluminum concentration (Van Landeghem *et al.*, 1998).

Control of the aluminum content of the dialysate and the replacement of aluminum-containing phosphate binders with calcium salts have resulted in a progressive and definite decrease in the prevalence of so-called pure ARBD expressed by vitamin D-resistant osteomalacia (Ballanti *et al.*, 1996; Monier-Faugere and Malluche, 1996). However, recent literature surveys (Table 5.1) indicate that a distinct accumulation of aluminum in bone is still noted in a considerable number of patients. It is unclear to what extent the introduction of new treatment modalities (such as vitamin D or erythropoietin) may, in the long term, alter the toxic potential of accumulated aluminum on the bone level. It has also been hypothesized that with the introduction of erythropoietin, even relatively low concentrations of circulating aluminum may, in addition to other etiological factors, contribute to the development of adynamic bone disease associated with a relative hypoparathyroidism (Smans *et al.*, 1996); a bone disorder which has been increasingly identified during the last few years (Malluche and Monier-Faugere, 1992; Sherrard *et al.*, 1993). Here, the underlying mechanism may consist of an increased transferrin-mediated uptake of aluminum by the parathyroid gland secondary to the erythropoietin-induced relative iron deficiency. Indeed, it has been demonstrated that in patients with relative iron depletion secondary to the use of erythropoietin treatment, aluminum will have a higher affinity for transferrin which will lead to a preferential accumulation of aluminum in transferrin-receptor expressing tissues such as the parathyroid gland (Smans *et al.*, 1995) and the osteoblast (Kasai *et al.*, 1991). This may result in an increased toxic effect of aluminum on these tissues which may be expressed by the development of hypoparathyroidism-associated adynamic bone disease.

Table 5.1 Current status of bone aluminum accumulation/toxicity in dialysis patients

---

In 268 Canadian dialysis patients 85 still had a bone surface Aluminon® staining >25% (Sherrard *et al.*, 1993).

In 209 Saudi-Arabian hemodialysis patients 61% had variable degrees of bone aluminum toxicity (Huraib *et al.*, 1993).

In Brazilian patients 74 out of 96 patients (77%) had aluminum overload (extent of stainable aluminum > 20%) (Jorgetti *et al.*, 1994).

In the United States of America, in 1995, over 25% of the patients still had a >30% positive staining for aluminum (Monier-Faugere and Malluche, 1996).

Acute intoxications have repeatedly been reported in recent years (Simoes *et al.*, 1994; Burwen *et al.*, 1995; Caramelo *et al.*, 1995; D'Haese and De Broe 1996a).

Anemia and resistance to erythropoietin therapy

The aluminum-associated anemia is typically microcytic. Here, the presence of microcytosis with normal serum ferritin levels suggests that aluminum intoxication may be the causative factor. Several mechanisms by which aluminum leads to microcytic anemia have been postulated. These include the interference of aluminum with both porphyrin and heme synthesis, disturbances in erythroid maturation, and increased hemolysis (Drüeke, 1994). Evidence has been presented in the literature for the hematopoietic toxicity of aluminum to be transferrin-mediated, either by preventing the site-specific loading of iron to transferrin or, alternatively, by the unloading of transferrin-bound iron on to specific cell receptors (Drüeke, 1990). More detailed studies are required, however, to define further the exact role of aluminum in the development of this hematological disorder. Recently, a partial or even total resistance to the hematopoietic action of recombinant human erythropoietin characterized by an increase in erythrocyte porphyrin content has been reported in dialysis patients with concomitant aluminum intoxication (Rosenlöf *et al.*, 1990). Here, interference with heme synthesis has been suggested, as a consequence of aluminum's ability to bind to transferrin, thus preventing iron incorporation into heme.

Aluminum encephalopathy

The first supporting evidence for aluminum as an etiological agent for dialysis encephalopathy was the demonstration that brain aluminum levels, as well as other tissue aluminum levels, were significantly higher in patients on dialysis who died of a neurological syndrome of, at that time an unknown cause, as compared to the concentrations found in a group of uremic patients on dialysis who died of other causes. (Alfrey *et al.*, 1976). Further evidence was provided by studies showing that areas having a high incidence of dialysis encephalopathy also had high aluminum levels in the municipal water supplies used to prepare the dialysate. In most cases, neurological disturbances are accompanied by other aluminum-related abnormalities such as fracturing osteomalacia and anemia.

Early-onset 'chronic' dialysis encephalopathy is characterized by intermittent speech disturbances and dyspraxia. Serum aluminum levels, in general, will exceed 100 μg/l and EEG findings will be abnormal. As the disease progresses the speech disturbances become more severe and eventually the patient becomes completely mute. Additional findings include twitching, myoclonic jerks, motor apraxia, seizures, and personality changes. In the absence of adequate treatment (see below) death usually occurs within 6 months following the onset of the disease (Alfrey, 1978). Some similarities in neurochemistry, neuropathology and cerebral function to patients with Alzheimer disease have been reported (Farran *et al.*, 1990). With the introduction of an adequate water-treatment systems, aluminum monitoring programs, and the partial replacement of aluminum-containing phosphate binders classical aluminum neurotoxicity is now extremely rare. However, acute forms of aluminum neurotoxicity from three different causes, have repeatedly been reported in the literature. These include dialysis performed with highly, mostly accidentally contaminated dialysates (Simoes *et al.*, 1994), the concomitant administration of citrate and aluminum (Bakir *et al.*, 1986), and desferrioxamine treatment (Barata *et al.*, 1996). In these patients serum aluminum levels mostly rise to above 300 μg/l, and the most common symptoms include obtundation, auditory and visual neurotoxicity, coma, and seizures. EEG patterns are similar to those found in chronically intoxicated patients. Although several theories have been advanced to explain how aluminum exerts its toxicity, at this time the mechanism by which acute and chronic aluminum neurotoxicity occurs in dialysis patients is unknown (Alfrey and Froment, 1990; Fraser and Arieff, 1994).

Other disorders related to aluminum accumulation in dialysis patients

In addition to the above disorders aluminum accumulation has been associated with joint pain, proximal musculoskeletal weakness, and dialysis-related arthropathy (Netter *et al.*, 1990). A toxic effect of aluminum on the myocardium has also been suggested (London *et al.*, 1989). In view of the association between trace metals other than aluminum and the development of uremic heart failure, further studies are required to establish a definite etiological role for aluminum (Pehrsson and Lins, 1983; Sjogren *et al.*, 1996). Even though the liver is an important storage organ for aluminum, no direct toxic effects have been described in the adult dialysis population. Perhaps the lysosomal sequestration of aluminum within this organ prevents the element from exerting its deleterious effect (Verbueken *et al.*, 1984). However, in children on parenteral nutrition contaminated with aluminum, accumulation of aluminum in the liver was associated with cholestatic liver disease (Klein 1989). This may result from reduced bile flow and increased serum bile-acid concentration and glucuronyl transferase activity as shown in experimental rat studies (Klein 1989; Klein *et al.*, 1989). Furthermore, it has been suggested that patients with an increased body load of aluminum are more prone to bacterial sepsis (Davenport *et al.*, 1991), and that the element may promote oxygen-radical formation via either inhibition of the activity of superoxide dismutase (Shainkin-Kestenbaum *et al.*, 1989) or by catalyzing the vanadium-mediated oxidation of NADH (Adler *et al.*, 1995). Because of the limited data, however, these findings require further investigation and should be interpreted with caution.

Diagnosis of aluminum overload/toxicity

Because bone is the major storage organ for aluminum and since it exerts its most important toxic action at this site, the histological, histochemical, and chemical examination of a bone biopsy must still be considered as the 'gold standard' for the diagnosis of aluminum overload/toxicity. However, bone biopsy is an invasive procedure that can only be performed by trained medical staff. Moreover, bone biopsy examination and data interpretation are complex. Thus reliance on bone biopsy for the routine diagnosis of aluminum overload/toxicity is impractical.

Among the non-invasive diagnostic tools available, regular monitoring of serum aluminum levels ranks as the easiest and most cost-effective. The determination of baseline serum aluminum concentrations holds a certain diagnostic value; however, these mainly reflect recent exposure and, as such, offer the greatest value for the early detection of incipient aluminum loading (Savory *et al.*, 1983; D'Haese *et al.*, 1990*b*). It is important, in the interpretation of baseline serum aluminum values that the iron status be taken into account, in view of the recent observations by Van Landeghem *et al.* (1998) which demonstrate a distinct bone-aluminum accumulation despite low serum aluminum values in iron-overloaded patients.

A valuable, non-invasive diagnostic alternative is the desferrioxamine (DFO) test. Desferrioxamine is a chelating agent that liberates aluminum from its body stores. The aluminum–DFO complex, aluminoxamine, enters the blood compartment from these sites. A substantial increment in the serum aluminum level (ΔSAl) 44 hours after DFO (5 mg/kg given IV during the last hour of a dialysis session) may indicate the presence of aluminum overload. Moreover, a ΔSAl threshold of 50 μg/l may, in combination with a serum iPTH measurement, differentiate between aluminum overload/increased risk for toxicity and ARBD (D'Haese *et al.*, 1995*b*).

Treatment of aluminum overload/toxicity

Aluminum in the blood is about 80–90% bound to transferrin. This protein binding is the primary reason why aluminum is so poorly removed during dialysis even when concentrations are high. The administration of DFO will not only increase the absolute serum aluminum concentration but will also increase it in the form of the dialyzable aluminoxamine (mol. wt, 583 Da): this can be easily removed by high-performance dialyzers either combined or not with hemoperfusion (Vasilakakis *et al.*, 1992). DFO treatment although still the only available method for removing aluminum in dialysis patients, is effective in reversing aluminum-related diseases (see above).

The therapeutic use of this chelator can cause various, often fatal, side-effects (Boelaert and de Locht, 1992). Limited epidemiological studies have pointed towards a greater incidence of these side-effects, in particular mucormycosis with higher doses and/or more frequent administration of the chelator. Therefore, as for the DFO test and following the recommendations made at '*The Consensus Conference on the Diagnosis and Treatment of Aluminium Overload*', a dose as low as 5 mg/kg should also be used in the treatment of aluminum overload/toxicity. At this dose the chelation capacity for aluminum is not significantly inferior compared to when higher doses are used (Verpooten *et al.*, 1992). However, in severely intoxicated patients where the serum aluminum level after DFO-treatment may rise to above 300 μg/l, it has been observed that the patients' neurological state has worsened even when doses of DFO as low as 5 mg/kg have been administered in the conventional way (i.e. during the last hour of dialysis followed by removal of the chelates 44 hours later). These side-effects could be minimized when DFO is given 5 hours before the start of the dialysis session (Barata *et al.*, 1996). Using this latter strategy, maximal aluminum chelation is obtained, whereas the exposure to circulating aluminoxamine, ferrioxamine, and unchelated DFO is limited (Verpooten *et al.*, 1992). Based on these data, updated strategies for both the diagnosis and treatment of aluminum overload/toxicity have recently been described (D'Haese *et al.*, 1995*b*; Barata *et al.*, 1996).

Prevention of aluminum overload/toxicity

In practice, aluminum accumulation cannot be totally prevented in uremic patients. However, appropriate measures can minimize the risk of aluminum overload. Water used for preparing dialysis solutions, final dialysis fluids, as well as the patients' serum aluminum levels should all be monitored periodically. Efforts should be undertaken to keep the aluminum content of the dialysis fluids below 3 or even 2 μg/l. The administration of aluminum, in any form, to the patient groups identified as being at increased risk for aluminum toxicity (children, diabetic patients, parathyroidectomized patients, etc.) should be avoided whenever possible. When aluminum is given the concomitant ingestion of citrate in any form, including fruit juices and effervescent analgesics, must be avoided. Replacement of Al(OH)$_3$ by calcium carbonate is a valuable alternative, but it can not be used in all patients because of gastrointestinal intolerance or hypercalcemia.

Silicon

Silicon (mol. wt, 28 Da) is, next to oxygen, the second most abundant element in nature. It constitutes 28% of the earth's crust, and mainly occurs in its oxygenated form as silica (SiO$_2$) or various silicate complexes (SiO$_4^{4-}$). Silicon, which is essentially a non-metal, is frequently used in the ceramic industries and for the manufacture of semiconductors. The organic silicon-based polymers, the so-called silicones (polymeric chains containing alternately linked silicon and oxygen atoms), are widely used for industrial as well as clinical and pharmaceutical purposes.

Metabolism of silicon

Dietary silicon is present in most vegetables either in its silica or silicate form, often in appreciable amounts (up to 10% of the dry mass) (Epstein, 1994). It is rapidly absorbed by the intestine. At physiological pH, in blood and extravascular fluid, the element is supposed to circulate unbound to proteins, most probably as silicic acid (Birchall 1986; D'Haese *et al.*, 1995c). In humans and in animals renal excretion is the major route of silicon elimination; the renal clearance being around 90 ml/min. After an injection of radioactive silicon (Si–31) a rapid accumulation of the element has been noted in various organs, but this rapidly declines to values in equilibrium with the plasma concentration thus indicating a steady-state exchange between plasma and tissues (Adler *et al.*, 1986a). Hence, in subjects with normal renal function no organs seem to act as storage sites for the element, with the exception of bone. Bone has been found to have some capacity to retain silicon; which may be relevant in view of the suggested essential role silicon has for growth and development, bone calcification, and the formation of glycosaminoglycan complexes in connective tissues (Carlisle, 1972; Schwarz 1973). The element has also been identified in mitochondrial granules in the liver, kidney, and spleen (Mehard and Volcani, 1976), but its function in this context has not been demonstrated so far.

Silicon/silicones in dialysis patients

The literature dealing with the accumulation of silicon in dialysis patients is somewhat confusing with regard to the nomenclature used. Here a clear-cut differentiation should be made between the accumulation of the inorganic (*silica, silicates*, etc.) and organic (*silicones*) silicon-containing compounds, both of which may accumulate in dialysis patients but originate from totally different sources and exert different toxic effects.

Accumulation of silicon in dialysis patients

Due to the abundancy of silicon and the absence of adequate renal function, which is the main excretory pathway of silicon, an accumulation of silicon may reasonably be expected in subjects with chronic renal failure. Indeed, increased serum silicon levels in these subjects which correlate with the creatinine clearance have been reported in the literature (Table 5.2) (Berlyne *et al.*, 1985; Dobbie and Smith, 1986; Adler and Berlyne, 1986*b* Gitelman *et al.*, 1992*a, b*; D'Haese *et al.*, 1995*c*). In dialysis patients, serum silicon levels are dependent on the concentration gradient between the silicon present in the dialysis fluid and the ultrafiltrable amount of the element (>98%) in serum. Silicon crosses into the extracellular compartment during dialysis, the net effect being a greatly increased serum level (Table 5.2). Contamination of the dialysis fluids appears to be due to the use of silicon-contaminated concentrates (D'Haese *et al.*, 1995*c*) or reverse-osmosis membranes of the water-treatment installations that inadequately remove silicon during the water-purification process (Gitelman *et al.*, 1992*b*; D'Haese *et al.*, 1995*c*). With regard to the latter, silicon is not removed from tap water by deionization or by a charcoal column, but solely by reverse osmosis (D'Haese *et al.*, 1995*c*). Inadequate removal of silicon by reverse-osmosis membranes is also associated with the inadequate removal of aluminum (D'Haese *et al.*, 1996*a*). In addition to the use of contaminated dialysis fluids, the dietary intake of silicon from tap water also seems to contribute to the serum silicon accumulation in dialysis patients (Dobbie and Smith, 1986; D'Haese *et al.*, 1995*a*). Dramatic variations in serum silicon levels may be expected from center to center and from country to country, (Dobbie and Smith, 1986; Gitelman *et al.*, 1992*b*; D'Haese *et al.*, 1995*a*).

With regard to the clinical relevance of the increased serum silicon levels in uremic patients, little is known at the present time. There is some concern that exposure to large amounts of silicon adversely affects the health status of end-stage renal failure patients. Indeed, based on what is currently known of silicon's biological role, alterations in the matrix metabolism of connective tissue, bone, and skin might reasonably be expected in the presence of hypersilicemia (Carlisle, 1972, Dobbie and Smith, 1982). Furthermore, silicon's suggested role in the production of oxygen radicals (Shainkin-Kestenbaum *et al.*, 1990) may play a part in the development of a variety of important well-known clinical complications such as inflammatory processes, cell damage, and the promotion of carcinogenic processes. On the other hand, high silicon concentrations in drinking water have been associated with protection against the toxic effects of aluminum (Dobbie and Smith, 1982; Birchall *et al.*, 1989).

Accumulation of silicones in dialysis patients

Due to the widespread use of silicones in medical devices (blood lines, pump tubings, etc.) the risk of introducing these substances through extracorporeal blood circuits is real. Silicones have long been presumed to be inert and biocompatible, but are now well-recognized inducers of particular pathologic entities. Silicone inclusions originating from silicone tubing, torn off under the shearing stress of roller pumps, were reported in the early 1980. Silicone-filled macrophages or giant cells were observed in the spleen, liver, heart, lungs, and thoracic and abdominal lymph nodes (Bommer *et al.*, 1981*a*, *b*; Parfrey *et al.*, 1981; Leong *et al.*, 1982; Kossovsky *et al.*, 1990). Accumulation of silicones in hemodialysis patients may, in addition to granulomatous inflammation, also lead to the development of more complex clinicopathologic entities such as splenomegaly (Bommer *et al.*, 1981), various degrees of hepatic inflammation and fibrosis, granulomatous hepatitis (Parfrey *et al.*, 1981; Leong *et al.*, 1982), and giant cell myocarditis (Kossovsky *et al.*, 1990). Although the use of silicone-based tubings in dialysis instrumentation has been dramatically reduced during recent years, the potential for the accumulation of these substances should still be considered in hemodialysis patients.

Table 5.2 Serum silicon levels and renal function

	Concentration, μg/l Mean $\pm$ SD (n)	Reference
Normal renal function	161 $\pm$ 44 (15)	D'Haese *et al.*, 1995*c*
	140 $\pm$ 14 (?)	Fahal *et al.*, 1993
	150 $\pm$ 85 (18)	Gitelman *et al.*, 1992*b*
	220 $\pm$ 80 (?)	Hosokawa *et al.*, 1987
	602 $\pm$ 126 (50)	Dobbie and Smith 1986
	265 $\pm$ 82 (23)	Adler *et al.*, 1986
	275 $\pm$ 91 (17)	Berlyne *et al.*, 1985
Preterminal renal failure	2581 $\pm$ 864 (15)	D'Haese *et al.*, 1995*c*
	1280 $\pm$ 760 (16)	Gitelman *et al.*, 1992*a*
	1296 $\pm$ 336 (21)	Dobbie and Smith 1986
	520 $\pm$ 276 (36)	Adler *et al.*, 1986
	480 $\pm$ 269 (10)	Berlyne *et al.*, 1985
Hemodialysis	3813 $\pm$ 1744 (1267)	D'Haese *et al.*, 1995*a*
	1599 $\pm$ 611 (33)	Fahal *et al.*, 1993
	4600 $\pm$ 2039[a] (26)	Gitelman *et al.*, 1992*b*
	624 $\pm$ 204 (54)	Hosokawa *et al.*, 1987
	60 $\pm$ 196[b] (18)	Dobbie and Smith, 1986
	up to 4172 $\pm$ 476[b] (16)	
	839 $\pm$ 127 (5)	Berlyne *et al.*, 1985
CAPD	1408 $\pm$ 683 (225)	D'Haese *et al.*, 1995*c*
	1900 $\pm$ 6000 (25)	Gitelman *et al.*, 1992*b*

[a] Mean $\pm$ SD serum silicon concentrations noted in two different dialysis centers.
[b] Mean $\pm$ SD serum silicon concentration in the center which had those patients with the lowest silicon levels vs. that with patients having the highest concentrations. Four centers were studied.

Strontium

Strontium (mol. wt, 88) is a member of the alkaline earth elements. In its chemical characteristics it resembles calcium and barium and has properties intermediate between these two elements. In the geosphere, strontium is ranked fifteenth in order of elemental crustal abundance. From a biological point of view the compounds consisting of strontium and phosphate are of most interest, since, chemically, they are closely related to calcium phosphate in calcified tissues. Industrially, the element is used in ceramics, greases, plastics, permanent magnets, and iron castings. In medicine, both stable and radioactive strontium have been used as markers for calcium metabolism, whereas the radioactive strontium-89 isotope has been applied in the palliative treatment of bone metastases. The divalent strontium salt, S12911, has recently been proposed as a potential therapeutic agent in the management of osteopenic disorders (Blumsohn *et al.*, 1994; Sips and van der Vijgh, 1994; Grynpas *et al.*, 1996).

Strontium in dialysis patients

The information in the literature regarding strontium accumulation/toxicity in dialysis patients is rather limited. In view of (a) the striking physicochemical similarities with calcium, (b) strontium's potential to accumulate in dialysis patients (Mauras *et al.*, 1986; Schrooten *et al.*, 1996) (c) the reported interference with vitamin D biosynthesis and calcium absorption (Omdahl and DeLuca, 1972), and (d) the effects on bone formation, mineralization, and resorption in experimental studies (Grynpas and Marie, 1990; Grynpas *et al.*, 1996), the lack of information on the effects of strontium on bone metabolism in dialysis patients is surprising. Indeed, in the dialysis population, alterations in vitamin D synthesis and calcium absorption, which in turn may alter bone metabolism, are common. In view of this, the recent observations that strontium levels in bone are increased in osteomalacia is intriguing (D'Haese *et al.*, 1996*b*). Moreover, recent experimental work indicates that when chronic renal-failure rats are given strontium they may develop osteomalacia (Cabrera *et al.*, 1996 and Schrooten *et al.*, 1998*a*). These preliminary observations require further experimental evidence in order to define the exact role of strontium in the development of this particular disorder. However, they might be indicative of an unidentified disease entity within the dialysis population. This is also supported by data from a multicenter study, indicating that strontium levels in serum vary dramatically from center to center and from country to country (Schrooten *et al.*, 1998*b*). As for silicon, these variations seem to be due to regional differences in the strontium content of dialysis fluids but they may also depend on a number of other factors (Schrooten *et al.*, 1998*b*). This variability together with the potential effects of strontium on bone, may necessitate the monitoring of the strontium status in the dialysis population as well as the determination of its concentration in dialysis fluids and tap water. Here, the recent availability of accurate and precise methodologies for the routine determination of strontium will be important tools (Barto *et al.*, 1995; D'Haese *et al.*, 1997).

Conclusions

The issue of aluminum overload/toxicity is now well recognized and should not be considered a past phenomenon within the current dialysis population. Acute intoxications still occur on a regular basis, and chronic accumulation of the element may in the long term result in the development of subtle disorders at the level of the parathyroid glands, the osteoblast, hemopoiesis, and resistance to erythropoietin. Regular control of serum and dialysate aluminum levels is still required and will allow the early identification of both patients and centers at risk. In the diagnosis of aluminum overload/toxicity the desferrioxamine test is a useful non-invasive tool. Also, the chelator is still the only available agent for the treatment of aluminum toxicity. However, it should be used at low doses following well-defined administration schedules in order to reduce the risk for often fatal side-effects.

In contrast to aluminum, the clinical relevance of silicon and strontium overload in dialysis patients is unknown, but potentially their accumulation may have adverse effects in bone.

References

Abreo, K., Jangula, J., Jain, S. K., Sella, M., and Glass, J. (1991). Aluminum uptake and toxicity in cultured mouse hepatocytes. *Journal of the American Society of Nephrology*, **1**, 1299–304.

Adler, A. J., and Berlyne, G. M. (1986*a*). Silicon metabolism. II. Renal handling in chronic renal failure patients. *Nephron*, **44**, 36–9.

Adler, A. J., Etzion, Z., and Berlyne G. M. (1986*b*). Uptake, distribution, and excretion of [31]silicon in normal rats. *American Journal of Physiology*, **251**, E670–3.

Adler, A., Caruso, C., and Berlyne, G. M. (1995). The effect of aluminum on the vanadium-mediated oxidation of NADH. *Nephron*, **69**, 34–40.

Alfrey, A. C. (1978). Dialysis encephalopathy syndrome. *Annual Review of Medicine*, **29**, 93–8.

Alfrey, A. C. (1989). Trace elements and regular dialysis. In *Replacement of renal function by dialysis* (ed. J. F. Maher), pp. 996–1003 Kluwer. Academic Publishers, Dordrecht.

Alfrey, A. C., and Froment D. C. (1990). Dialysis encephalopathy. In *Aluminum in renal failure*. (ed. M. E. De Broe and J. W. Coburn), pp. 249–57. Kluwer Academic Publishers, Dordrecht.

Alfrey, A. C., LeGendre, G. R., and Kaehny, W. D. (1976). The dialysis encephalopathy syndrome—possible aluminum intoxication. *New England Journal of Medicine*, **294**, 184–8.

Andress, D. L., Maloney, N. A., Endres, D. B., and Sherrard, D. J. (1986). Aluminum-associated bone disease in chronic renal failure: high prevalence in a long-term dialysis population. *Journal of Bone* and Mineral Research, **5**, 391–8.

Bakir, A. A., Hryhorczvk, D. O., Berman, E., Dunea, G. (1986). Acute fatal hyperaluminemic encephatopathy in undialyzed and recently dialyzed uremic patients. *Trans American Society of Artificial Internal Organs*, **32**, 171–76.

Ballanti, P., Martin Wedard, B., and Bonucci, E. (1996). Frequency of adynamic bone disease and aluminum storage in Italian uraemic patients—retrospective analysis of 1429 iliac crest biopsies. *Nephrology, Dialysis, Transplantation* **11**, 663–7.

Barata, J. D., D'Haese, P. C., Pires, C., Lamberts, L. V., Simoes, J., and De Broe, M. E. (1996). Low-dose (5 mg/kg) desferrioxamine treatment in acutely intoxicated haemodialysis patients using two drug administration schedules. *Nephrology, Dialysis, Transplantation* **11**, 125–32.

Barto, R., Sips, A. J. A. M., van de Vijgh, W. J. F., and Coen Netelenbos, J. (1995). Sensitive method for analysis of strontium in human and animal plasma by graphite furnace atomic absorption spectrophotometry. *Clinical Chemistry*, **41**, 1159–63.

Berlyne, G., Dudek, E., Adler, A. J., Rubin, J. E., and Seidman, M. (1985). Silicon metabolism: the basic facts in renal failure. *Kidney International*, **28**, S175–7.

Birchall, J. D. (1986). The toxicity of aluminum and the effect of silicon on its bioavailability. In Silicon biochemistry, Ciba Foundation Symposium, No. 121 (ed. D. Evered and M. O'Connor), pp. 73–9. John Wiley, New York.

Birchall, J. D., Exley, C., Chappell, J. S., and Philips, M. J. (1989). Acute toxicity of [26]aluminum to fish eliminated in silicon–rich acid waters. *Nature*, **338**, 146–8.

Blumenthal, N. C., and Posner, A. S. (1984). *In vitro* model of aluminum–induced osteo-malacia: inhibition of hydroxyapatite formation and growth. *Calcified Tissue International*, **36**; 439.

Blumsohn, A., Morris, B., and Eastell, R. (1994). Stable strontium absorption as a measure of intestinal calcium absorption: comparison with the double–radiotracer calcium absorp-tion test. *Clinical Science*, **87**, 363–8.

Boelaert, J. R., and de Locht, M. (1992). Side-effects of desferrioxamine in dialysis patients. *Nephrology, Dialysis, Transplantation*, S–1, 44–7.

Bommer, J., Ritz, E., and Waldherr, R. (1981*a*). Silicone-induced splenomegaly. Treatment of pancytopenia by splenectomy in a patient on hemodialysis. *New England Journal of Medi-cine*, **305**, 1077–9.

Bommer, J., Ritz, E., Waldherr, R., and Gastner, M. (1981*b*). Silicone cell inclusions causing multi-organ foreign body reaction in dialysed patients. *Lancet*, **i**, 1314 (Letter).

Burwen, D. I., Olsen, M. O., Bland, L. A., Arduino, M. J., Reid, M. H., and Jarvis, W. R. (1995). Epidemic aluminum intoxication in hemodialysis patients traced to use of an aluminum pump. *Kidney International*, **48**, 469–74.

Cabrera, W., D'Haese, P. C., Nouwen, E. J., Schrooten, I., Goodman, W. G., and De Broe, M. E. (1996). Strontium-induced osteomalacia. A new disease entity in the dialysis population? Experimental evidence for a causal role. *Journal of the American Society of Nephrology*, **7**, 1788 (Abstract).

Candy, J. M., Oakley, A. E., Klinowski, J; *et al.* (1986). Aluminosilicates and senile plaque for-mation in Alzheimer's disease. *Lancet*, **i**, 354–57.

Cannata, J. B., Briggs, J. D., Junor, B. J. R., Fell, G. S., and Beastall, G. (1983). Effect of acute alu-minium overload on calcium and parathyroid hormone metabolism. *Lancet*, **i**, 501–3.

Cannata, J. B., Alaizola, I. R., Gomez-Alonso, C., Menéndeze-Fraga, P., Alonso–Suarez, M., and Diaz-Lopez, J. (1993). Serum aluminum transport and aluminum uptake in chronic renal failure: role of iron and aluminum metabolism. *Nephron*, **65**, 141–6.

Caramelo, C. A., Cannata, J. B., Rodeles, M. R., *et al.* (1995). Mechanisms of aluminum-induced microcytosis: lessons from accidental aluminium intoxication. *Kidney International*, **47**, 164–8.

Carlisle, E. M. (1972). Silicon as an essential element for the chick. *Science*, **178**, 619–21.

Davenport, A., Davison, A. M., Will, E. J., Newton, K. E., and Toothill, C. (1991). Aluminium mobilization following renal transplantation and the possible effect on susceptibility to bacterial sepsis. Quarterly Journal of Medicine, **79**, 407–23.

De Broe, M. E., and Coburn, J. W. (ed.) (1990). *Aluminum and renal failure.* Kluwer Academic, Dordrecht.

De Broe, M. E., D'Haese, P. C., Coutteneye, M. M., Van Landeghem, G. F., and Lamberts, L. V. (1993). New insights and strategies in the diagnosis and treatment of aluminum overload in dialysis patients. *Nephrology, Dialysis, Transplantation*, **8**, 47–50.

D'Haese, P. C., Lamberts, L. V., Liang, L; Boone, L. P., Van Waeleghem, J. -P., De Broe, M. E. (1990a). Contribution of parenteral and dialysate solutions to the aluminum accumulation in dialysis patients. *Blood Purification*, 8, 359–62 (Letter to the Editor).

D'Haese, P. C., and De Broe, M. E. (1994). Aluminum toxicity. In *Handbook of dialysis*, (ed. J. T. Daugirdas and T. S. Ing), pp. 522–36. Little, Brown, New York.

D'Haese, P. C., and De Broe, M. E. (1996a). Adequacy of dialysis: trace elements in dialysis fluids. *Nephrology, Dialysis, Transplantation*, 11 (Suppl. 2), 92–7.

D'Haese, P. C., Clement, J. P., Elseviers, M. M., Lamberts, L. V., Van de Vyver, F. L., and De Broe, M. E. (1990b). Value of serum aluminium monitoring in dialysis patients: a multicentre study. *Nephrology, Dialysis, Transplantation* 5, 45–53.

D'Haese, P. C., Couttenye, M.-M., Goodman, W. G., *et al.* (1995b). Use of the low-dose desferrioxamine test to diagnose and differentiate between patients with: aluminum-related bone disease/increased risk for toxicity/aluminum overload. *Nephrology, Dialysis, Transplantation*, 10, 1874–84.

D'Haese, P. C., Shaheen, F. A., Huraib, S. O., *et al.* (1995c). Increased silicon levels in dialysis patients due to high silicon content in the drinking water, inadequate water treatment procedures, and concentrate contamination: a multicentre study. *Nephrology, Dialysis, Transplantation*, 10, 1838–44.

D'Haese, P. C., Couttenye, M.-M., Lamberts, L. V., Goodman, W. G., and De Broe, M. E. (1995b). Increased strontium levels in bone of dialysis patients with osteomalacia. *Journal of the American Society of Nephrology*, 6, 935 (Abstract).

D'Haese, P. C., Cabrera, W. E., Lamberts, L. V., *et al.* (1996b). Bone strontium levels are increased in dialysis patients with osteomalacia. *Nephrology, Dialysis, Transplantation*, 11, 42 (Abstract).

D'Haese, P. C., Van Landeghem, G. F., Lamberts, L. V., Bekaert, V. A., Schrooten, I., and De Broe, M. E. (1997). Measurement of strontium in serum, urine, bone and soft tissues by Zeeman atomic absorption spectrometry. *Clinical Chemistry*, 43, 121–28.

Dobbie, J. W., and Smith, M. J. B. (1982). The silicon content of biological fluids. *Scottish Medical Journal*, 27, 17–19.

Dobbie, J. W., and Smith, M. J. B. (1986). Urinary and serum silicon in normal and uraemic individuals. In *Silicon biochemistry*, Ciba Foundation Symposium, No. 121 (ed. D. Evered and M. O'Connor), pp. 194–213. John Wiley, New York.

Drüeke, T. B. (1990). Other clinical syndromes associated with aluminum. In *Aluminum in renal failure*. (ed. M. E. De Broe and J. W. Coburn), pp. 259–65. Kluwer Academic, Dordrecht.

Drüeke T. B. (1994). Aluminum and microcytic anaemia. *Life Chemistry Reports*, 11, 231–34.

Edwardson, J. A., Moore, P. B., Ferrier, I. N., *et al.* (1993). Effect of silicon on gastrointestinal absorption of aluminum. *Lancet*, 342, 211–12.

Epstein, E. (1994). The anomaly of silicon in plant biology. *Proceedings of the National Academy of Sciences*, 91, 11–17.

Fahal, I. H., Ahmad, R., Bell, G. M., Birchall, J. D., and Roberts, N. B. (1993). Profile of serum silicon in aluminum-overloaded patients on regular haemodialysis treatment. *Journal of Analytical Atomic Spectrometry, Spectrom*, 8, 911–13.

Farrar, G., Altmann, P., Welch, S., *et al.* (1990). Defective gallium-transferrin binding in Alzheimer disease and Down syndrome: possible mechanism for accumulation of aluminum in brain. *Lancet*, 335, 747–50.

Fraser, C. L., and Arieff, A. I. (1994). Metabolic encephalopathy as a complication of renal failure: mechanisms and mediators. *New Horizons*, 2, 518–26.

Gitelman, H. J., Alderman, F., and Perry, S. J. (1992a). Renal handling of silicon in normals and patients with renal insuficiency. *Kidney International*, 42, 957–9.

Gitelman, H. J., Alderman, F., and Perry, S. J. (1992*b*). Silicon accumulation in dialysis patients. *American Journal of Kidney Diseases*, 14, 140–3.

Goodman, W. G. (1990). Pathophysiologic mechanisms of aluminum toxicity: aluminum-induced bone disease. In *Aluminum in renal failure* (ed. M. E. De Broe and J. W. Coburn), pp. 87–108. Kluwer Academic Dordrecht.

Grynpas, M. D., and Marie, P. J. (1990). Effects of low doses of strontium on bone quality and quantity in rats. *Bone*, 11, 313–19.

Grynpas, M. D., Hamilton, E., Cheung, R., *et al.* (1996). Strontium increases vertebral bone volume in rats at a low dose that does not induce detectable mineralization defect. *Bone*, 18, 253–9.

Hosokawa, S., Morinaga, M., Nishitani, H., Maeda, T., and Yoshida, O. (1987). Silicon in chronic hemodialysis patients. *Transactions of the American Society of Artificial Internal Organs*, 23, 260–4

Huraib, S., Souqqiyeh, Z., Aswad, S., and Al-Swailem, R. (1993). Pattern of renal osteodystrophy in haemodialysis patients in Saudi Arabia. *Nephrology, Dialysis, Transplantation*, 8, 603–8.

Jorgetti, V., Ricco Soeiro, N. M., Mendes, V., *et al.* (1994). Aluminum-related osteodystrophy and desferrioxamine treatment: role of phosphorus. *Nephrology, Dialysis, Transplantation*, 9, 668–74.

Kasai, K., Hori, M. T., and Goodman, W. G. (1991). Transferrin enhances the antiproliferative effect of aluminum on osteoblast-like cells. *American Journal of Physiology, Endocrinology and Metabolism*, 260, E537–43.

Klein, G. L. (1989). Aluminum in parenteral products: medical perspective on large and small volume parenterals. *Journal of Parenteral Science and Technology*, 43, 120–4.

Klein, G. L., Lee, T. C., Heyman, M. B., and Rassin, D. K. (1989). Altered glycine and taurine conjugation of bile acids following aluminum administration to rats. *Journal of Pediatric Gastroenterology and Nutrition*, 9, 361–4.

Kossovsky, N., Cole, P., and Zackson, D. A. (1990). Giant cell myocarditis associated with silicone. An unusual case of biomaterials pathology discovered at autopsy using X-ray energy spectroscopic techniques. *American Journal of Clinical Pathology*, 93, 148–52.

Leong, A. S. Y., Disney, A. P., and Gove, D. W. (1982). Spallation and migration of silicone from blood-pump tubing in patients on hemodialysis. *New England Journal of Medicine*, 306, 135–40.

London, G. R., de Vernejoul, M.-C., Fabiani, F., *et al.* (1989). Association between aluminum accumulation and cardiac hypertrophy in hemodialyzed patients. *American Journal of Kidney Diseases*, 13, 75–83.

Malluche, H. H., and Monier-Faugere, M.-C. (1992). Risk of adynamic bone disease in dialyzed patients. *Kidney International*, 42, S62–7.

Mauras, Y., Ang, K. S., Simon, P., Tessier, B., Cartier, F., and Allain, P. (1986). Increase in blood plasma levels of boron and strontium in hemodialyzed patients. *Clinica Chimica Acta*, 156, 315–20.

Mehard, C. W., and Volcani, B. E. (1976). Silicon-containing granules of rat liver, kidney and spleen mitochondria. *Cell and Tissue Research*, 174, 315–27.

Mladenovic, J. (1988). Aluminum inhibits erythropoiesis *in vitro*. *Journal of Clinical Investigation*, 81, 1661–5.

Monier-Faugere, M.-C., and Malluche, H. H. (1996). Trends in renal osteodystrophy: a survey from 1983 to 1995 in a total of 2248 patients. *Nephrology, Dialysis, Transplantation*, 11, 111–20.

Morrissey, J., Rothstein, M., Mayor, G., and Slatopolsky, E. (1983). Suppression of parathyroid hormone secretion by aluminum. *Kidney International*, 23, 699–704.

Netter, P., Kessler, M., Gaucher, A., and Bannwarth, B. (1990). Does aluminum have a patho-genic role in dialysis associated arthropathy? *Annals of the Rheumatic Diseases*, **49**, 573–5.

Omdahl, J. L., and DeLuca, H. F. (1972). Rachitogenic activity of dietary strontium. I. Inhib-ition of intestinal calcium absorption and 1,25-dihydroxycholecalciferol synthesis. *Jour-nal of Biological Chemistry*, **247**, 5520–6.

Parfrey, P. S., O'Driscoll, J. B., and Paradinas, F. J. (1981). Refractile material in the liver of haemodialysis patients. *Lancet*, i, 1101–2 (Letter).

Pehrsson, S. K., and Lins, L.-E. (1983). The role of trace elements in uremic heart failure. *Nephron*, **34**, 93–8.

Rosenlöf, K., Fyhrquist, F., and Tenhunen, R. (1990). Erythropoietin, aluminum, and anaemia in patients on haemodialysis. *Lancet*, **335**, 247–49.

Salusky, I. B., Foley, J., Nelson, P., and Goodman, W. G. (1991). Aluminum accumulation during treatment with aluminum hydroxide and dialysis in children and young adults with chronic renal disease. *New England Journal of Medicine*, **324**, 527–31.

Savory, J., Berlin, A., Courtoux, C., Yeoman, B., and Wills, M. (1983). Summary report of an international workshop on 'The role of biological monitoring in the prevention of aluminum toxicity in man: aluminum analysis in biological fluids'. *Annals of Clinical and Laboratory Science*, **13**, 444–51.

Schrooten, I., Cabrera, W., Goodman, W. G., Dawre, S., Lamberts, L. V., Marijnissen, R., Dorr-iné, W., De Broe, M. E., D'Haese, P. C. (1998*a*). Strontium causes osteomalacia in chronic renal failure rats. *Kidney International* (In press).

Schrooten, I., D'Haese, P. C., Elseviers, M. M., Lamberts, L. V., De Broe, M. E. (1998*b*). Strontium-induced osteomalacia (OM). A new disease entity in patients with end-stage renal failure in dialysis. An epidemiological survey. *Nephrology, Dialysis, Transplantation*, **13**, 188 (Abstract).

Schwarz, K. (1973). A bound form of silicon in glycosaminoglycans and polyuronides. *Proceed-ings of the National Academy of Science of the United States of America*, **70**, 1608–12.

Shainkin-Kestenbaum, R., Adler, A. J., Berlyne, G. M., and Caruso, C. (1989). Inhibition of superoxide dismutase by aluminum. *Clinical Science*, **77**, 463–6.

Shainkin-Kestenbaum, R., Adler, A. J., and Berlyne, G. M. (1990). Inhibition of superoxide dismutase by silicon. *Journal of Trace Elements and Electrolytes in Health and Disease*, **4**, 97–9.

Sherrard, D. J., Hercz, G., Pei, Y., *et al.* (1993). The spectrum of bone disease in end-stage renal failure—an evolving disordere. *Kidney International*, **43**, 436–42.

Simoes, J., Barata, J. D., D'Haese, P. C., and De Broe, M. E. (1994). Cela n'arrive qu'aux autres (letter). *Nephrology, Dialysis, Transplantation*, **9**, 67–8.

Sips, A. J. A. M., and van der Vijgh, J. F. (1994). Strontium. In *Handbook on metals in clinical and analytical chemistry* (ed. H. G. Seiler, A. Sigel, and H. Sigel), pp. 577–85. Marcel Dekker; New York.

Sjogren, B., Ljunggren, K. G., Almkvist, O., Frech, W., Basun, H. (1996). A follow-up study of five cases of aluminosis. *International Archives of Occupational and Environmental Health*, **68**, 161–64.

Smans, K. A., D'Haese, P. C., Van Landeghem, G. F., Lamberts, L. V., and De Broe, M. E. (1995). Aluminum transferrin (AlTf) but not Alcitrate (Alcit) uptake by the parathyroid gland (PTG) may contribute to the development of hypoparathyroidism associated with adynamic bone disease (ABD). *Journal of the American Society of Nephrology*, **6**, 940 (Ab-stract).

Smans, K. A., Van Landeghem, G. F., D'Haese, P. C., Couttenye, M. M., and De Broe, M. E. (1996). Is there a link between erythropoietin therapy and adynamic bone disease? *Nephrology, Dialysis, Transplantation*, **11**, 1248–9.

Tomson, C. R. V., and Ward, M. K. (1989). Aluminum toxicity in renal failure. In *Replacement of renal function by dialysis* (ed. J. F. Maher), pp. 1004–17. Kluwer Academic, Dordrecht.

Van de Vyver, F. L., D'Haese, P. C., and De Broe, M. E. (1990). The metabolism of aluminum. In *Aluminum in renal failure*. (ed. M. E. De Broe and J. W. Coburn), pp. 27–39. Kluwer Academic, Dordrecht.

Van Landeghem, G. F., D'Haese, P. C., Lamberts, L. V., De Broe, M. E. (1994). A quantitative HPIEC-ETAAS hybrid technique for studying the protein binding and speciation of aluminum. *Analytical Chemistry*, **66**, 216–22.

Van Landeghem, G. F., D'Haese, P. C., Lamberts, L. V., and De Broe, M. E. (1997). Competition of iron and aluminum for transferrin: the molecular basis for aluminum deposition in iron-overloaded dialysis patients. *Journal of Experimental Nephrology*, **5**, 239–45.

Van Landeghem, G. F., D'Haese, P. C., Lamberts, L. V., *et al.* (1998). A distinct bone aluminum accumulation/toxicity in the presence of low serum aluminum values may be explained by the effect of iron on the speciation of aluminum. *Clinical Nephrology* (In Press).

Vanuytsel, J. L., D'Haese, P. C., Couttenye, M. M., and De Broe, M. E. (1992). Higher serum aluminum levels in iron-depleted dialysis patients. *Nephrology, Dialysis, Transplantation*, **7**, 177 (Letter).

Vasilakakis, D. M., D'Haese, P. C., Lamberts, L. V., Lemoniatou, E., Digenis, P. N., and De Broe, M. E. (1992). Removal of aluminoxamine and ferrioxamine by charcoal hemoperfusion and hemodialysis. *Kidney International*, **41**, 1400–7.

Verbueken, A. H., Van de Vyver, F. L., Van Grieken, R. E., *et al.* (1984). Ultrastructural localization of aluminum in patients with dialysis-associated osteomalacia. *Clinical Chemistry*, **30**, 763–8.

Verpooten, G. A., D'Haese, P. C., Boelaert, J. R., Becaus, I., Lamberts, L. V., and De Broe, M. E. (1992). Pharmacokinetics of aluminoxamine and ferrioxamine and dose finding of desferrioxamine in haemodialysis patients. *Nephrology, Dialysis, Transplantation*, **7**, 931–8.

Zanen, A. L., Adriaansen, H. J., van Bommel, E. F. H., Posthuma, R., and de Jong, G. M. Th. (1996). 'Oversaturation' of transferrin after intravenous ferric gluconate (Ferrlecit® in haemodialysis patients. *Nephrology, Dialysis, Transplantation*, **11**, 820–4.

ß$_2$-Microglobulin amyloidosis

Michel Jadoul and Charles van Ypersele de Strihou

Introduction

ß$_2$-Microglobulin amyloidosis (ß2mA) is a now well-characterized complication of long-term dialysis. Assenat *et al.* (1980) first reported the presence of amyloid deposits in carpal tunnel biopsies from hemodialysis (HD) patients. This 'dialysis-related amyloidosis' (DRA) was renamed ß$_2$-microglobulin amyloidosis after Gejyo *et al.* (1985) demonstrated that ß2m is the major component of DRA deposits. It subsequently became apparent that the prevalence of ß2mA increased both with age at the onset of dialysis and with the duration of the treatment (van Ypersele *et al.*, 1991)

Our understanding of this crippling complication has improved markedly over the last 10 years. In this chapter, we review the clinical characteristics of ß2mA, the available diagnostic tools, the risk factors for the development of the disease, and briefly summarize current pathophysiological concepts. We finally review the preventive strategies and the management of established ß2mA.

Clinical characteristics

ß2mA has a marked affinity for joint tissues (cartilage, capsule, synovium). Hence, its clinical picture usually includes the carpal tunnel syndrome (CTS), chronic invalidating arthralgias associated with amyloid bone cysts, leading occasionally to bone fractures from enlarging cysts. Finally, amyloid deposits may be found, usually in minute amounts, in various organs.

Carpal Tunnel Syndrome

The CTS is usually the first manifestation of ß2mA (van Ypersele *et al.*, 1988). It may be observed as early as 3–5 years after the onset of dialysis. Its prevalence rises thereafter and becomes clinically significant after >7 years HD, reaching about 100% after >20 years HD (Charra *et al.*, 1988; van Ypersele *et al.*, 1988; Bardin, 1996). The symptoms are no different from those observed in non-HD patients: paresthesias of the palmar surfaces of the first 3–4 fingers, with eventual sensory and motor loss (wasting of the thenar muscles especially). The pain typically exacerbates at night and during HD sessions, as well as by tapping over the palmar surface of the wrist (Tinel's sign) or forcing flexion of the wrist (Phalen's sign) (van Ypersele *et al.*, 1988; Bardin, 1996). Sooner or later it involves both hands. The differential diagnosis includes uremic neuropathy and cervical root compression (Bardin, 1996). Electromyography will confirm the diagnosis. Occasionally, amyloid deposits are associated with an ulnar nerve compression, manifested by paresthesias of the palmar surface of the 4th–5th fingers, the so-called Guyon's syndrome (Borgatti *et al.*, 1991).

Histological examination of the material removed during surgery reveals mainly fibrous tissue. ß2m amyloid deposits are identified in approximately 70% of the cases (van Ypersele *et al.*, 1988). Very often they are small. Their absence in 30% of patients may be ascribed either to sampling problems or to the fact that ß2mA is not the only etiology of the CTS in HD patients (van Ypersele *et al.*, 1988): the vascular access and microcrystalline wrist arthritis have been incriminated (Bardin, 1996), and it should not be forgotten that the CTS is not uncommon especially in middle-aged women. It is clear from most pathological studies that the median nerve is compressed mainly by fibrous tissue and only very rarely by the amyloid deposit itself. ß2mA-related CTS should be strongly suspected in long-term (>7 years) HD patients, especially when its symptoms are associated with chronic arthralgias. Its management is discussed below.

Amyloid arthropathy: the peripheral joints

As mentioned earlier, ß2mA has a strong affinity for peripheral joints. The first deposits appear in the cartilage. They extend subsequently to the synovia, the joint capsules, and the attached tendons. The deposits, initially paucicellular, are eventually surrounded by macrophages (Argilés *et al.*, 1994). The former stage is usually asymptomatic, whereas the latter is characterized by symptoms of articular inflammation.

The prevalence of arthralgias rises with HD duration. In Charra *et al.*'s series (1988), shoulder pain and stiffness was noted as early as 5 years after HD onset, affecting 50% and 100% of patients after 13 and 19 years HD, respectively. Arthralgias are usually insidious at the onset. Thereafter, they follow a chronic, progressive course. Articular involvement is usually bilateral (Brown *et al.*, 1986), usually starting in the shoulders, extending later to the hips, knees, wrists, etc. The pain may exacerbate at night or during HD sessions (van Ypersele *et al.*, 1988). Joint mobility becomes restricted as the disease progresses (Bardin, 1996).

Joint swelling is not a constant finding but joint effusions may develop and are usually of the low inflammatory type (Bardin, 1996), unless hemarthrosis develops as observed in a minority of patients (Cary *et al.* 1986). Synovial fluid aspiration may yield small synovial fragments in which ß2m amyloid deposits may be recognized (Muñoz-Gómez *et al.*, 1987). Chronic tenosynovitis of the finger flexors is also frequently observed (Bardin *et al.*, 1985; Bardin, 1996). It is associated with mobility restriction, pain, and palmar swelling, and, in some patients, trigger fingers.

The differential diagnosis of arthralgias in HD patients is wide: it includes infection, microcrystalline deposits of calcium phosphate or uric acid, and erosive enthesopathy associated with severe hyperparathyroidism (Bardin, 1996). Monoarticular involvement will suggest infection or microcrystalline deposition. Still, septic arthritis may be polyarticular in HD patients, with low-grade or no fever. Needle aspiration of synovial fluid with a leukocyte count (high in the case of infection) and fluid culture will yield the correct diagnosis. The acute flares of calcium phosphate or uric acid deposits around joints are distinct from the chronic arthralgias of amyloid arthropathy. The enthesopathies of severe hyperparathyroidism usually coexist with other signs of severe hyperparathyroidism, an indication for subtotal parathyroidectomy.

Unusual manifestations of ß2mA include subcutaneous ß2m amyloid masses with a periarticular location (elbow, knee, hip) (Brancaccio *et al.*, 1988; Reese *et al.*, 1988; Floege *et al.*, 1989; Fernández *et al.*, 1990).

Amyloid arthropathy: the spine

In 1984 Kuntz *et al.* first described a destructive spondylarthropathy developing in long-term HD patients. Radiological signs include severe narrowing of the intervertebral spaces, especially at the cervical level, erosions and geodes of the vertebral plates without significant osteophytosis. Clinical signs are usually limited to moderate pain which is relieved by analgesics. This syndrome, subsequently recognized as common in long-term HD patients, is not solely due to amyloid deposits since, in a few typical cases, no ß2mA was found at histology (Bindi and Chanard, 1990; Deforges-Lasseur *et al.*, 1993). It is probably of multifactorial origin: age, mechanical stress, and/or severe hyperparathyroidism are probably involved (Bindi and Chanard, 1990). The main differential diagnosis is infectious discitis, whose clinical presentation is usually more acute with fever and an increased serum C-reactive protein level. Magnetic resonance imaging will show normal disc signals in T1 and T2 sequences in destructive spondylarthropathy, in contrast to the low T1, high T2 signals in infectious discitis (Maruyama *et al.*, 1992).

Another unusual type of spinal complication, directly related to ß2mA, occurs in long-term HD: amyloid masses develop in the epidural space and joints of the cervical spine, especially the atlanto-occipital joint (Allain *et al.*, 1988; Kröner *et al.*, 1991; Koch, 1992). They eventually result in subacute or acute neurological compression, with quadriparesis or occipital nerve neuralgia.

Bone fractures

ß2m amyloid invades not only cartilage, synovia, and capsules but also the adjacent bones. The development of bone cysts (whose radiological differential diagnosis is reviewed below) may eventually culminate in pathological fractures, especially at the femoral neck (Huaux *et al.*, 1985; van Ypersele *et al.*, 1988; Campistol *et al.*, 1990; Koch, 1992). Other locations include the scaphoid bone and the C1–C2 junction.

Systemic (non-osteoarticular) manifestations

ß2m amyloid deposits are also found in various organs. They are detected much later than in the joints but their prevalence is not well characterized. Deposits are usually found in blood vessel walls (Gal *et al.*, 1994). Their small size explains why they are usually asymptomatic. More rarely, larger ß2m amyloid deposits within visceral organs of long-term HD patients are responsible for symptoms: these include heart failure with pulmonary hypertension, gastrointestinal tract bleeding, bowel perforation, infarction or pseudo-obstruction, chronic diarrhea, macroglossia, or lingual nodules (Maher *et al.*, 1988; Choi *et al.*, 1989; Guccion *et al.*, 1989; Sethi *et al.*, 1989; Shinoda *et al.*, 1989; Zhou *et al.*, 1991; Ikegaya *et al.*, 1995; Lutz *et al.*, 1995; Araki *et al.*, 1996). In the latter cases, HD duration ranged from 12 to 19 (median 14) years.

Diagnostic tools

The 'gold standard': histology

The 'gold standard' for the diagnosis of all types of amyloidosis remains the histological examination of affected tissues. Unfortunately, joint biopsy remains an invasive procedure not devoid of risk. In patients with gross clinical evidence of joint effusion, joint puncture (with Congo Red staining of small synovial fragments contained in the synovial fluid) has been proposed as a less invasive, but sensitive alternative: this proved positive in 6/7 (86%) tested samples in patients in whom ß2mA was virtually certainly present (Muñoz-Gómez *et al.*, 1987).

Overall, histology of affected tissues (mainly joints) remains unavailable in most patients suspected of ß2mA, whereas biopsies of non-osteoarticular structures (including subcutaneous fat and rectum) have proven insensitive (Hardouin *et al.*, 1987; Varga *et al.*, 1987; Koch, 1992).

Still, the definition of the sensitivity and specificity of other diagnostic tools relies necessarily on histological evidence.

The prevalence of histological ß2mA in the joints appears much higher than suspected on clinical grounds: up to 20–30% of patients are affected within 2–3 years HD, and more than 90% beyond 7 years HD, both in peripheral joints (Jadoul *et al.*, 1997*a*) and vertebrae (Ohashi *et al.*, 1992).

Unfortunately, pathological examination is limited first by sampling problems: indeed, ß2mA is not evenly distributed among different joints as there appears to be a preferential involvement of sternoclavicular joints and cervical vertebrae compared with shoulders or dorsal vertebrae (Ohashi *et al.*, 1992; Jadoul *et al.*, 1997*a*). Second, pathology does not allow an adequate quantitation of overall amyloid deposits.

The prevalence of histological systemic (non-osteoarticular) ß2mA remains ill-defined. It develops after >10 years HD. The review of all postmortem reports of systemic ß2mA shows preferential involvement of some organs (Table 6.1)—heart, 80%; gastrointestinal tract, 78%; lungs, 59%; liver, 41%; kidneys, 33%. Spleen involvement is very unusual, 5% (Casey *et al.*, 1986; Fuchs *et al.*, 1987; Noël *et al.*, 1987; Ogawa *et al.*, 1987; Theaker *et al.*, 1987; Maher *et al.*, 1988; Sethi *et al.*, 1989; Campistol *et al.*, 1990; Athanasou *et al.*, 1991; Zhou *et al.*, 1991; Ohashi *et al.*, 1992; Gal *et al.*, 1994; Lutz *et al.*, 1995; Araki *et al.*, 1996).

Attention should be paid to the fact that ß2m amyloid is not unusual in the prostate of patients with normal renal function. This localization is clearly the result of different pathophysiological mechanisms (Cross *et al.*, 1992).

Table 6.1   Organ involvement in patients with visceral ß2mA

	Ratio of positive/tested cases (%)
Heart	24/30 (80)
Gastrointestinal tract	21/27 (78)
Lungs	16/27 (59)
Liver	11/27 (41)
Kidneys	7/21 (33)
Spleen	1/18 (5)

For review of available post-mortem reports, see references in the text.

Skeletal radiographs

Bone cysts have been recognized from 1985 on as a hallmark of ß2mA. The radio-logical pattern in ß2mA is similar to that observed in osteoarticular AL amyloidosis (Maldague *et al.*, 1996). It includes swelling of soft tissues, with a preserved or widened joint space, and cystic defects in the juxta-articular bones. These characteristics are helpful in the differential diagnosis with other arthropathies such as osteoarthritis or synovitis.

The joints preferentially involved are the wrists, shoulders, and hips (van Ypersele *et al.*, 1988). Bone cysts increase in size and number over time (Fig. 6.1), together with displacement of fat pads (reflecting the soft-tissue swelling) (Fig. 6.2). Skeletal radio-graphs may allow a specific diagnosis of bone ß2mA, provided that strict criteria are applied (van Ypersele *et al.*, 1991; Maldague *et al.*, 1996). These include the radiological assessment of each lesion and of their anatomical distribution. Individual lesions should be taken into account, provided that their size exceeds 10 mm (hip, shoulder) or 5 mm (wrist). These defects have to be located outside areas prone to show synovial inclusions, such as the femoral neck, and outside the weight-bearing area of the acet-abulum. A normal joint space adjacent to the bone defect is required in order to exclude osteoarthritic bone cysts (Fig. 6.3). When defects of an adequate size affect a weight-bearing area or usual sites of synovial inclusions, only defects whose diameter increases by >30%/year are considered significant (Fig. 6.4) (van Ypersele *et al.*, 1991; Maldague *et al.*, 1996).

At least two joints should be involved for ß2mA to be diagnosed (van Ypersele *et al.*, 1991). When the two affected joints are the wrists, at least two significant bone defects must be detected in one of them.

These criteria allow, in our experience, a specific diagnosis of ß2mA. Unfortu-nately, their sensitivity is limited.

Ultrasonography

Capsulosynovial ('soft tissue') swelling precedes the development of bone cysts in ß2mA. This is demonstrated by the early displacement of the fat pad, prior to the appearance of typical bone cysts in the shoulder (van Ypersele *et al.*, 1988).

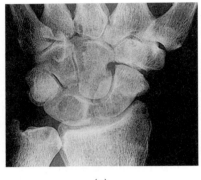

(a)

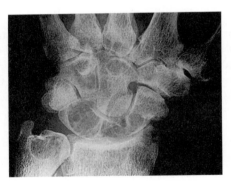

(b)

Fig. 6.1 Evolution of typical ß2mA bone defects of the wrist in a 52-year-old male, over a 5-year period. (a) After 11 years of dialysis, typical bone defects in the navicular, the lunate, the proximal angle of the hamate, and the distal end of the ulna. (b) Five years later (16 years of dialysis), increase in the size of each of the previous bone defects and the development of new defects in the hamate, the capitatum, the distal radius, and the proximal end of metacarpals 3, 4, and 1. (Reproduced from Maldague *et al.*, 1996, with permission.)

Technical developments now permit an accurate assessment of capsules and tendons by joint ultrasonography (US), thus yielding a potentially promising, more sensitive tool for ß2mA diagnosis.

Several cross-sectional studies have reported a thickening of shoulder tendons/hip capsules in HD patients at high risk of, or with histologically documented ß2mA. Using a high-frequency, linear-array transducer in 49 HD patients, Jadoul *et al.* (1993) observed a correlation between supraspinatus shoulder tendon (SST) and femoral neck capsule (FNC) thickness, and HD duration. The number of thickened tendons/capsules per patient also increased with HD duration. The thickness of one (or more) tendon/capsule exceeded the upper limit of normal in two-thirds of HD patients. In another study, shoulder tendons proved thicker in 10 long-term HD patients with proven, symptomatic DRA than in 17 younger HD patients (McMahon *et al.*, 1991). These findings have been repeatedly confirmed (Kay *et al.*, 1992; Cardinal *et al.*, 1995).

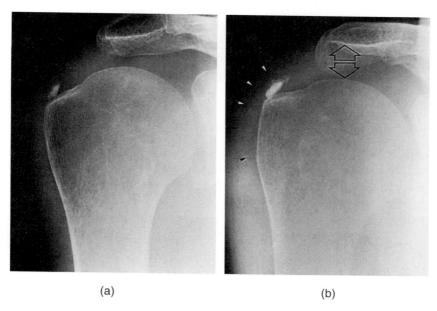

(a)   (b)

Fig. 6.2 Progressive swelling of shoulder soft tissues is reflected by lateral displacement of the subdeltoid fat pad (arrowheads) and a concurrent widening of the subacromial space (vertical empty arrows). Unrelated calcification in the supraspinatus tendon. (Reproduced from Maldague *et al.*, 1996, with permission.)

A longitudinal study of a series of 16 patients followed for an average of 21 ± 4 months suggests that ultrasound (US) may allow the monitoring of ß2mA. In nine patients dialyzed for >60 months at initial US, the SST thickness rose by an average of 1.2 mm within a mean interval of 21 months. By contrast, in seven patients on HD for <60 months at initial US, and thus at lower risk of ß2mA, SST thickness did not change significantly (Jadoul *et al.*, 1993).

The sensitivity and specificity of the ultrasonographic diagnosis of ß2mA is yet to be fully defined. Available data appear promising, with figures ranging from 79 to 100% for sensitivity in two series of symptomatic patients (Kay *et al.*, 1992; Jadoul *et al.*, 1993) and of 100% for specificity in a small series (Kay *et al.*, 1992) of asymptomatic patients with no histological evidence of ß2mA. Larger studies, including a substantial proportion of early (asymptomatic) cases with ß2mA, combining US and histological evaluation are now required.

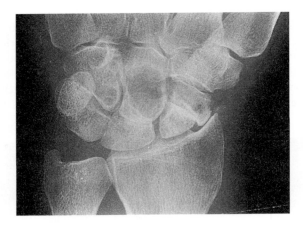

Fig. 6.3 Differential diagnosis of ß2mA-related cystic defects of the wrists. Degenerative subchondral cysts of the capitate, the proximal part of the hamate, and the distal scaphoid with typical focal joint space narrowing of the radionavicular and capitatolunate joint spaces, secondary to a navicular pseudarthrosis with carpal instability. (Reproduced from Maldague *et al.*, 1996, with permission.)

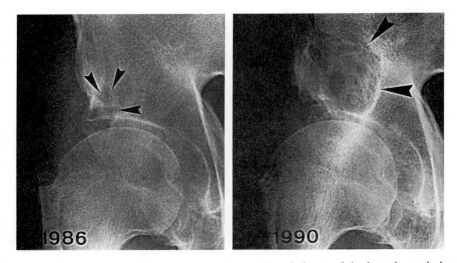

Fig. 6.4 ß2mA-related rapid enlargement of a subchondral cyst of the lateral acetabulum. This patient also developed typical ß2mA lesions in the wrists. (Reproduced from Maldague *et al.*, 1996, with permission.)

Several pitfalls and limitations should be carefully taken into account in the ultrasonographic evaluation of joints. Measurements should be obtained outside irregularities of bone outline, perpendicular to the bone surface. Anechogenic effusions should not be confused with tissue thickening. Transient thickening may further be observed in cases of tendinitis, synovitis. Measurement may be impossible in a little less than 10% of joints as a consequence of major periarticular calcifications, the inability to hold the position, etc. (Jadoul *et al.*, 1993, 1996*b*).

Finally, intra- and interobserver measurement differences average 0.5 ± 0.4 mm and 0.6 ± 0.5 mm, respectively, for the SST, and 0.5 ± 0.6 mm and 1.2 ± 0.8 mm, respectively, for the FNC, so that borderline abnormalities should be interpreted with caution (Jadoul *et al.*, 1993).

Overall, US appears to be a promising, non-invasive method for ß2mA diagnosis and monitoring.

Serum amyloid P component (SAP) and ß2m scintigraphy

SAP scintigraphy

SAP, a non-fibrillar plasma glycoprotein synthesized by the liver, undergoes non-covalent calcium–dependent binding to almost all types of amyloid fibrils. This avidity has been used in scintigraphic studies with $[^{123}\text{I}]$SAP, first in a mouse model of systemic amyloidosis and then in the various types of human amyloidosis (Hawkins *et al.*, 1990).

In a cross-sectional study of 38 long-term HD patients, $[^{123}\text{I}]$SAP accumulated at all sites ($n = 16$) of histologically proven ß2mA and many sites of clinically suspected ß2mA. The scintigraphic pattern correlated with HD duration, with no uptake in six short-term HD patients (Nelson *et al.*, 1991). Wrist uptake was predominant. Surprisingly, however, splenic uptake was observed in 12 of the 38 long-term HD patients, although histological ß2mA is highly uncommon at that site and, when present, is minimal. In contrast, hip uptake was infrequent (3/38) and shoulder uptake was not detected in 7/19 cases with clinical manifestations. Overall, the specificity and sensitivity of the method appear limited: splenic uptake is probably an artefact, whereas the lack of hip or shoulder uptake probably reflects methodological problems. A more recent study of SAP scintigraphy in AL amyloidosis supports a cautious evaluation of the diagnostic potential of SAP scintigraphy (Hachulla *et al.*, 1996).

A further limit of SAP scintigraphy accrues from the fact that SAP binds not just to ß2mA but to all types of amyloid. It does not allow the distinction to be made between ß2mA and other amyloidoses, including that associated with age.

SAP scintigraphy has been advocated in order to quantify the amount of deposited amyloid. There is, as yet, little histological evidence supporting this claim, a not surprising conclusion when the difficulties related to histological quantitation and the variability of the sensitivity of the scintigraphic method are taken into consideration (Jadoul *et al.*, 1997*b*).

ß2m scintigraphy

ß2m labeled with I-131 has also been utilized in scintigraphic studies. Sensitivity for the detection of large amyloid deposits appears excellent in 42 long-term HD patients (Floege *et al.*, 1990). Tracer enrichment was demonstrated in resected amyloid tissue and isolated amyloid fibrils. Specificity is also adequate, since no uptake has been

documented in short-term HD patients or HD patients with inflammatory conditions, so that tracer uptake is not due to non-specific binding of ß2m to HLA-rich
cells.

The overall ß2mA scintigraphic images appear reproducible; the test appears more
sensitive than clinical or radiological evaluation for ß2mA (Floege *et al.*, 1990). The
diagnostic value of ß2mA scintigraphy for small, incipient amyloid deposits remains
to be documented. It should be pointed out that this method cannot be utilized in
patients with a significant renal function, as ß2m is readily excreted by the kidney.

The use of I-131 for ß2m scintigraphy is limited by the substantial radiation exposure. Preliminary results with [111]Indium–DTPA-labeled ß2m have been recently presented. Advantages include lower radiation exposure, easier labeling, better optical
resolution, and stable images. Sensitivity seems better than with I-131 scintigraphy,
with visualization of uptake in smaller joints (Schaeffer *et al.*, 1996). Histological valid-
ation of these observations is now required.

Risk factors for ß2mA

The clinical and histological identification of ß2mA in cohorts of patients on dialysis
has permitted an assessment of the various factors involved in the development of this
complication.

1. *Dialysis modality*: ß2mA has been reported in patients given various types of renal
   replacement therapies including HD, CAPD (Jadoul *et al.*, 1990), and hemofiltration (Renaud *et al.*, 1988). The size of the different cohorts of patients treated solely
   with each modality proved sufficient to assess other factors such as treatment
   duration and age only in patients on hemodialysis. The available indirect clinical
   evidence (prevalence of CTS) suggests that the prevalence of ß2mA is similar in
   CAPD and HD patients (Benz *et al.*, 1988). This is confirmed by the recent observation that the prevalence of amyloid deposits recognized on pathological examination of joints obtained at autopsy is not significantly different in hemodialysis and
   peritoneal dialysis patients (Jadoul *et al.*, 1997*c*).
2. *Duration of dialysis*: this has rapidly emerged as a critical factor in the clinical manifestation of ß2mA. In Charra *et al.*'s large series (1988), the prevalence of CTS
   requiring surgery rises with hemodialysis duration from 10 to 50 and 100% of the
   patients after 9, 14, and 20 years of hemodialysis, respectively. The prevalence of
   radiological signs of ß2mA detected in a multicenter study (van Ypersele *et al.*,
   1991) increases from 10 to 20 and 50% in patients on Cuprophan hemodialysis for
   8, 11, and 15 years, respectively. Similarly, the prevalence of histological evidence of
   joint ß2mA increases from 20 to 30% after 2–3 years HD to > 90% after > 7 years
   HD (Ohashi *et al.*, 1992; Jadoul *et al.*, 1997*a*).
3. *Age at the onset of dialysis*: independently of dialysis duration, age at the onset of dialysis has been identified as a significant risk factor for the development of ß2mA
   detected by radiological, clinical, histological, or scintigraphic criteria (van Ypersele *et al.*, 1991; Schaeffer *et al.*, 1992; Jadoul *et al.*, 1997*a*).
4. *HD membrane*: ß2mA has been reported in a few patients with long-standing renal

failure (Zingraff *et al.*, 1990) prior to renal replacement therapy, thus demonstrating that the HD membrane is not a prerequisite for its development. Still, the fact that the highest prevalence of ß2mA is observed in patients on long-term hemodialysis raises the question of a potential role of HD membrane-type as a risk factor for ß2mA. Several studies relying on different clinical endpoints have thus been performed. Current evidence suggests that, indeed, high-flux biocompatible membranes such as polyacrylonitrile (AN69) significantly delay ß2mA development.

There have been two types of investigation performed: cross-sectional comparisons of two groups of patients with similar duration of HD on two types of membranes and longitudinal studies of two groups treated consistently with different types of HD membranes; the first type assesses only prevalence, whereas the second evaluates the incidence of ß2mA.

Chanard *et al.*, 1986 relied on CTS operation as a marker of ß2mA. In a cross-sectional study they compared 11 patients with CTS and 13 patients without CTS. Dialysis duration was equivalent in both groups, i.e. approximately 10.5 years. The CTS group differed from the non-CTS group by a significantly ($p < 0.001$) longer duration of low-flux, bioincompatible, Cuprophan and a shorter duration of high-flux, biocompatible, AN69 dialysis. In a subsequent longitudinal study of 85 patients on HD for more than 5 years the same group demonstrated that the actuarial risk of CTS operation was higher ($p < 0.012$) in the 54 Cuprophan-treated than in the 31 AN69-treated patients (Chanard *et al.*, 1989). van Ypersele *et al.* (1991) relied on radiological evidence of ß2mA. In a longitudinal multicenter study of 221 patients on HD for ≥ 5 years, the onset of typical amyloid bone cysts as well as CTS surgery was evaluated. The rigorous radiological criteria for ß2mA outlined above were used by a single team of radiologists who reviewed all radiographs obtained during the follow-up of each patient. Actuarial survival curves without CTS were not significantly different between Cuprophan and AN69 patients. In contrast, the actuarial risk of amyloid bone cysts was 5.5 higher in Cuprophan than AN69 patients. Both membrane type ($p < 0.004$) and age at the onset of therapy ($p < 0.007$) were significant, independent risk factors (van Ypersele *et al.*, 1991). These conclusions were confirmed by a Japanese cross-sectional study: the Cuprophan/ AN69 duration ratio was higher in 12 patients with cysts than in 18 patients without, despite a similar overall HD duration (Miura *et al.*, 1992). Küchle *et al.* (1996) recently reported that high-flux polysulfone HD is associated with a much lower risk of DRA development than Cuprophan HD. Patients on Cuprophan HD for an average of 40 months were randomly assigned to further HD either on Cuprophan or on high-flux polysulfone for an additional 72 months. During the latter period, 8/10 Cuprophan patients developed the CTS and bone cysts, versus none among the 10 polysulfone patients. Two cross-sectional studies claimed that AN69 HD did not influence the prevalence of radiological cysts (Brunner *et al.*, 1990; Kessler *et al.*, 1992). However, neither study relied on adequate criteria for amyloid bone cysts. In addition, selection criteria to include patients in a specific membrane group were so inappropriate in one study that some AN69-group patients had been dialyzed for a longer duration on Cuprophan than on AN69 (Brunner *et al.*, 1990). Finally, neither study considered the role of age.

Pathophysiology

A variety of biological events have been identified in the genesis of ß2mA. We will now review them in order to provide a better understanding of the clinical characteristics of the complication.

Role of ß2m retention

Long-term ß2m retention appears to be prerequisite for ß2mA development, although a critical threshold has not been demonstrated. Several factors determine serum ß2m levels in patients treated by dialysis.

1. *ß2m production* unrelated to HD is known to increase markedly in 'immunoinflammatory' states such as AIDS, systemic lupus erythematosus, rheumatoid arthritis, viral hepatitis, and interferon–alpha treatment (van Ypersele and Jadoul, 1996). As yet, however, clinical data have not supported the hypothesis that these conditions enhance ß2mA development.
2. *The influence of residual renal function* on serum ß2m levels has been recently highlighted. ß2m is normally catabolized by the kidney. Even a minimal residual renal function is associated with lower serum ß2m levels (Kabanda *et al.*, 1994). For instance, serum ß2m levels are twice as high in HD patients with a GFR of < 1 ml/min than in those with a GFR of 4–5 ml/min. (McCarthy *et al.*, 1994).
3. *Age of the patient* is another determinant of ß2m levels. Recently, Kabanda *et al.* (1994) identified, in a large cross-sectional study, that age was negatively correlated to serum ß2m levels, independently of residual renal function (Fig. 6.5).
4. *Duration of hemodialysis* has been proposed as a significant determinant of serum ß2m levels in a large cross-sectional analysis (Charra *et al.*, 1988). This conclusion was not confirmed in another study which, unlike the former one, took into account age and renal function in a stepwise, multiple regression analysis (Kabanda *et al.*, 1994).
5. *Metabolic acidosis* has been recently identified as a possible stimulus for ß2m production *In vitro*, a low pH (5.1) lowers ß2m cellular expression of cultured human myeloid cells and increases ß2m release in the supernatant, possibly as the result of ß2m dissociation from the cell surface. *In vivo*, the serum ß2m level is inversely correlated with the serum bicarbonate concentration both in chronic and terminal renal failure. Furthermore, the shift from acetate to bicarbonate dialysate raises blood pH and lowers serum ß2m level (Sonikian *et al.*, 1996). Pending confirmation, these results suggest that metabolic acidosis may enhance ß2m production.
6. *The dialysis modality including membrane type* also influences serum ß2m levels. The available evidence demonstrates that serum ß2m levels are 30% lower in patients treated by CAPD or HD with high-flux biocompatible membranes, such as AN69 or polysulfone, than in patients undergoing low-flux bioincompatible Cuprophan dialysis (Mrowka and Schiffl, 1993; van Ypersele and Jadoul, 1996). This difference reflects the ability of both high-flux and peritoneal membranes to clear ß2m more effectively. Indeed, ß2m removal is nil with Cuprophan, whereas it is

significant with CAPD and high–flux HD membranes, as a result of their increased porosity and sometimes adsorptive capacity.

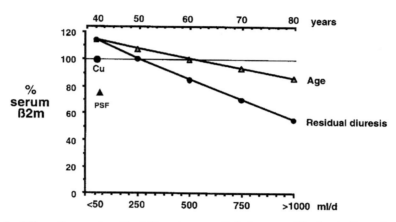

Fig. 6.5 Effect of age and residual diuresis on predialysis serum ß2m levels. Stepwise regression analysis of 112 patients identified age and residual diuresis as significant, independent determinants of serum ß2m. Mean predialysis serum ß2m value of 38.9 mg/l was taken as 100% at 60 years of age and 250 ml/min residual diuresis. For comparison purposes the mean predialysis serum ß2m observed with polysulfone was expressed as a percentage of the mean values with cuprophane. (Reproduced from van Ypersele de Strihou *et al.*, 1996, with permission.)

It is thus more the porosity than the biocompatibility of the membrane that determines serum ß2m levels (van Ypersele *et al.*, 1994).

However, some studies have suggested that the bioincompatibility of HD membranes stimulates ß2m synthesis and/or release. Available *in-vitro* data remain conflicting. The increased release demonstrated in some studies (Zaoui *et al.*, 1990) is of marginal significance when compared with daily ß2m synthesis. *In-vivo* studies of ß2m turnover have failed to detect a significant effect of membrane type (van Ypersele *et al.*, 1994). This latter conclusion should, however, be viewed with caution as the number of studies, as well as that of investigated patients, is small, interindividual variations in the data substantial, and the number of assumptions underlying the mathematical models, multiple and often unsubstantiated. Should some membrane types enhance ß2m production, the relevance of this phenomenon would seem limited when compared with the substantial clearance of ß2m by some HD membranes (van Ypersele *et al.*, 1994).

Whatever the ability of dialysis membranes to remove ß2m, it always fails to meet daily ß2m production whether normal (3 mg/kg per day) or enhanced (4.35 mg/kg per day). Indeed, as hemodialysis is intensified, the serum ß2m level decreases, which in turn reduces ß2m mass removal by HD. Even daily hemofiltration with AN69 removes less than 1000 mg/week (Canaud *et al.*, 1992). It may thus be calculated that a patient dialyzed with Cuprophan will accumulate 400 g ß2m within 4 years (increased ß2m production) or 8 years (normal ß2m production). Under the same condition, a patient dialyzed with AN69, a membrane with a high clearing capacity for ß2m, would retain 400 g after 8 and 14 years, respectively, according to ß2m production (van Ypersele *et al.*, 1994). These calculations assume the absence of an extrarenal clearance of ß2m. Although kinetic studies have suggested the existence, in normal subjects, of a very small non-renal catabolism, this pathway is yet to be identified. Whether or not such a pathway exists, these calculations underline the fact that patients on dialysis continuously accumulate ß2m, thus contributing to the progression of ß2mA over time.

Role of ß2m modification

After the demonstration (Gejyo *et al.*, 1985; Gorevic *et al.*, 1986) that DRA deposits contain ß2m fibrils, the factors responsible for ß2m fibril formation have been actively sought. Connors *et al.* (1985) have provided evidence that under stringent conditions ß2m amyloid fibrils could be formed *in vitro* from intact ß2m. These experiments have, up to now, not been reproduced. Investigators have thus considered the possibility that ß2m had to be modified in order to precipitate as fibrils.

Linke *et al.* (1989) have isolated from ß2mA deposits, not only native ß2m but also truncated peptides with a shortened amino-terminal sequence. The non-random site of cleavage suggests *in-vivo* proteolysis rather than purification artifacts. They propose that the proteolytic transformation of a hydrophilic precursor molecule into a more hydrophobic amyloidogenic peptide is a prerequisite for ß2mA just, as for other types of amyloid.

Several reports have identified an isoform of ß2m with a more acidic pI (acidic ß2m) in the serum, ultrafiltrate, and deposits of HD patients (Ogawa *et al.*, 1988; Odani *et al.*, 1990). Deamidation at amino-acid position 17 has been suggested as the main factor contributing to a more acidic pI and a lower molecular weight. Its relevance is, however, questioned as modified ß2m is not specific for long-term HD patients or amyloid deposits (Argilés *et al.*, 1995). More recently, Miyata *et al.* (1993) have demonstrated that a fraction of 'acidic' ß2m is due to progressive glycation of the molecule. A significant fraction (10%) of acidic ß2m consists of Amadori products and a smaller one (1%) of advanced glycation end products (AGEs) (Miyata *et al.*, 1996*a*). Both Amadori products and AGEs are formed by non-enzymatic, glycoxidation linking proteins with sugar-derived aldehydes. Interestingly, AGE modification is an irreversible process which damages the protein. More recently, some molecular structures of ß2m AGEs have been identified (carboxymethyllysine, pentosidine, deoxyglucosone, and imidazolone) and their circulating levels measured (Miyata *et al.*, 1996*b*, Niwa *et al.*, 1997). Whether AGE modification enhances amyloid fibril precipitation remains to be demonstrated. Of note, pentosidine crosslinks proteins, a characteristic possibly relevant in the formation of fibrils.

More interesting, however, is the demonstration that AGE-modified ß2m is endowed with a chemotactic power, attracts monocytes, and stimulates the derived macrophages to release proinflammatory cytokines (Miyata *et al.*, 1994). Since amyloid deposits are initially asymptomatic and devoid of monocytes, it is possible that progressive glycoxidation of deposited amyloid eventually attracts macrophages, resulting in a local inflammatory reaction expressed clinically by arthralgias and the carpal tunnel syndrome.

Hopefully, further studies will unravel the role of ß2m glycoxidation both in the initial formation of amyloid fibrils and subsequently in the inflammatory, clinically relevant, stage. The role of dialysis membranes in the clearing of AGEs should be delineated and might also contribute to the development of an adequate prevention of ß2mA.

ß2mA, an inflammatory disorder?

Early observations have pointed to an inflammatory component in ß2mA. Sethi *et al.* (1988*a*) reported that the serum level of the C-reactive protein, an acute-phase react-ant, is higher in HD patients with than in those without DRA. The rapid relief of DRA complaints after renal transplantation (see below) has also been ascribed to the anti-inflammatory properties of steroids. Taken together with some clinical charac-teristics of arthralgias (e.g. nocturnal exacerbation), these observations suggest two stages in ß2mA. The first is asymptomatic and diagnosed mainly by pathology. The second is symptomatic, accompanied by an inflammatory reaction. Within this con-text, it is noteworthy that macrophages accumulate around ß2mA deposits in the late, symptomatic phase of the disease (Argilés *et al.*, 1994). As discussed above this might result from the potent chemotactic ability for monocytes of AGE-ß2m. AGE-ß2m is further able to stimulate macrophages to secrete TNF-alpha, IL-1ß, and IL-6 in a dose-dependent manner. This property appears highly specific of AGE-ß2m as neither truncated ß2m nor deamidated, nor early Amadori ß2m share this capacity (Miyata *et al.*, 1996*a*). Finally, cytokine release might contribute to progressive bone loss and bone cysts (Miyata *et al.*, 1996*c*).

Why this affinity of ß2mA for osteoarticular structures?

Initially, the peculiar affinity of ß2mA for osteoarticular tissues was attributed to hyperparathyroidism, aluminum, or iron overload. More than 10 years later, none of these factors remains incriminated in the pathogenesis of ß2mA (van Ypersele and Jadoul, 1996). The preferential accumulation of ß2m in osteoarticular structures appears to be linked with the biochemical composition of such tissues. Homma *et al.* (1989) have demonstrated a preferential collagen-binding affinity of ß2m, dependent on both ß2m concentrations and the amount of collagen in the *in-vitro* preparations. Interestingly, Hou *et al.* (1997) have recently demonstrated *in vitro* that AGE-modified collagen has an enhanced ß2m binding capacity. Thus advanced glycation might con-tribute to ß2mA not only through alterations of ß2m but also through modification of joint collagen.

More recently, some extracellular matrix components such as glycosaminoglycans have been reported to be closely associated with fibrils in several types of amyloidosis. Athanasou *et al.* (1995*a*, *b*) observe, with various histochemical and immunohisto-chemical methods, a close association between the localization of highly sulfated glycosaminoglycans (especially keratan sulfate) and both senile and ß2m amyloid deposits, in cartilage, synovium, and heart.

The fact that glycosaminoglycans expression on articular cartilages changes with the onset of arthritic changes and age might contribute to the influence of the patients' age on the development of ß2mA.

Prevention and treatment of ß2mA

Prevention of ß2mA

The best therapy of ß2mA is undoubtedly a successful renal transplantation (TP). Unfortunately, most patients at high risk of ß2mA (e.g. older patients) are often less likely to benefit from renal TP. The prevention of ß2mA in such cases will have to rely on dialytic strategies.

Role of the dialysis modality

ß2mA has been reported in patients whatever their 'dialysis' modality, including CAPD, hemofiltration, and HD. No large-scale comparison of the incidence and pre-valence of ß2mA with each of these modalities is as yet available. The technical sur-vival on CAPD remains rather short and the cost of hemofiltration high, so that long-term survivals are presently observed mainly in patients on hemodialysis.

Role of HD membrane type

As discussed earlier, the use of high-flux membranes such as AN69 delays the devel-opment of ß2mA. Thus, their use is recommended in patients who are unlikely to be suitable candidates for renal TP (e.g. older patients, especially as age increases the risk of ß2mA) and in those likely to wait for many years on HD for a successful graft (e.g. hyperimmunized patients or patients who have no or little access to TP). As the 'membrane effect' appears mainly linked to the ability to clear ß2m, this characteristic should be considered in membrane prescription. ß2m removal is achieved both by convection (highest for polysulfone and AN69) and adsorption (highest for AN69 and polymethylmethacrylate): both parameters have to be included in the evaluation (van Ypersele *et al.*, 1994).

Palliative treatment

Medical treatment

Chronic arthralgias are best treated by paracetamol/dextropropoxyphene (as non-steroidal anti-inflammatory drugs entail a substantial risk of gastrointestinal tract complication in such fragile patients). Although intra-articular steroids are helpful especially when a single joint is very painful, their transient effectiveness and the risk of infectious complications limit their long-term usefulness. If first-line therapies fail, low-dose oral prednisone (0.1 mg/kg) may prove effective. In a recent, prospective open trial in 27 HD patients with severe, symptomatic ß2mA, a dramatic reduction in the number of painful joints was observed shortly after starting prednisone, with a recurrence of pain within 24 hours of interruption (Bardin, 1994). However, as seven patients died, apparently from prednisone-unrelated causes, within a mean follow-up of 10 months, additional data are needed to define better (e.g. by a randomized study) the safety of this regimen.

Surgical treatment

Early surgery is recommended after CTS diagnosis in HD patients as the relentless course of β2mA may otherwise lead to serious, irreversible neuromuscular impairment. CTS surgery may be performed either classically or endoscopically (Okutsu *et al.*, 1993), although the experience with the latter procedure in HD patients remains limited. Recurrences have been reported (Brown *et al.*, 1986), but should be rare if the surgeon is experienced and meticulously removes the tissue compressing the nerve.

Pathological femoral fractures or spinal cord compression are obvious indications for joint prosthesis or vertebral fusion, respectively (Campistol *et al.*, 1990; Goutallier *et al.*, 1994).

Severe shoulder arthralgias may benefit from various endoscopic or surgical procedures. Okutsu *et al.* (1991) have performed endoscopic resection of the coracoacromial ligament in 48 shoulders of 29 long-term HD patients with intolerable shoulder pain. Shoulder pain is relieved in all patients and the improvement persists during follow-up (10–25 months, average 17.5 months). Takenaka *et al.* (1992) have performed arthroscopic synovectomy in eight patients with shoulder pain: transient relief (≤ 12 months) is observed in most patients. Open surgery, performed by the same group in five patients with humeral cysts, including curettage of cysts and ceramic implantation together with resection of hypertrophied synovium and masses, has led to pain relief throughout follow-up (12 months). More information on the long-term follow-up of such interventions is needed.

Dialytic treatment

Small, uncontrolled, and, up to now, unconfirmed studies have reported a subjective improvement of arthralgias in a few patients switched from Cuprophan HD to high-flux HD or CAPD (Laurent *et al.*, 1985; Hardouin *et al.*, 1988). Similarly, Nakazawa *et al.* (1993) have used a selective β2m adsorbent for hemoperfusion connected in series with an AN69 dialyzer in an effort to reduce the serum β2m level. Serum β2m level is lowered by 20% during the use of the device. Articular symptoms improved in two out of three treated patients but recurred after interruption of the treatment. Here again, controlled studies are required. Whatever their result, the cost of the device is likely to preclude its widespread use.

Renal transplantation

Renal transplantation should be urgently considered in all patients with β2mA who are suitable candidates.

A striking, almost immediate improvement of β2mA joint symptoms and signs has been observed by all teams soon after a successful TP (Sethi *et al.*, 1988*b*; Jadoul *et al.*, 1989; Mourad and Argilés, 1996; Tan *et al.*, 1996). Although this beneficial short-term effect has been ascribed to the high doses of steroids used, it lasts in the long-term despite the reduction and, sometimes, the interruption of steroid treatment. In addition, the progression of ß2mA deposits is stopped as demonstrated by the lack of progression of typical amyloid bone cysts after a successful TP (Jadoul *et al.*, 1989; Bardin *et al.*, 1995; Mourad and Argilés, 1996; Tan *et al.*, 1996).

Much more controversial is the issue of the potential regression of ß2mA deposits after a successful TP. On the one hand, radiological bone cysts do not regress after a successful TP (Jadoul *et al.*, 1989; Mourad and Argilés, 1996), a fact attributed to the actual persistence of the ß2mA deposits demonstrated in one case (Jadoul *et al.*, 1996), or alternatively, to a very slow turnover of bone amyloid deposits. Actual ß2mA deposits persist for up to 10 years after a successful TP (Bardin *et al.*, 1995; Jadoul *et al.*, 1996). In the absence of sequential quantitative biopsies, however, the possibility of partial regression of ß2mA cannot be formally excluded. The unusually rapid recurrence of ß2mA signs after the resumption of HD for graft failure confirms that regression is very limited at best (Mourad and Argilés, 1996).

On the other hand, Tan *et al.* (1996) have recently claimed that labeled SAP uptake fell 3–5 years after successful transplantation, whereas it increased in similar patients still maintained on HD for the same duration. These data are taken as evidence of significant ß2mA regression. Such a conclusion hinges both on the specificity of the method and on its ability to quantitate amyloid deposits. As mentioned earlier, neither of these assumptions is satisfactorily validated (Jadoul *et al.*, 1997*b*). Overall, both the clinicoradiological and the scintigraphic approach provide interesting information, apparently contradictory at this stage. Their reconciliation will probably require an alternative approach to solve the problem of ß2mA regression.

Conclusions

ß2mA is a major complication of long-term HD. The understanding of its pathogenesis has progressed substantially since the identification of the disease. These advances will hopefully lead to clinical proposals to prevent and manage this disease more effectively.

References

Allain, T. J., Stevens, P. E., Bridges, L. R., and Phillips, M. E. (1988). Dialysis myelopathy: quadriparesis due to extradural amyloid of ß2 microglobulin origin. *British Medical Journal*, **296**, 752–3.

Araki, H., Muramoto, H., Oda, K., Koni, I., Mabuchi, H., and Mizukami, Y. (1996). Severe gastrointestinal complications of dialysis-related amyloidosis in two patients on long-term hemodialysis. *American Journal of Nephrology*, **16**, 149–53.

Argilés, À., Mourad, G., Kerr, P. G., García, M., Collins, B., and Demaille, J. G. (1994). Cells surrounding haemodialysis-associated amyloid deposits are mainly macrophages. *Nephrology, Dialysis, Transplantation*, **9**, 662–7.

Argilés, À., García-García, M., Derancourt, J., Mourad, G., and Demaille, J. G. (1995). Beta 2 microglobulin isoforms in healthy individuals and in amyloid deposits. *Kidney International*, **48**, 1397–405.

Assenat, H., Calemard, E., Charra, B., Laurent, G., Terrat, J. C., and Vanel, T. (1980). Hémo-dialyse. Syndrome du canal carpien et substance amyloïde. *La Nouvelle Presse Médicale*, **24**, 1715.

Athanasou, N. A., Ayers, S., Rainey, A. J., Oliver, D. O., and Duthie, R. B. (1991). Joint and systemic distribution of dialysis amyloid. *Quarterly Journal of Medicine*, **78**, 205–14.

Athanasou, N. A., Puddle, B., and Sallie, B. (1995a). Highly sulphated glycosaminoglycans in articular cartilage and other tissues containing ß2 microglobulin dialysis amyloid deposits. *Nephrology, Dialysis, Transplantation*, **10**, 1672–8.

Athanasou, N. A., West, L., Sallie, B., and Puddle, B. (1995b). Localized amyloid deposition in cartilage is glycosaminoglycans-associated. *Histopathology*, **26**, 267–72.

Bardin, T. (1994). Low-dose prednisone in dialysis-related amyloid arthropathy. *Revue du Rhumatisme (English edition)*, **61** (Suppl. 9), 97S–100S.

Bardin, T. (1996). Arthropathy and carpal tunnel syndrome of ß2-microglobulin amyloidosis. In *Dialysis amyloid* (ed. C. van Ypersele and T. B. Drüeke), pp. 71–97. Oxford University Press.

Bardin, T., Kuntz, D., Zingraff, J., Voisin, M.-C., Zelmar, A., and Lansaman, J. (1985). Synovial amyloidosis in patients undergoing long-term hemodialysis. *Arthritis and Rheumatism*, **28**, 1052–8.

Bardin, T., Lebail-Darné, J. L., Zingraff, J., *et al.* (1995). Dialysis arthropathy: outcome after renal transplantation. *American Journal of Medicine*, **99**, 243–8.

Benz, R. L., Siegfried, J. W., and Teehan, B. P. (1988). Carpal tunnel syndrome in dialysis patients: comparison between continuous ambulatory peritoneal dialysis and hemo-dialysis populations. *American Journal of Kidney Diseases*, **9**, 473–6.

Bindi, P., and Chanard, J. (1990). Destructive spondyloarthropathy in dialysis patients: an overview. *Nephron*, **55**, 104–9.

Borgatti, P. P., Lusenti, T., Franco, V., Anelli, A., and Brancaccio, D. (1991). Guyon's syndrome in a long-term haemodialysis patient. *Nephrology, Dialysis, Transplantation*, **6**, 734–5.

Brancaccio, D., Gallieni, M., Padovese, P., Anelli, A., Coggi, G., and Uslenghi, C. (1988). Dialysis amyloidosis with massive popliteal deposition of ß2-microglobulin amyloid. *Lancet*, **i**, 802.

Brown, E. A., Arnold, I. R., and Gower, P. E. (1986). Dialysis arthropathy: complication of long-term treatment with haemodialysis. *British Medical Journal*, **292**, 163–6.

Brunner, F. P., Brynger, H., Ehrich, J. J. H., *et al.* (1990). Case control study on dialysis arthropathy: the influence of two different dialysis membranes: data from the EDTA Registry. *Nephrology, Dialysis, Transplantation*, **5**, 432–6.

Campistol, J. M., Solé, M., Muñoz-Gómez, J., Riba, J., Ramón, R., and Revert, L. (1990). Pathological fractures in patients who have amyloidosis associated with dialysis. *Journal of Bone and Joint Surgery*, **72-A**, 568–74.

Canaud, B., Assounga, A., Kerr, P., Aznar, R., and Mion, C. (1992). Failure of a daily haemofiltration programme using a highly permeable membrane to return ß2-microglobulin concentrations to normal in haemodialysis patients. *Nephrology, Dialysis, Transplantation*, **7**, 924–30.

Cardinal, E., Buckwalter, K. A., Braunstein, E. M., Raymond-Tremblay, D., and Benson, M. D. (1995). Amyloidosis of the shoulder in patients on chronic hemodialysis: sonographic findings. *American Journal of Roentgenology*, **166**, 153–6.

Cary, N. R. B., Sethi, D., Brown, E. A., Erhardt, C. C., Woodrow, D. F., and Gower, P. E. (1986). Dialysis arthropathy: amyloid or iron? *British Medical Journal*, **293**, 1392–4.

Casey, T. T., Stone, W. J., DiRaimondo, C. R., *et al.* (1986). Tumoral amyloidosis of bone of beta-2-microglobulin origin in association with long-term hemodialysis. *Human Pathology*, **17**, 731–8.

Chanard, J., Lavaud, S., Toupance, O., Roujouleh, H., and Melin, J. P. (1986). Carpal tunnel syndrome and type of dialysis membrane used in patients undergoing long-term hemodialysis. *Arthritis and Rheumatism*, **118**, 153–65.

Chanard, J., Bindi, P., Lavaud, S., Toupance, O., Maheut, H., and Lacour, F. (1989). Carpal tunnel syndrome and type of dialysis membrane. *British Medical Journal*, **298**, 867–8.

Charra, B., Calemard, E., and Laurent, G. (1988). Chronic renal failure treatment duration and mode: their relevance to the late dialysis periarticular syndrome. *Blood Purification*, **6**, 117–24.

Choi, H.-S. H., Heller, D., Picken, M. M., Sidhu, G. S., and Kahn, T. (1989). Infarction of intestine with massive amyloid deposition in two patients on long-term hemodialysis. *Gastroenterology*, **96**, 230–4.

Connors, L. H., Shirahama, T., Skinner, M., Fenves, A., and Cohen, A. S. (1985). In vitro formation of amyloid fibrils form intact ß2-microglobulin. *Biochemical and Biophysical Research Communications*, **131**, 1063–8.

Cross, P. A., Bartley, C. J., and McClure, J. (1992). Amyloid in prostatic corpora amylacea. *Journal of Clinical Pathology*, **45**, 894–7.

Deforges-Lasseur, C., Combe, C., Cernier, A., Vital, J. M., and Aparicio, M. (1993). Destructive spondyloarthropathy presenting with progressive paraplegia in a dialysis patient. Recovery after surgical spinal cord decompression and parathyroidectomy. *Nephrology, Dialysis, Transplantation*, **8**, 180–4.

Fernández, E., Baró, P., Montoliu, J., Campistol, J. M., and Solé, M. (1990). Dialysis-associated amyloidosis presenting as a tumour in the elbow. *Nephrology, Dialysis, Transplantation*, **5**, 237–8.

Floege, J., Brandis, A., Nonnast-Daniel, B., *et al.* (1989). Subcutaneous amyloid-tumor of beta-2-microglobulin origin in a long-term hemodialysis patient. *Nephron*, **53**, 73–5.

Floege, J., Durchert, W., Brandis, A., *et al.* (1990). Imaging of dialysis-related amyloid (AB-amyloid) deposits with [131]I-ß2-microglobulin. *Kidney International*, **38**, 1169–76.

Fuchs, A., Jagirdar, J., and Schwartz, I. S. (1987). Beta-2-microglobulin amyloidosis (Aß2M) in patients undergoing long-term hemodialysis. *American Journal of Clinical Pathology*, **88**, 302–7.

Gal, R., Korzets, A., Schwartz, A., Rath-Wolfson, L., and Gafter, U. (1994). Systemic distribution of ß2-microglobulin-derived amyloidosis in patients who undergo long-term hemodialysis. *Archives of Pathology and Laboratory Medicine*, **118**, 718–21.

Gejyo, F., Yamada, T., Odani, S., *et al.* (1985). A new form of amyloid protein associated with chronic hemodialysis was identified as ß2-microglobulin. *Biochemical and Biophysical Research Communications*, **129**, 701–6.

Gorevic, P. D., Munoz, P. C., Casey, T. T., *et al.* (1986). Polymerization of intact ß2-microglobulin in tissue causes amyloidosis in patients on chronic hemodialysis. *Proceedings of the National Academy of Sciences*, **83**, 7908–12.

Goutallier, D., Piat, Ch., Kuntz, D., *et al.* (1994). Surgical treatment of destructive spondylarthropathy in haemodialysis patients. A review of ten interbody fusion procedures in eight hemodialysis patients. *Revue du Rhumatisme* (English Edition), **61** (Suppl. 9), 101S–4S.

Guccion, J. G., Redman, R. S., and Winne, C. E. (1989). Hemodialysis-associated amyloidosis presenting as lingual nodules. *Oral Surgery, Oral Medicine, Oral Pathology*, **68**, 619–23.

Hachulla, E., Maulin, L., Deveaux, M., *et al.* (1996). Prospective and serial study of primary amyloidosis with serum amyloid P component scintigraphy: from diagnosis to prognosis. *American Journal of Medicine*, **101**, 77–87.

Hardouin, P., Flipo, R. M., Lecomte-Houcke, M., Foissac-Gegoux, P., and Delcambre, B. (1987). Amylose des hémodialysés. Recherche d'une diffusion générale par biopsie rectale. (Letter) *La Presse Médicale*, **16**, 445–6.

Hardouin, P., Flipo, R. M., Foissac-Gegoux, P., Dumont, A., Duquesnoy, B., and Delcambre, B. (1988). Dialysis-related ß2 microglobulin—amyloid arthropathy. Improvement of clinical symptoms after a switch of dialysis membranes. *Clinical Rheumatology*, 7, 41–5.

Hawkins, P. H., Lavender, J. P., and Pepys, M. B. (1990). Evaluation of systemic amyloidosis by scintigraphy with ^{123}I-labeled serum amyloid P component. *New England Journal of Medicine*, 323, 508–13.

Homma, N., Gejyo, F., Isemura, and Arakawa, M. (1989). Collagen-binding affinity of beta-2-microglobulin, a preprotein of hemodialysis-associated amyloidosis. *Nephron*, 53, 37–40.

Hou, F. F., Chertow, G. M., Kay, J., *et al.* (1997). Interaction between ß2-microglobulin and advanced glycation end products in the development of dialysis related-amyloidosis. *Kidney International*, 51, 1514–19.

Huaux, J. P., Noël, H., Malghem, J., Maldague, B., Devogelaer, J. P., and Nagant de Deuxchaisnes, C. (1985). Erosive azotemic osteoarthropathy: possible role of amyloidosis. *Arthritis and Rheumatism*, 28, 1075–6.

Ikegaya, N., Kobayashi, S., Hishida, A., Kaneko, E., Furuhashi, M., and Maruyama, Y. (1995). Colonic dilatation due to dialysis-related amyloidosis. *American Journal of Kidney Diseases*, 25, 807–9.

Jadoul, M., Malghem, J., Pirson, Y., Maldague, B., and van Ypersele de Strihou, C. (1989). Effect of renal transplantation on the radiological signs of dialysis amyloid osteoarthropathy. *Clinical Nephrology*, 32, 194–7.

Jadoul, M., Noël, H., and van Ypersele de Strihou, C. (1990). ß2-m amyloidosis in a patient treated exclusively by CAPD. *American Journal of Kidney Diseases*, 15, 86–88.

Jadoul, M., Malghem, J., Vande Berg, B., and van Ypersele de Strihou, C. (1993). Ultrasonographic detection of thickened joint capsules and tendons as marker of dialysis-related amyloidosis: a cross-sectional and longitudinal study. *Nephrology, Dialysis, Transplantation*, 8, 1104–9.

Jadoul, M., Noël, H., Malghem, J., Galant, C., and van Ypersele de Strihou, C. (1996a). Histological beta-2-microglobulin amyloidosis 10 years after a successful renal transplantation. *American Journal of Kidney Diseases*, 27, 888–90.

Jadoul, M., Vande Berg, B., and Malghem, J. (1996b). Ultrasonography of the joints. In *Dialysis amyloid* (ed. C. van Ypersele and T. B. Drüeke), pp. 136–44, Oxford University Press.

Jadoul, M., Garbar, C., Noël, H., *et al.* (1997a). Histological prevalence of ß2-microglobulin amyloidosis in hemodialysis: a prospective post-mortem study. *Kidney International*, 51, 1928–32.

Jadoul, M., Drüeke, T., Zingraff, J., and van Ypersele de Strihou, C. (1997b). Does dialysis-related amyloidosis regress after transplantation? *Nephrology, Dialysis, Transplantation*, 12, 655–7.

Jadoul, M., Garbar, C., Vanholder, R., *et al.* (1997c). High prevalence of histological ß2 microglobulin amyloidosis in CAPD patients. *Nephrology, Dialysis, Transplantation*, 12, A175.

Kabanda, A., Jadoul, M., Pochet, J. M., Lauwerys, R., van Ypersele de Strihou, C., and Bernard, A. (1994). Determinants of the serum concentrations of low molecular weight proteins in patients on maintenance hemodialysis. *Kidney International*, 45, 1689–96.

Kay, J., Benson, C. B., Lester, S., *et al.* (1992). Utility of high-resolution ultrasound for the diagnosis of dialysis-related amyloidosis. *Arthritis and Rheumatism*, 35, 926–32.

Kessler, M., Netter, P., Azoulay, E., Mayeux, D., and Péré, P. (1992). Dialysis-associated arthropathy: a multicentre survey of 171 patients receiving haemodialysis for over 10 years. *British Journal of Rheumatology*, 31, 157–62.

Koch, K. M. (1992). Dialysis-related amyloidosis. *Kidney International*, 41, 1416–29.

Kröner, G., Stäbler, A., Seiderer, M., Moran, J. E., and Gurland, H. J. (1991). ß2 microglobulin-related amyloidosis causing atlantoaxial spondylarthropathy with spinal-cord compression in haemodialysis patients: detection by MRI. *Nephrology, Dialysis, Transplantation*, S2, 91–5.

Küchle, D., Fricke, H., Held, E., and Schiffl, H. (1996). High-flux hemodialysis postpones clinical manifestation of dialysis-related amyloidosis. *American Journal of Nephrology*, 16, 484–8.

Kuntz, D., Naveau, B., Bardin, T., Drüeke, T., Treves, R., and Dryll, A. (1984). Destructive spondyloarthropathy in hemodialysed patients. A new syndrome. *Arthritis and Rheumatism*, 27, 369–75.

Laurent, G., Charra, B., Calemard, E., Uzan, M., Vanel, T., and Terrat, J. C. (1985). Amélioration par la dialyse péritonéale continue ambulatoire des douleurs abarticulaires accompagnant le syndrome du canal carpien des hémodialysés. *La Presse Médicale*, 14, 2105–6.

Linke, R. P., Hampl, H., Lobeck, H., *et al.* (1989). Lysine-specific cleavage of ß2-microglobulin in amyloid deposits associated with hemodialysis. *Kidney International*, 36, 675–81.

Lutz, A. E., Schneider, U., Ehlerding, G., Frenzel, H., Koch, K. M., and Kühn, K. (1995). Right ventricular cardiac failure and pulmonary hypertension in a long-term dialysis patient—unusual presentation of visceral ß2-microglobulin amyloidosis. *Nephrology, Dialysis, Transplantation*, 3, 269–71.

McCarthy, J. T., Williams, A. W., and Johnson, W. J. (1994). Serum ß2-microglobulin concentration in dialysis patients: importance of intrinsic renal function. *Journal of Laboratory and Clinical Medicine*, 123, 495–505.

McMahon, L. P., Radford, J., and Dawborn, J. K. (1991). Shoulder ultrasound in dialysis related amyloidosis. *Clinical Nephrology*, 35, 227–32.

Maher, E. R., Hamilton Dutoit, S., Baillod, R. A., Sweny, P., and Moorhead, J. F. (1988). Gastrointestinal complications of dialysis related amyloidosis. *British Medical Journal*, 297, 265–6.

Maldague, B., Malghem, J., and Vande Berg, B. (1996). Radiology of dialysis amyloidosis. In *Dialysis amyloid* (ed. C. van Ypersele and T. B. Drüeke), pp. 98–135, Oxford University Press.

Maruyama, H., Gejyo, F., and Arakawa, M. (1992). Clinical studies of destructive spondyloarthropathy in long-term hemodialysis patients. *Nephron*, 61, 37–44.

Miura, Y., Ishiyama, T., Inomata, A., *et al.* (1992). Radiolucent bone cysts and the type of dialysis membrane used in patients undergoing long-term hemodialysis. *Nephron*, 60, 268–73.

Miyata, T., Oda, O., Inagi, R., *et al.* (1993). ß-2 microglobulin modified with advanced glycation end products is a major component of hemodialysis-associated amyloidosis. *Journal of Clinical Investigation*, 92, 1243–51.

Miyata, T., Inagi, R., Iida, Y., *et al.* (1994). Involvement of ß2-microglobulin modified with advanced glycation end products in the pathogenesis of hemodialysis-associated amyloidosis. *Journal of Clinical Investigation*, 93, 521–8.

Miyata, T., Iida, Y., Ueda, Y., *et al.* (1996a). Monocyte/macrophage response to ß2-microglobulin modified with advanced glycation end products. *Kidney International*, 49, 538–50.

Miyata, T., Yasuhiko, U., Iida, Y., *et al.* (1996b). Accumulation of albumin-linked and free-form pentosidine in the circulation of uremic patients with end-stage renal failure: renal implications in the pathophysiology of pentosidine. *Journal of the American Society of Nephrology*, 7, 1198–206.

Miyata, T., Notoya, K., Yoshida, K., *et al.* (1996c). Advanced glycation end products enhance osteoclast-induced bone resorption in cultured mouse unfractionated bone cells and in rats implanted subcutaneously with devitalized bone particles. *Journal of the American Society of Nephrology*, 7, 260–70.

Mourad, G., and Argilés, A. (1996). Renal transplantation relieves the symptoms but does not reverse ß2-microglobulin amyloidosis. *Journal of the American Society of Nephrology*, 7, 798–804.

Mrowka, C., and Schiffl, H. (1993). Comparative evaluation of ß2-microglobulin removal by different hemodialysis membranes: a six-year follow-up. *Nephron*, 63, 368–9.

Muñoz-Gómez, J., Gómez-Pérez, R., Solé-Arques, M., and Llopart-Buisán, E. (1987). Synovial fluid examination for the diagnosis of synovial amyloidosis in patients with chronic renal failure undergoing haemodialysis. *Annals of the Rheumatic Diseases*, **46**, 324–6.

Nakazawa, R., Azuma, N., Suzuki, M., *et al.* (1993). A new treatment for dialysis-related amyloidosis with ß2-microglobulin adsorbent column. *International Journal of Artificial Organs*, **16**, 823–9.

Nelson, S. R., Hawkins, P. N., Richardson, S., *et al.* (1991). Imaging of haemodialysis-associated amyloidosis with ^{123}I-serum amyloid P component. *Lancet*, **338**, 335–8.

Niwa, T., Katsuzaki, T., Miyazaki, S., *et al.* (1997). Amyloid ß2-microglobulin is modified with imidazolone, a novel advanced glycation end product, in dialysis-related amyloidosis. *Kidney International*, **51**, 187–94.

Noël, L. H., Zingraff, J., Bardin, T., Atienza, C., Kuntz, D., and Drüeke, T. (1987). Tissue distribution of dialysis amyloidosis. *Clinical Nephrology*, **27**, 175–8.

Odani, H., Oyama, R., Titani, K., Ogawa, H., and Saito, A. (1990). Purification and complete amino acid sequence of novel beta-2-microglobulin. *Biochemical and Biophysical Research Communications*, **168**, 1223–6.

Ogawa, H., Saito, A., Hirabayashi, N., and Hara, K. (1987). Amyloid deposition in systemic organs in long-term hemodialysis patients. *Clinical Nephrology*, **28**, 199–204.

Ogawa, H., Saito, A., Oda, O., Nakajima, M., and Chung, T. G. (1988). Detection of novel ß2-microglobulin in the serum of hemodialysis patients and its amyloidogenic predisposition. *Clinical Nephrology*, **32**, 158–63.

Ohashi, K., Hara, M., Kawai, R., *et al.* (1992). Cervical discs are most susceptible to beta-2-microglobulin amyloid deposition in the vertebral column. *Kidney International*, **41**, 1646–52.

Okutsu, I., Ninomiya S., Takatori, Y., *et al.* (1991). Endoscopic management of shoulder pain in long-term haemodialysis patients. *Nephrology, Dialysis, Transplantation*, **6**, 117–19.

Okutsu, I., Hamanaka, I., Ninomiya, S., Takatori, Y., Shimizu, K., and Ugawa, Y. (1993). Results of endoscopic management of carpal-tunnel syndrome in long-term haemodialysis versus idiopathic patients. *Nephrology, Dialysis, Transplantation*, **8**, 1110–14.

Reese, W., Hopkovitz, A., and Lifschitz, M. D. (1988). ß2 microglobulin and associated amyloidosis presenting as bilateral popliteal tumours. *American Journal of Kidney Diseases*, **12**, 323–5.

Renaud, H., Fournier, A., and Morinière, Ph. (1988). Erosive osteoarthropathy associated with ß2-microglobulin amyloidosis in a uraemic patient treated exclusively by long-term haemofiltration with biocompatible membranes. *Nephrology, Dialysis, Transplantation*, **3**, 820–2.

Schaeffer, J., Ehlerding, G., Burchert, W., Floege, J., Shaldon, S., and Koch, K. M. (1992). Relationship of scintigraphically proven dialysis-related amyloidosis (DRA) to age and time on hemodialysis (HD). *Journal of the American Society of Nephrology*, **3**, 392 (Abstract).

Schaeffer, J., Floege, J., and Koch, K. M. (1996). Whole-body scintigraphy. In: *Dialysis amyloid* (ed. C. van Ypersele and T. B. Drüeke), pp. 145–55, Oxford University Press.

Sethi, D., Muller, B. R., Brown, E. A., Maini, R. N., and Gower, P. E. (1988*a*). C-reactive protein in haemodialysis patients with dialysis arthropathy. *Nephrology, Dialysis, Transplantation*, **3**, 269–71.

Sethi, D., Brown, E. A., Maini, R. N., and Gower, P. E. (1988*b*). Renal transplantation for dialysis arthropathy. *Lancet*, **ii**, 448–9.

Sethi, D., Cary, N. R. B., Brown, E. A., Woodrow, D. F., and Gower, P. E. (1989). Dialysis-associated amyloid: systemic or local? *Nephrology, Dialysis, Transplantation*, **4**, 1054–9.

Shinoda, T., Komatsu, M., Aizawa, T., *et al.* (1989). Intestinal pseudo-obstruction due to dialysis amyloidosis. *Clinical Nephrology*, **32**, 284–9.

Sonikian, M., Gogusev, J., Zingraff, J., *et al.* (1996). Potential effect of metabolic acidosis on ß2-microglobulin generation: *in vivo* and *in vitro* studies. *Journal of the American Society of Nephrology*, **7**, 350–6.

Takenaka, R., Fukatsu, A., Matsuo, S., Ishikawa, K., Toriyama, T., and Kawahara, H. (1992). Surgical treatment of hemodialysis-related shoulder arthropathy. *Clinical Nephrology*, **38**, 224–30.

Tan, S.-Y, Irish, A., Winearls, C. G., *et al.* (1996). Long term effect of renal transplantation on dialysis-related amyloid deposits and symptomatology. *Kidney International*, **50**, 282–9.

Theaker, J. M., Raine, A. E. G., Rainey, A. J., Hervyet, A., Clark, A., and Oliver, D. O. (1987). Systemic amyloidosis of ß2-microglobulin type: a complication of long term haemodialysis. *Journal of Clinical Pathology*, **40**, 1247–51.

van Ypersele de Strihou, C. (1996). ß2-Microglobulin amyloidosis: effect of ESRF treatment modality and dialysis membrane type. *Nephrology, Dialysis, Transplantation*, **11** (Suppl. 2), 147–9.

van Ypersele de Strihou, C., and Jadoul, M. (1996). Prevention and treatment of ß2-microglobulin amyloidosis. In *Dialysis amyloid* (ed. C. van Ypersele and T. B. Drüeke), pp. 261–76, Oxford University Press.

van Ypersele de Strihou, C., Honhon, B., Vandenbroucke, J. M., Huaux, J. P., Noel, H., and Maldague, B. (1988). Dialysis amyloidosis. In: *Advances in nephrology*, Vol. 117 (ed. J. P. Grünfeld, J. F. Bach, and J. L. Funck-Brentano), pp. 401–22. Year Book Medical Publishers, **117**.

van Ypersele de Strihou, C., Jadoul, M., Malghem, J., Maldague, B., Jamart, J., and the Working Party on Dialysis Amyloidosis (1991). Effect of dialysis membrane and patient's age on signs of dialysis related amyloidosis. *Kidney International*, **39**, 1012–19.

van Ypersele de Strihou, C., Floege, J., Jadoul, M., and Koch, K. M. (1994). Amyloidosis and its relationship to different dialysers. *Nephrology, Dialysis, Transplantation*, **9** (Suppl. 2), 156–61.

Varga, J., Idelson, B. A., Felson, D., Skinner, M., and Cohen, A. S. (1987). Lack of amyloid in abdominal fat aspirates from patients undergoing long-term hemodialysis. *Archives of Internal Medicine*, **147**, 1455–7.

Zaoui, P. M., Stone, W. J., and Hakim, R. M. (1990). Effects of dialysis membranes on beta2-microglobulin production and cellular expression. *Kidney International*, **38**, 962–8.

Zhou, H., Pfeifer, U., and Linke, R. (1991). Generalized amyloidosis from ß2-microglobulin, with caecal perforation after long-term haemodialysis. *Virchows Archiv für pathologische Anatomie und Physiologie und für klinische Medizin*, **419**, 349–53.

Zingraff, J. J., Noël, L. H., Bardin, T., *et al.* (1990). ß2-Microglobulin amyloidosis in chronic renal failure. *New England Journal of Medicine*, **323**, 1070–1.

7

Acquired cystic disease and renal tumors in long-term dialysis patients

Isao Ishikawa

Acquired cystic disease

Introduction

Advances in dialysis treatment have prolonged the lives of many dialysis patients, but long-term dialysis has led to a new set of complications, such as beta-2 microglobulin-induced amyloidosis, renal osteodystrophy, and aluminum intoxication; as well as acquired cystic disease and renal cell carcinoma (Dunnill *et al.*, 1977; Ishikawa, 1991*b*). Autopsy examination (Dunnill *et al.*, 1977) and diagnostic imaging (Ishikawa *et al.*, 1980) have revealed acquired cystic disease of the diseased kidney and its complications. In 1977, Dunnill *et al.* described the very important observation that 14 cases with acquired cysts, including six accompanied by renal tumors, were found among 30 autopsy cases—one of the patients had died due to metastasis of a renal cell carcinoma. In 1980, Ishikawa *et al.* reported the findings, using computed tomographic scanning of the diseased kidneys, in 96 of their patients undergoing dialysis due to chronic glomerulonephritis. The renal volume of bilateral diseased kidneys was 110 ± 38 ml/1.48 m^2 at the middle of the first year after the start of dialysis, 73 ± 18 ml at the second year, and 55 ± 18 ml at the third year. After 3 years' dialysis, the renal volume in some of the patients increased because of the development of acquired cysts. The incidence of acquired cysts was 44% in patients with less than 3 years' dialysis and 79% in those more than 3 years' dialysis. Furthermore, three renal cell carcinomas were found in their 96 dialysis patients. Since these hallmark descriptions appeared, many cross-sectional studies were conducted, (Bommer *et al.*, 1980; Hughson *et al.*, 1980; Levine *et al.*, 1984; Narasimhan *et al.*, 1986; Matson and Cohen, 1990), and long-term follow-up studies were undertaken thereafter. Longitudinal 10-year and 15-year follow-up studies were conducted in 96 dialysis patients (Ishikawa *et al.*, 1990; Ishikawa *et al.*, 1997) and a 7-year follow-up study was performed in 30 dialysis patients by Levine *et al.* (1991). These studies revealed that long-term dialysis causes cystic changes in the diseased kidney and that the progression of these changes aggravates the kidney disease (Ishikawa *et al.*, 1980; Grantham and Levine, 1985). Enlarged kidneys due to acquired cysts tend to be more susceptible to renal cell carcinoma (MacDougall *et al.*, 1990; Ishikawa, 1991*b*).

This chapter reviews recent findings, mainly regarding acquired renal cystic disease and renal tumors, in patients on dialysis for more than 10 years. Certain related conclusions, drawn by various investigators, are also reviewed. These include the assertions that the incidence of renal cell carcinoma in dialysis patients is not high (Chandhoke *et al.*, 1992), that the prognosis in renal cell carcinoma is not poor, and that routine screening for renal cell carcinoma is not necessary in dialysis patients (Chandhoke *et al.*, 1992; Sarasin *et al.*, 1995). Data on these topics will be presented in this chapter.

Definition of acquired renal cystic kidney

Acquired renal cystic disease is defined as the presence of more than one to five cysts per kidney (depending on the source) in a patient with non-cystic kidney disease, or displacement of more than 25% of renal parenchyma by the acquired cysts (Ishikawa, 1991*b*).

Pathology of acquired renal cystic disease

The gross findings for diseased kidneys after more than 10 years' hemodialysis are vastly different from patient to patient, ranging from severely contracted kidneys without acquired cysts to kidneys enlarged due to extensive cystic changes. The kidney weight in acquired renal cystic disease is usually lower than that of the normal kidney (20–100 g/kidney), but it is sometimes greater than that of normal kidney, occasionally being as much as 1094 (Kessler *et al.*, 1991) to 1250 g (Gehrig *et al.*, 1985).

The diameter of 94.4% of all acquired cysts is less than 0.6 cm (Ishikawa *et al.*, 1988), which is below the sensitivity of computed tomography (Fig. 7.1). The remaining small number of cysts are usually less than 2 cm in diameter, although exceptional cysts 3–5 cm in diameter are also found (Fig. 7.2). In severe cystic change the kidney resembles a cluster of grapes. The cysts contain a clear to pale yellow fluid and, in places, a red-brown to black fluid. In cross-section, very little atrophic parenchyma but innumerable cysts are present throughout the kidneys (Fig. 7.1). In less severe cystic change, the cysts are situated mainly in the cortical area (Dunnill *et al.*, 1977). Microscopically, the cyst lining cells comprise a thin-layered, single epithelium in most cysts, although hyperplastic multilayered epithelia or papillary proliferative epithelia are found in a few cysts (in 30% of the cases) (Hughson *et al.*, 1980) (Fig. 7.3). Solid tumor, tubular or papillary adenoma (Dunnill *et al.*, 1977) (in 5–25% of the cases), and renal cell carcinoma (1.5% of the cases) (Ishikawa, 1985*b*) are sometimes present in these kidneys (Fig. 7.1). The pathology of end-stage renal disease reveals the effects of dynamic processes (Dunnill *et al.*, 1977; Hughson *et al.*, 1980), and the end-stage kidney does not denote a resting organ. Several findings support this assertion: staining for epidermal growth factor (EGF), epidermal growth factor receptor (EGFR), vimentin, cytokeratin, and insulin-like growth factor-1 (IGF-1) is seen in lining epithelial cells, proliferating cells of atypical cysts, adenoma, and renal cell carcinoma (Horiguchi and Ishikawa, 1993) and c-*erb*-B2 protein staining is also found in the lining epithelial cells (Herrera, 1991). Acquired cysts are positive for proliferative cell nuclear antigen. The proliferative index in single-layered epithelia is 3.61%, 9.1% in the hyperplastic epithelia, and 13.7% or 8.67% in renal cell carcinoma, in contrast to the index of 0.22 to 0.33% in normal tubular epithelia (Nadasdy *et al.*, 1995). Renal cell carcinoma comprises the clear cell subtype and the granular or mixed cell subtype. Coexisting clear (non-papillary) and mixed (papillary) renal cell carcinomas are found in the same kidney in some cases (Ishikawa and Kovacs, 1993). The tumors are often multifocal and bilateral (Dunnill *et al.*, 1977), and this tendency is prominent in patients on long-term hemodialysis.

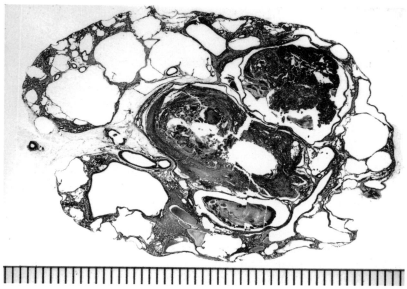

Fig. 7.1 Cut section of acquired cystic kidney complicated with renal cell carcinoma in a 31-year-old man on hemodialysis for 15 years and 9 months due to chronic glomerulonephritis. Note that almost all renal cysts are less than 6 mm in diameter (the scale denotes mm).

Epithelial lining cells are derived from proximal tubular cells; immunohistochemical studies using lectin have revealed that cyst epithelia are mainly positive for proximal tubular markers, such as tetragonolobus lotus lectin (Ishikawa *et al.*, 1989*a*). The cyst to serum ratio for sodium is near 1, that for creatinine around 7, and that for beta-2 microglobulin near 0 (Ishikawa, 1985*a*; 1986). The excretion of para-aminohippurate and gentamicin into cysts (Ishikawa *et al.*, 1989*b*) is also suggestive that acquired cysts are derived from proximal tubular cells. Cysts are multiple interconnected cavities (Mickisch *et al.*, 1984; Vandeursen *et al.* 1991) and communicate with glomeruli (Feiner *et al.*, 1981; Vandeursen *et al.*, 1991).

Characteristics of acquired cystic disease

The most important factor for the development of acquired cystic disease is the duration of uremia or of dialysis (Ishikawa *et al.*, 1980) (Fig. 7.2). The prevalence of acquired

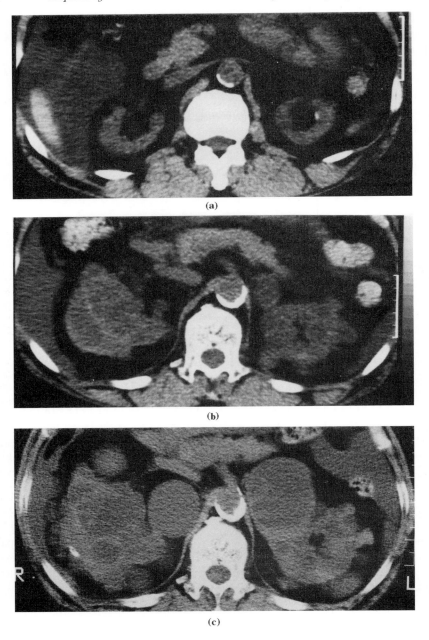

(a)

(b)

(c)

Fig. 7.2 Development of acquired renal cystic disease in a 59-year-old male patient on continuous ambulatory peritoneal dialysis due to chronic glomerulonephritis. After 4 years of dialysis the bilateral kidney volume by computed tomography was (a) 174 ml. After (b) 6 years, and (c) 11 years of dialysis, severe cystic changes with rather large cysts appeared (bilateral kidney volume, 811 ml and 1605 ml, respectively).

cystic disease is dependent on the duration of hemodialysis, being 12% in the pre-dialysis periods, 44% after less than 3 years of dialysis, 79% after more than 3 years, and 90% after more than 10 years (Ishikawa, 1991*b*). Thus almost all hemodialysis patients who are on dialysis for more than 10 years have acquired cystic disease of the kidneys. A secondary factor is a sex difference in the prevalence and severity of acquired cystic disease, with male patients showing a higher incidence and greater severity of acquired cystic disease (Ishikawa *et al.*, 1985). A 10-year follow-up study of 96 hemodialysis patients revealed that the kidney volume increased 2.7 times in 33 male patients but did not change in 24 female patients (Ishikawa *et al.*, 1990). In 21 male patients the kidney volume was 196 ± 218 ml at the 10-year follow-up and 225 ± 213 ml at the 15-year follow-up, the increase rate being 1.26 ± 0.39 (p<0.02). On the other hand, in female patients it was 78 ± 51 ml at the 10-year follow-up and 117 ± 91 ml at the 15-year follow-up (increase rate, 1.43 ± 0.45) (p<0.01) (Ishikawa *et al.*, 1997).

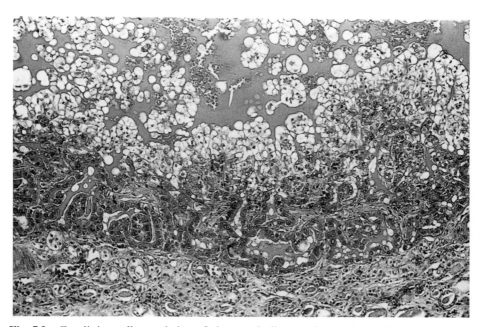

Fig. 7.3   Cyst lining cells consisting of phenotypically granular or clear cells have started to grow with papillary configuration. The 47-year-old male patient had been on hemodialysis for 10 years and 6 months. (Hematoxylin and eosin, 250 ×.)

Neither the age nor the underlying disease in hemodialysis patients affects the development and severity of acquired cystic disease (Ishikawa *et al.*, 1980), though diabetic nephropathy retards the development of acquired cystic disease. The modality of dialysis treatment used does not affect the relationship to acquired cysts: the incidence of acquired cystic disease in continuous ambulatory peritoneal dialysis patients is the same as that in hemodialysis patients (Ishikawa *et al.*, 1991*a*).

Acquired cystic disease in transplant recipients

A notable finding is the regression of acquired cystic disease after successful renal transplantation (Ishikawa *et al.*, 1983), i.e. almost all acquired cysts in male patients on dialysis disappear within one to several months, even within 2 weeks according to more recent experience (Fig. 7.4). Acquired renal cysts are reversible and regress if the etiology, that is the uremic condition, is eliminated. This is a very important observation since it suggests the pathogenesis of acquired cysts.

However, the regression of acquired renal cysts in transplant recipients is not complete, and the prevalence of acquired renal cysts is 37–50% in renal transplant recipients (Ishikawa *et al.*, 1991*b*). Acquired renal cystic disease in transplant recipients is fundamentally different from that in dialysis patients as there are only a few cysts in the atrophic kidneys and there is no enlargement of the native kidneys if graft function is good.

A follow-up study in 61 renal graft recipients of acquired cysts of the native kidney revealed that there were no acquired renal cysts in 32 (52.5%) recipients, that the numbers of cysts did not change in 9 (14.8%) recipients, that the number of cysts decreased in 9 (14.8%) recipients, and that it increased in 11 (18%) recipients who had a longer follow-up after transplantation (Ishikawa *et al.*, 1991*b*). These newly developed cysts may differ from acquired renal cysts in dialysis patients (Ishikawa *et al.*, 1991*b*). The prevalence of acquired cysts was 57% in transplant recipients treated with cyclosporin and 8% in the recipients treated without cyclosporin, suggesting that this drug might be a cystogen (Lien *et al.*, 1993). Of course, acquired cysts develop after long-standing uremia due to chronic rejection (Ishikawa *et al.*, 1989*c*) not only in native kidneys but also in the graft, but complications of acquired cysts such as perirenal bleeding or renal neoplasm are rare. Acquired cysts develop in the native kidney more frequently than in the graft (Ishikawa *et al.*, 1989*c*).

Complications of acquired cystic disease

Renal cell carcinoma and retroperitoneal bleeding are the two major complications of acquired cystic disease (Ishikawa, 1991*a*). Other minor complications are cyst infection, amelioration of anemia, and matrix stone formation. Renal cell carcinoma is described later.

Retroperitoneal bleeding (hematoma)

Since a summary of 46 cases complicated with retroperitoneal bleeding from the rupture of acquired cysts appeared in 1990 (Ishikawa *et al.*, 1990) a further 26 cases have been reported. Among them were rare cases with bilateral retroperitoneal bleeding in one hemodialysis patient (Herms *et al.*, 1993) and one transplant recipient (Oliveras *et al.*, 1993), and a hemoperitoneum due to cyst rupture in a patient on continuous ambulatory peritoneal dialysis. The risk factors for rupture of acquired cysts are similar to those for renal cell carcinomas in dialysis patients (Ishikawa, 1991*b*), i.e. male gender, long-term hemodialysis, and enlarged kidneys due to acquired cysts. Levine *et al.* (1987) followed 30 patients for 7 years and observed a large perinephric

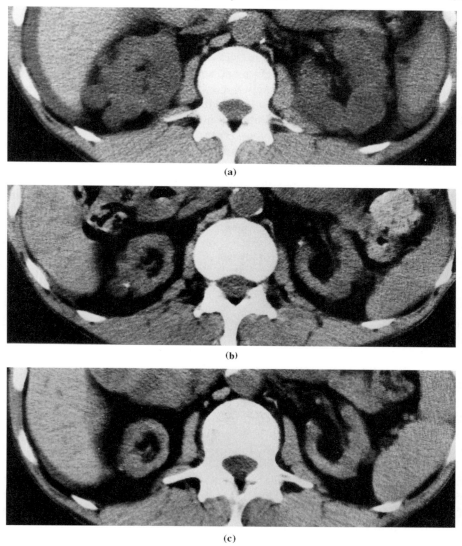

(a)

(b)

(c)

Fig. 7.4 Regression of acquired renal cystic disease after successful renal transplantation in a 45-year-old man who had been on continuous ambulatory peritoneal dialysis for 8 years and 9 months (bilateral kidney volume: 558 ml) (a) before transplantation (b) Two weeks (182 ml) and (c) 4 weeks (163 ml) after transplantation almost all acquired renal cysts have disappeared and the native kidneys have become contracted.

hematoma in four cases (13%) and renal cell carcinomas in two. We followed 96 patients for 15 years and noted renal cell carcinomas in six and retroperitoneal bleeding in three. Patients with acquired renal cystic diseases have an increased prevalence of retroperitoneal bleeding.

Erythrocytosis

The direct relationship between the development and presence of acquired cysts and the amelioration of renal anemia is not yet clarified (Ishikawa, 1985*b*; 1991*a*). The frequency of acquired cysts is increased and amelioration of anemia is observed in long-term dialysis patients. However, it is not necessary to postulate a direct cause and consequence relationship between acquired cysts and the amelioration of anemia. Patients with multiple cysts were reported to show high concentrations of serum erythropoietin and hemoglobin in one report (Edmunds *et al.*, 1991), whereas no relationship was found between acquired cysts and anemia in other studies (Glicklich *et al.* 1990). Furthermore, high hemoglobin concentrations are observed in long-term dialysis patients with atrophic kidneys without acquired cysts. Therefore, we speculate that there are many signals to fibroblasts around the proximal peritubular interstitium stimulating the production of erythropoietin, and that cystic changes constitute one of those signals.

In an investigation into the effect of human recombinant erythropoietin administration, one of the growth factors, no effect on the development or progression of acquired cysts was seen (Ishikawa *et al.*, 1996*b*).

Etiology of acquired cystic disease

The mechanisms of renal cyst formation have been investigated mainly in experimental animals or through experiments using *in-vitro* tubular epithelia, which are composed of proliferated tubular cells and fluid accumulated within distended cavities with remodeling of the extracellular matrix (Grantham, 1993). The proliferation of tubular epithelia stimulated by the activation of a proto-oncogene and/or EGF, causes hyperplasia of tubular cells and cyst formation. Increased sensitivities for EGF (Moskowitz *et al.*, 1995) and other mitogens, including iron-containing mitogens, may stimulate cyst formation. High proliferative activities of tubular cells and cyst-lining epithelia are already documented, and there is an overexpression of the c-*erb*-B2 protein and IGF-1. Klotz *et al.* (1991) found renal cell-specific growth factor activity in the serum of dialysis patients that was different from that of EGF, platelet-derived growth factor (PDGF), and basic fibroblast growth factor (bFGF). Carone *et al.* (1994) could not show the displacement of Na–K-ATPase from the basolateral to apical side in acquired cystic disease which Wilson *et al.* (1991) found in experimental animals. Apoptosis of tubules and extracellular matrix is not described as being a feature of acquired cystic disease at present. Furthermore, the relationship between the mechanism of cyst development and tumor formation has not been clarified, though the sequence of events from cyst to adenoma to renal cell carcinoma is postulated.

A hypothesis that a decreased androgen to estrogen ratio and an elevation of estrogen are related to cyst formation was proposed as an explanation for the male preponderance in acquired cystic disease (Concolino *et al.*, 1993). However, this has yet to be proven.

Many other hypotheses (Ishikawa, 1991*a*); e.g. those implicating ischemia, tubular obstruction due to oxalate or beta-2 microglobulin, polyamine, silicon, and vanadium

(Marco-Franco *et al.*, 1991), have been proposed in addition to the uremic metabolite theory (Ishikawa, 1991*a*), that endogenous growth factors, found at higher levels in males, induce cysts.

Diagnosis of acquired cystic disease

The clinical diagnosis of acquired cystic disease is based on either sonographic examination or computed tomographic scanning (Ishikawa, 1991*b*). One clinically important aspect of the evaluation, when acquired cystic disease is diagnosed, is the determination of the severity of cystic changes and the presence or absence of renal cell carcinoma. A differential diagnosis between hemorrhagic cyst and renal cell carcinoma is sometimes necessary if plain computed tomographic scanning is used. This modality is preferred when retroperitoneal bleeding is suspected, since the positional relationship of the bleeding site and the kidney can be determined and the amount of bleeding estimated.

Treatment of acquired cystic disease

Long-term dialysis patients have a high incidence of acquired cystic disease, but the acquired cystic disease *per se* is not the object of treatment (Ishikawa, 1991*b*). Only when a complication is found is treatment necessary. Treatment for renal cell carcinoma is described later. When retroperitoneal bleeding is diagnosed, conservative treatments, analgesics, and blood transfusion are started to control pain and to maintain blood pressure; if the blood pressure is not easily maintained, embolization or nephrectomy is then considered. Infected acquired cysts, though rare, often necessitate nephrectomy. Matrix stones that cause flank pain require only conservative treatment because they pass spontaneously. Rarely, erythrocytosis makes it necessary to administer an angiotensin-converting enzyme inhibitor or theophylline.

Renal tumor (renal cell carcinoma) in long-term dialysis patients

Relationship to acquired cystic disease

Renal cell carcinoma occurs in 1.5% of all dialysis patients (Ishikawa, 1991*b*), but develops in 5% of patients who receive hemodialysis for more than 10 years. A sequence of events which may occur is tubular epithelia to cyst lining cells, to hyperplastic epithelia, to adenoma, and finally to renal cell carcinoma. The pathological descriptions by Dunnill *et al.* (1977) and Hughson *et al.* (1980) support this concept; a single kidney with acquired cystic kidney often presents a range of pathological findings from cysts to adenocarcinoma. All pathological findings for epithelial cells suggest that they are mainly derived from proximal tubules, and that the risk factors for patients developing acquired cysts and developing renal cell carcinoma are the same (Ishikawa, 1991*b*). Kidneys enlarged due to acquired cysts are more likely to develop renal cell carcinoma (MacDougall *et al.*, 1990; Ishikawa, 1991*b*). These indirect lines of evidence suggest a sequence or continuum proceeding from cysts to renal cell carcinoma (Ishikawa, 1991*a*).

However, renal cell carcinoma may occur by chance (Chandhoke *et al.*, 1992). Renal cell carcinoma is seen in patients with chronic renal failure before dialysis, and renal cell carcinoma may develop in kidneys without acquired cysts (Ishikawa and Shinoda, 1983). Takahashi *et al.* (1993) found 349 renal cell adenomas, as defined by Thoenes *et al.* (1990), in 41 out of 50 pathological cases, with the number of adenomas increasing according to the duration of hemodialysis. However, acquired renal cystic disease was found in twelve cases (24%). They concluded that acquired cystic disease is not related to renal cell tumors. Miller *et al.* (1989) also stated that there is little relationship between acquired cysts and renal cell tumors.

The two lines of thought might be reconciled by Ishikawa and Shinoda's observation (1983) that there are two types of renal cell carcinoma, with those in older, short-term dialysis patients being unrelated to, and those in younger, long-term dialysis patients being related to, acquired cysts. A recent hypothesis regarding renal cell carcinoma in the general population, which may be applicable to that in dialysis patients, asserts that most common non-papillary (clear) renal cell carcinomas develop as a carcinoma from the outset, whereas papillary (mixed-cell subtype) renal tumors develop as a papillary adenoma, with subsequent transition to renal cell carcinoma (papillary carcinoma) (Kovacs, 1993). Long-term dialysis patients might show an increased risk of developing papillary tumors: papillary adenoma and papillary adenocarcinoma (Ishikawa and Kovacs 1993). Therefore, it is reasonable, at present, to think that there are two types of renal cell carcinoma in dialysis patients, but further cytogenetic studies are necessary to test this hypothesis.

Incidence of renal cell carcinoma in dialysis patients

There are many arguments as to whether the incidence of renal cell carcinoma in dialysis patients is higher than that in the general population, since there have been no carefully controlled studies to examine incidence in these two populations matched for age, gender, and diagnostic methods (Chandhoke *et al.*, 1992). Therefore, some investigators believe that the incidence of renal cell carcinoma is not high in dialysis patients; as, for example, stated clearly by Chandhoke *et al.* (1992) based on the autopsy data presented by Hajdu and Thomas (1967). However, it is generally agreed that there are many cases of renal cell carcinomas among young patients on long-term dialysis. There are also many non-fatal cases of renal cell carcinoma in our experience (Ishikawa, 1996).

The prevalence of renal cell carcinoma in Japan, based on the literature, is 75 per 4118 dialysis patients, which is the equivalent of 1821 per 100 000 dialysis patients. According to screening studies using sonographic examination, including that by Tosaka *et al.* (1990), the prevalence is 28–137 renal cell carcinomas per 100 000 dialysis patients, or 13- to 65-fold higher than in the general population. Terasawa *et al.* (1994) found, again using sonographic examination, 41 renal cell carcinomas in 1603 dialysis patients, in contrast to only 22 in 27 933 individuals in the general population, i.e. 32-fold higher in dialysis patients than in the general population.

The incidence rate of renal cell carcinoma, based on our 10-year follow-up studies in dialysis patients, is 402 renal cell carcinomas (Ishikawa *et al.*, 1990), compared with three renal cell carcinomas per year per 100 000 population (Fujimoto and Hanai, 1992), suggesting a rate 134 times higher than that in the general population. Furthermore, Port *et al.* (1989) reported a 4 fold increased prevalence or incidence of renal cell carcinoma in dialysis patients relative to that in the general population: Gardner and Evan (1984) a 7-fold, MacDougall *et al.* (1987) a 50-fold, and Levine (1992) a 3- to 6- fold increase.

A questionnaire study performed in 1992 (Ishikawa, 1993*b*) revealed that the renal cell carcinoma frequency in dialysis patients was 125 cases per year per 100 000 dialysis patients, compared with three cases per year per 100 000 of the population, i.e. 40 times higher than that in the general population. In a more controlled comparison, the incidence of this carcinoma, as based on a 1994 questionnaire study (Ishikawa, 1996), was 18 times higher in male patients and 15 times higher in female patients compared with the general population when age and gender were matched. In that study, the incidence of renal cell carcinoma was raised 1400-fold in 25- to 30-year-old male dialysis patients and 650-fold in 30- to 35-year-old female dialysis patients.

These data, with the exception of the autopsy data presented by Hajdu and Thomas (1967), support the generalization that the prevalence or incidence of renal cell carcinoma is about 20 times higher than that in the general population. It seems indisputable that renal cell carcinoma in dialysis patients is qualitatively different from that in the general population, given the higher prevalence of this carcinoma in patients with than without acquired cysts, the relationship of 80% of these carcinomas to acquired cystic disease, and their markedly high incidence in young patients.

Questionnaire studies in Japan

Questionnaire studies on renal cell carcinoma performed every 2 years between 1982 and 1994 revealed a progressive increase: there were 34 cases in 1982, and 37, 48, 115, 130 (Ishikawa, 1993*a*), 184 (Ishikawa, 1993*b*), and 273 (Ishikawa, 1996) every 2 years from 1984 to 1994 (Table 7.1). In total, the 821 patients consisted of 665 male patients and 156 female patients, with a male: female ratio of 4.3 (Ishikawa, 1996). The questionnaire return rate was 74% in 1982 and 60% in 1994. The 273 patients with renal cell carcinomas reported in 1994 had a mean age of 53.5 ± 11.3 years, their mean duration of hemodialysis was 118.2 ± 71.0 months, and 138 (50.9%) out of 271 patients had more than 10 years' hemodialysis. The renal cell carcinoma was first suspected based on the symptoms in 26 (9.5%), and based on screening results in 234 patients without symptoms (sonography in 128 and computed tomographic scanning in 106). Thus, in dialysis patients this carcinoma is typically a symptomless tumor and screening is necessary for its diagnosis. Accompanying acquired renal cystic disease was found in 224 (82.7%) of 271 patients. The underlying disease was chronic glomerulonephritis in 212 (78%) patients, diabetic nephropathy in 12, nephrosclerosis in 9, autosomal dom-inant polycystic kidney disease in 8, and others and unknown in 32. The mean diameter of the tumor was 4.0 ± 2.7 cm, but many tumors were less than 4 cm. The pathological findings were reported in 210 patients (76.9%), and the cellular type, described in 194 patients, consisted of clear-cell subtype in 105 patients, granular-cell subtype in 42, and mixed-cell subtype in 47. Granular-and mixed-cell subtypes were

Table 7.1. Renal cell carcinoma in dialysis patients (questionnaire studies in Japan)

	1982[a]	1984	1986	1988	1990	1992	1994	Total
Number of renal cell carcinoma (cases)	34	37	48	115	130	184	273	821
Male	25	31	40	91	112	150	216	665
Female	9	6	8	24	18	34	57	156
M : F	2.8 : 1	5.2 : 1	5.0 : 1	3.8 : 1	6.2 : 1	4.4 : 1	3.8 : 1	4.3 : 1
Mean age (years)[b] (no. of patients)	47.9 ± 15.6	49.7 ± 11.1	50.5 ± 10.0	51.4 ± 11.7	52.6 ± 10.9	53.8 ± 11.8 (183)	53.5 ± 11.3 (272)	52.6 ± 11.6 (818)
Mean duration of hemodialysis (months) (no. of patients)	49.4 ± 32.8	73.6 ± 46.3	83.9 ± 45.2	94.6 ± 54.5	106.1 ± 61.2	111.0 ± 64.3 (183)	118.2 ± 71.0 (271)	104.5 ± 64.4 (815)
Presence of ARCD (%)	23/32 (71.9)	20/32 (62.5)	39/46 (84.8)	92/115 (80.0)	102/124 82.3%	142/179 (79.3)	224/271 (82.7)	642/799 (80.4)
Tumor size (cm) (no. of patients)	4.25 ± 3.21	4.90 ± 3.99	5.39 ± 3.78	4.58 ± 3.44	4.22 ± 2.53	4.70 ± 3.20 (166)	4.00 ± 2.70 (242)	4.40 ± 3.10 (741)
Number of patients with metastases (%)	7/33 (21.2)	8/33 (24.2)	10/48 (20.8)	17/106 (16.0)	19/126 (15.1)	29/182 (15.9)	35/269 (13.0)	125/797 (15.7)
Number of hemodialysis patients (at the year and month)	42 223 (81.12)	53 017 (83.12)	66 310 (85.12)	80 553 (87.12)	88 534 (88.12)	116 303 (90.12)	123 000 (92.12)	

[a]Year of study; [b]mean ± SD. ARCD-acquired renal cystic disease.

observed more frequently in patients with more than 5 years' hemodialysis, suggesting that tumors of these subtypes are related to acquired cysts (Fig. 7.5).

As for the outcome at a mean follow-up of 1 year after the diagnosis of renal cell carcinoma, death due to renal cancer was observed in 18 patients (6.6%) and metastasis in 35 (13.0%). The rates of metastasis did not differ among tumors with different cell types. The annual incidence of renal cell carcinoma estimated based on the 1992 questionnaire was 123 cases per 100 000 dialysis patients, and it increased to 187 cases per 100 000 dialysis patients based on the 1994 questionnaire. This incidence was 444 cases per 100 000 patients on dialysis for more than 10 years and 117 cases per 100 000 patients on dialysis for less than 10 years, revealing that the former patient group was 3.8 times more likely than the latter to be diagnosed with renal cell carcinoma.

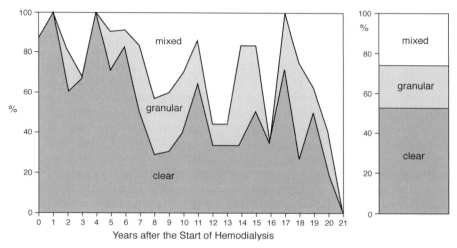

Fig. 7.5   A higher incidence of granular and mixed cell subtypes than of the clear-cell subtype is seen in long-term hemodialysis patients.

Sex differences in renal cell carcinoma in dialysis patients

The incidence of renal cell carcinoma in male patients is 3.8-fold higher than that in female patients based on our questionnaire study in Japan (Ishikawa, 1996). Of the 344 patients with this cancer who were on dialysis for more than 10 years, 289 were male and 55 were female. Thus the prevalence is 5.3-fold higher in males than in females. The male preponderance becomes more prominent with long-term dialysis.

Duration of hemodialysis and renal cell carcinoma

Annual incidence of renal cell carcinoma was estimated (Fig. 7.6) by the number of patients with renal cell carcinoma obtained from the 1994's questionnaire study (Ishikawa, 1996) and the number of dialysis patients from the Registry of Japanese Society for Dialysis Therapy at the end of 1992. These data suggest that long-term dialysis clearly increases the risk of renal cell carcinoma, especially after 5 years and again after 12 years of hemodialysis.

Symptoms of renal cell carcinoma in dialysis patients

Almost all dialysis patients with renal cell carcinoma are symptomless. When symptoms are present, the most frequent symptom is gross hematuria (68.0%), followed by abdominal pain, flank pain and/or back pain (11.5%), fever (9.8%), erythrocytosis (4.9%), and palpable tumor, accelerated erythrocyte sedimentation rate, and reduction of hematocrit (1.6% each) (Ishikawa, 1991*b*). Hypercalcemia and hypoglycemia have also been reported, and an erythropoietin-producing tumor (Murayama *et al.*, 1991) is described in the literature.

Histopathology and cytogenetics of renal cell carcinoma in dialysis patients

Bilateral renal cell carcinomas were seen in 11 out of 130 cases (8.5%) (Ishikawa, 1993*a*). Long-term dialysis tends to lead to renal cell carcinomas that are multifocal and bilateral, although Dunnill *et al.* (1977) described three types of renal tumor: tubular, papillary, and solid. Other classifications of renal cell carcinomas, have been proposed by Thoenes *et al.* (1990) and Kovacs (1993) based on data for the general population. Kovacs (1993) proposed that renal cell carcinomas could generally be classified into the two genetic types of non–papillary (clear) renal cell carcinomas: one shows loss of heterozygosity in tumor suppressor gene in the short arm of Chromosome 3 (3p) region and the other, less common, papillary renal cell tumor shows changes of chromosome number. Papillary renal cell adenoma presents mainly trisomy of Chromosomes 7 and 17 and loss of the Y chromosome; adenomas of this type undergo transition to papillary renal cell carcinoma when trisomy of Chromosomes 12, 16, and 20 occurs in addition to the original genetic changes. Therefore, Ishikawa and Kovacs (1993) reclassified renal cell tumors and carcinomas microscopically. Non–papillary renal cell carcinomas were found in 22 out of 43 dialysis patients (51%) and papillary renal tumors in 21 (49%) (Fig. 7.7). The incidence of papillary renal cell tumors was clearly increased compared with that of 4.8% of all renal cell carcinomas in the general population. Long-term hemodialysis patients with papillary renal cell tumors showed no difference in age, gender, or size of the tumor compared to those with non–papillary renal cell carcinomas. These data suggest that there are two cytogenetically different tumors of the kidney in dialysis patients and that many renal cell carcinomas in long-term dialysis patients are papillary renal cell tumors.

Ishikawa *et al.* (1996*a*) reported that non–papillary renal cell carcinomas in four dialysis patients showed structural changes in 3p, 5q, and 17p. Of the 4 patients, three showed loss of heterozygosity in 3p14 and 3p21. On the other hand, papillary renal cell carcinomas showed supernumerary chromosomes; trisomy of Chromosomes 12, 16, or X and loss of the Y chromosome in male patients (Fig. 7.8). One non–papillary renal cell carcinoma showed a normal karyotype. So far no increased incidence of trisomy of Chromosomes 7 or 17 in papillary renal cell tumors has been demonstrated in

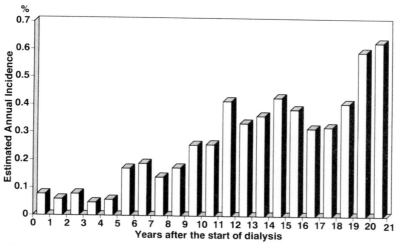

Fig. 7.6 Relationship between annual incidence of renal cell carcinoma and duration of hemodialysis.

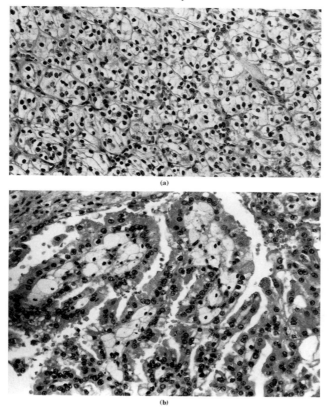

Fig. 7.7 Two types of renal cell carcinoma: (a) non-papillary clear-cell carcinoma in a 34-year-old man on hemodialysis for 5 years and 8 months, and (b) papillary tumor in a 64-year-old man on hemodialysis for 13 years. (Hematoxylin and eosin, 250 ×.)

dialysis patients, though it has been suggested to occur in the general population by Kovacs (1993) and Corless *et al.* (1996). The papillary renal cell carcinoma in the general population is often multifocal and related to cortical adenoma and a low-grade of tumor malignancy, and it tends to have central necrosis. These general characteristics of papillary renal cell carcinoma are very similar to those of renal cell carcinoma in dialysis patients.

We have described a 41-year-old male with papillary renal cell carcinoma showing a karyotype of 48, X, −Y, +5, +16, +20 (Ishikawa *et al.*, 1993) (Fig. 7.8). Thereafter, Yoshida *et al.* (1993) reported this carcinoma in a 47-year-old male on 8 years of hemodialysis showing 48, X, inv(X), t(7q: 19q), +del(10q), +16 (Fig. 7.8) and Matsumoto *et al.* (1995)

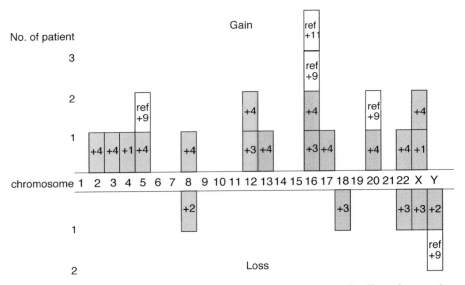

Fig. 7.8 Gains and losses of entire chromosomes in papillary renal cell carcinomas (open boxes, #9 and #11, indicate data from Ishikawa *et al.*, (1993) and Yoshida *et al.*, (1993)); tendency to develop trisomy of Chromosomes 5, 12, 16, 20 and loss of the Y chromosome. (Cited from (Ishikawa *et al.*, 1996*a*))

in a 40-year-old male on 9 years 6 months of hemodialysis showing a karyotype of 38, X, −Y, −1, −6, −8, −11, −14, −15, −22. The tumorigenesis, i.e. the pathway for the tumor development, was proposed by Ishikawa (1991*a*), Hughson *et al.* (1993), and Kovacs (1995) to be based on the structural and numeric changes of chromosomes.

Rare forms of renal cell carcinoma, oncocytoma (Makita *et al.*, 1991), sarcomatoid renal cell carcinoma (Suvarna *et al.*, 1994), and Bellini's duct tumor (Ito *et al.*, 1993) have been reported in dialysis patients. Urothelial carcinoma has also been reported in patients with acquired cysts (Chung-Park *et al.*, 1983).

Metastasis of renal cell carcinoma in dialysis patients

In their literature review Hughson *et al.* (1986) reported metastasis in 27% of renal cell carcinoma cases in dialysis patients. The questionnaire study performed in 1994 revealed that the metastasis rate was 13% at a mean follow-up of 1 year (Ishikawa, 1996). This may reflect an early detection of the renal cell carcinoma cases forming the object of the questionnaire study or a low incidence of metastasis of this carcinoma in dialysis patients. The rate was 55 (16.6%) in 331 patients with long-term dialysis for more than 10 years and 70 (15.2%) in 462 patients with less than 10 years' dialysis. The long-term dialysis patients did not have a high incidence of metastasis. The site distribution of the metastases was the same as that in the general population, typically with tumor embolization in the vena cava and metastasis to the bone, brain, skin, and lung. Pancreatic and lung metastases were found in one patient 5 years after nephrectomy. This suggests that careful long-term follow-up is necessary in dialysis patients after nephrectomy. It is not known, however, whether the prognosis in renal cell carcinoma in dialysis patients is poor or not, because there was no control study in which the histological subtype, stage, and grade of the renal cell carcinomas in the dialysis patients were matched with those in the general population.

Renal cell carcinoma in renal transplantation

The incidence of renal cell carcinoma in renal transplant recipients may be low, but the metastasis rate is high, compared to dialysis patients (Ishikawa, 1992a). Penn (1987) reported an increase in renal cell carcinoma of the native kidneys after cyclosporin therapy compared with conventional treatment. After successful renal transplantation, renal acquired cysts and hyperplastic cysts may regress (Ishikawa *et al.*, 1983), but it is not clear whether adenomas or small renal cell carcinomas regress or not. Data for 129 cases of renal cell carcinomas in renal transplant recipients were collected (Ishikawa, 1992a), and since then about 50 additional cases have been reported within the last few years. Dlugosz *et al.* (1989) reported five deaths from malignancy out of 222 deaths of transplant recipients: three were from metastatic renal cell carcinoma. Screening for renal malignancy may be necessary before and after renal transplantation.

Renal cell carcinoma in continuous ambulatory peritoneal dialysis patients

Since Ishikawa reviewed 10 cases of renal cell carcinoma in patients receiving continuous peritoneal dialysis (Ishikawa, 1992b), several other cases have been reported. The projected future increase in the number of long-term peritoneal dialysis patients will probably lead to an increased number of cases of renal cell carcinoma.

Pathogenetic mechanisms of acquired cyst and renal cell carcinoma

A current hypothesis posits that the uremia-related growth factors involved in compensatory hypertrophy of tubular epithelia due to nephron loss cause activation of proto-oncogenes leading to further chromosomal changes (Grantham, 1991; Ishikawa, 1991*a*; Hughson *et al.*, 1993; Kovacs, 1995). As a result, the two types of renal tumors develop: one being the non-papillary renal cell carcinoma due to structural chromosomal changes; the other being papillary adenocarcinoma arising from papillary adenoma derived from hyperplastic epithelium which is dependent on changes in chromosome numbers. It is already known that uremia causes sister chromatid exchange in peripheral blood lymphocytes (Cengiz *et al.*, 1988). However, the uremia-related growth factor(s) causing structural or numeric changes of chromosomes remain unclear.

Renal cell carcinoma in dialysis patients is often accompanied by other malignancies (Shikura *et al.*, 1991). Multiple cancers were found in 4 out of 35 patients (total of 40 malignancies, including nine renal cell carcinomas): three of four cases were double cancer and one was triple cancer including renal cell carcinoma, suggesting that immunosurveillance is impaired in dialysis patients with cancer.

Diagnosis of renal cell carcinoma in dialysis patients

Since less than 10% of renal cell carcinomas in dialysis patients are symptomatic, screening is needed to detect the tumor (Ishikawa, 1991*b*). If a solid mass is found, it is necessary to examine whether blood flow is present in the solid mass (Ishikawa, 1991*b*). For this purpose, bolus-enhanced, helical computed tomographic scanning is the best diagnostic modality. Gadolinium-enhanced, magnetic resonance imaging (Terens *et al.*, 1992) is also useful in evaluating the indications for operation. In an application of the recently developed sonographic angiography, 12 out of 13 tumors in dialysis patients showed enhancement (Takase *et al.*, 1994). If blood flow is depicted, whether as hypervascular or hypovascular by angiography, enhancement is also depicted by any of these modalities. Papillary cell tumor tends to be a hypovascular tumor, and non-papillary clear-cell tumor a hypervascular one.

When a mass in a short-term dialysis patient is seen protruding from the surface of the atrophic kidney with acquired cysts, it is relatively easy to make the diagnosis of renal cell carcinoma, but in a patient on long-term dialysis the solid mass is surrounded by multiple acquired cysts (Fig. 7.1), and it is therefore very difficult to make this diagnosis.

The most important differential diagnosis of renal cell carcinoma is that from hemorrhagic cysts. Blood flow is detectable by diagnostic imaging techniques in renal cell carcinoma (Ishikawa, 1991*b*).

Treatment of renal cell carcinoma in dialysis patients

A solid mass with blood flow is detectable using diagnostic imaging, and such a mass should be surgically treated regardless of the size (Ishikawa, 1991*b*). Some investigators (Grantham and Levine, 1985; Levine, 1992) recommend surgery if the tumor diameter is greater than 2 or 3 cm. Patients with a tumor measuring less than 2 cm should be followed every 6 months. In rare cases some renal cell carcinomas as small as 1.4 cm metastasized, and the growth of these tumors in dialysis patients can be either slow or rapid. Therefore we perform nephrectomy irrespective of the tumor size. If there is extensive enlargement of a kidney (weight more than 500 g) due to acquired cysts, nephrectomy may be indicated, even though the detection of a solid mass is not diagnostically conclusive (Ishikawa *et al.*, 1990). Unilateral nephrectomy on the affected side is recommended since bilateral nephrectomy causes severe hypotension and the patient's quality of life is impaired, even though the anemia is treated with recombinant erythropoietin. The contralateral kidney should be examined every 6 months as it sometimes develops renal cell carcinoma, but the incidence is not high enough to warrant bilateral nephrectomy.

Screening method for renal cell carcinoma in dialysis patients

Many investigators (Grantham and Levine, 1985; Matson and Cohen, 1990; Chandhoke *et al.*, 1992; Levine, 1992; Bretan, 1994; Sarasin *et al.*, 1995) agree that high-risk patients should be screened to detect renal cell carcinoma, especially after 3 years' hemodialysis. Ishikawa (1991*b*) recommends that all patients be screened after the start of hemodialysis because some renal cell carcinomas are detected in short-term dialysis patients without acquired cysts (Ishikawa and Shinoda, 1983). However, Levine (1992), Chandohoke *et al.* (1992), Sarasin *et al.* (1995), and others have stated that routine screening would not be justified based on cost–effect considerations. Chandhoke *et al.* (1992) reported that there is not a high incidence of renal cell carcinoma and that acquired cysts and renal cell carcinoma are found together only by chance. Sarasin *et al.* (1995) compared two screening methods using decision analysis. In one method all dialysis patients were screened at 3 years' dialysis and only those patients with acquired cysts were screened every year thereafter. In the second method only patients with symptoms were examined by imaging techniques. In the first method the number of deaths from cancer of 20-year-old dialysis patients, whose residual life span is 25 years, would be halved compared with those who were not screened, but the life span may be prolonged by 1.6 years. However, for 58-year-old patients, beginning dialysis with a life expectancy of 5 years, screening may prolong life expectancy by only 4 or 5 days. Therefore, routine screening for all dialysis patients is not justified in terms of cost-effectiveness. The benefit of screening depends on the incidence of metastatic renal cell carcinoma in dialysis patients and the general condition of the patients. Sarasin *et al.* (1995) agreed that screening may be of benefit in young dialysis patients, although to what degree is not clear. If the incidence of renal cell carcinoma we estimated is applied to decision analysis, the degree of benefit becomes higher.

At least those young dialysis patients with a high risk of renal cell carcinoma (male dialysis patients with more than 10 years' hemodialysis and enlarged kidneys due to extensive cystic changes) should be screened for renal cell carcinoma once a year using either sonography or computed tomographic scanning. Moreover, potential recipients of renal grafts should be screened before the operation and, if possible, 1 month postsurgery because it is easier to find renal cell carcinoma after the regression of acquired cysts (Ishikawa *et al.*, 1993).

Conclusions

This review of the literature pertaining to acquired renal cystic disease and renal tumors in long-term dialysis patients (more than 10 years' dialysis) revealed a number of trends, summarized as follows:

1. Acquired renal cystic disease is observed in 90% of patients who have been on hemodialysis for more than 10 years. Male patients present more extensive and earlier cystic changes than female patients. Renal cell carcinoma develops in 444 patients per year per 100 000 patients on hemodialysis for more than 10 years.
2. The incidence of renal cell carcinoma in male and female dialysis patients is 18-fold and 15-fold higher, respectively, than that in the general population. The incidence in male patients is four times higher than that in female patients and, compared with patients on hemodialysis for less than 10 years, patients on hemodialysis for more than 10 years show a 4-fold higher frequency.
3. Papillary renal cell tumors are related to acquired cysts and their incidence may be increased in long-term dialysis patients, whereas non-papillary clear-cell carcinoma may develop at any time after the start of hemodialysis.
4. A sequence of events from cyst to papillary adenoma to papillary renal cell carcinoma is proposed. Uremic metabolites and growth factors affect the tubular epithelia in an autocrine or paracrine manner and cause changes in the numbers of certain chromosomes. Non-papillary renal cell carcinoma initially develops as a carcinoma and may not be related to acquired cysts.
5. Young dialysis patients on hemodialysis for more than 10 years—as a high-risk group—should be screened annually using sonography or computed tomographic scanning. Before renal transplantation, all potential recipients should be examined for renal cell carcinoma because of its high metastatic rate.

References

Bommer, J., Waldherr, R., van Kaick, G., Strauss, L., and Ritz, E. (1980). Acquired renal cysts in uremic patients—in vivo demonstration by computed tomography. *Clinical Nephrology*, **14**, 299–303.

Bretan, P. N. Jr. (1994). Acquired renal cystic disease: is there a need for screening for renal cell carcinoma in patients with renal failure? *Seminars in Urology*, **7**, 89–92.

Carone, F. A., Nakamura, S., Caputo, M., Bacallao, R., Nelson, W. J., and Kanwar, Y. S. (1994). Cell polarity in human renal cystic disease. *Laboratory Investigation*, **70**, 648–55.

Cengiz, K., Block, A. M., Hossfeld, D. K., Anthone, R., Anthone, S., and Sandberg, A. A. (1988). Sister chromatid exchange and chromosome abnormalities in uremic patients. *Cancer Genetics and Cytogenetics*, **36**, 55–67.

Chandhoke, P. S., Torrence, R. J., Clayman, R.V., and Rothstein, M. (1992). Acquired cystic disease of the kidney: a management dilemma. *Journal of Urology*, **147**, 969–74.

Chung-Park, M., Ricanati, E., Lankerani, M., and Kedia, K. (1983). Acquired renal cysts and multiple renal cell and urothelial tumors. *Clinical Pathology*, **79**, 238–42.

Concolino, G., Santonati, A., Lubrano, C., Flammia, G. P., Ombres, M., and DiSilverio, F. (1993). Acquired cystic kidney disease: the hormonal hypothesis. *Urology*, **41**, 170–5.

Corless, C. L., Aburatani, H., Fletcher, J. A., Housman, D. E., Amin, M. B., and Weinberg, D. S. (1996). Papillary renal cell carcinoma, quantitation of chromosomes 7 and 17 by FISH, analysis of chromosomes 3p for LOH, and DNA ploidy. *Diagnostic Molecular Pathology*, **5**, 53–64.

Dlugosz, B. A., Bretan, P. N. Jr., Novick, A. C., *et al.* (1989). Causes of death in kidney transplant recipients: 1970 to present. *Transplantation Proceedings*, **21**, 2168–70.

Dunnill, M. S., Millard, P. R., and Oliver, D. (1977). Acquired cystic disease of the kidneys: a hazard of long-term intermittent maintenance haemodialysis. *Journal of Clinical Pathology*, **30**, 868–77.

Edmunds, M. E., Devoy, M., Tomson, C. R. V., *et al.* (1991). Plasma erythropoietin levels and acquired cystic disease of the kidney in patients receiving regular haemodialysis treatment. *British Journal of Haematology*, **78**, 275–7.

Feiner, H. D., Katz, L. A., and Gallo, G. R. (1981). Acquired cystic disease of kidney in chronic dialysis patients. *Urology*, **17**, 260–4.

Fujimoto, I., and Hanai, A. (1992). Japan, Osaka prefecture. In *Cancer incidence in five continents* (ed. D. M. Parkin, C. S. Muir, S. L. Whelan, Y. T. Gao, J. Ferlay, and J. Powell), pp. 498–501. International Agency for Research on Cancer, Lyon.

Gardner, K. D. Jr. and Evan, A. P. (1984). Cystic kidneys: an enigma evolves. *American Journal of Kidney Diseases*, **3**, 403–13.

Gehrig, J. J. Jr., Gottheiner, T. I., and Swenson, R. S. (1985). Acquired cystic disease of the end-stage kidney. *American Journal of Medicine*, **79**, 609–20.

Glicklich, D., Kutcher, R., Rosenblatt, R., and Barth, R. H. (1990). Time-related increase in hematocrit on chronic hemodialysis: uncertain role of renal cysts. *American Journal of Kidney Diseases*, **15**, 46–54.

Grantham, J. J. (1991). Acquired cystic kidney disease. *Kidney International*, **40**, 143–52.

Grantham, J. J. (1993). Fluid secretion, cellular proliferation, and the pathogenesis of renal epithelial cysts. *Journal of the American Society of Nephrology*, **3**, 1843–57.

Grantham, J. J., and Levine, E. (1985). Acquired cystic disease: replacing one kidney disease with another. *Kidney International*, **28**, 99–105.

Hajdu, S. I., and Thomas, A. G. (1967). Renal cell carcinoma at autopsy. *Journal of Urology*, **97**, 978–82.

Herms, S. P., Benkirane, H., Acosta, R. C., and Sampol, J. J. B. (1993). Enfermedad quistica renal adquirida, hemorragia renal espontanea bilateral y trasplante renal funcionante. Revision de la literatura y aportacion de un caso. *Actas Urologicas Espanolas*, **17**, 143–7.

Herrera, G. A. (1991). C-*erb* B-2 amplification in cystic renal disease. *Kidney International*, **40**, 509–13.

Horiguchi, T., and Ishikawa, I. (1993). Immunohistochemical study in acquired cystic disease of the kidney—expression of vimentin, epidermal growth factor, epidermal growth factor receptor and c-*erb* B2 gene product. *Japanese Journal of Nephrology*, **35**, 797–807. (Japanese).

Hughson, M. D., Hennigar, G. R., and McManus, J. F. A. (1980). Atypical cysts, acquired renal cystic disease, and renal cell tumors in end stage dialysis kidneys. *Laboratory Investigation*, **42**, 475–80.

Hughson, M. D., Buchwald, D., and Fox, M. (1986). Renal neoplasia and acquired cystic kidney disease in patients receiving long-term dialysis. *Archives of Pathology and Laboratory Medicine*, **110**, 592–601.

Hughson, M. D., Meloni, A. M., Dunn, T., Silva, F. G., and Sandberg, A. A. (1993). Tumorigenesis in the end-stage kidney. In *Proceedings of the fifth international workshop on polycystic kidney disease* (ed. P. A. Gabow and J. J. Grantham), pp. 94–7. Polycystic Kidney Research Foundation, Kansas City.

Ishikawa, I. (1985*a*). Unusual composition of cyst fluid in acquired cystic disease of the end-stage kidney. *Nephron*, **41**, 373–4.

Ishikawa, I. (1985*b*). Uremic acquired cystic disease of kidney. *Urology*, **26**, 101–8.

Ishikawa, I. (1986). Beta 2-microglobulin level of cyst fluid in uremic acquired cystic disease of the kidney. *Nephron*, **44**, 381.

Ishikawa, I. (1991*a*). Acquired cystic disease: mechanisms and manifestations. *Seminars in Nephrology*, **11**, 671–84.

Ishikawa, I. (1991*b*). Uremic acquired renal cystic disease, natural history and complications. *Nephron*, **58**, 257–67.

Ishikawa, I. (1992*a*). Acquired cysts and neoplasms of the kidneys in renal allograft recipients. *Contributions to Nephrology*, **100**, 254–68.

Ishikawa, I. (1992*b*). Acquired renal cystic disease and its complications in continuous ambulatory peritoneal dialysis patients. *Peritoneal Dialysis International*, **12**, 292–7.

Ishikawa, I. (1993*a*). Renal cell carcinoma in chronic hemodialysis patients—a 1990 questionnaire study in Japan. *Kidney International*, **43**, S167–S169.

Ishikawa, I. (1993*b*). Renal cell carcinoma in chronic hemodialysis patients—a 1992 questionnaire study. *Journal of Japanese Society for Dialysis Therapy*, **26**, 1355–62. (Japanese).

Ishikawa, I. (1996). Renal cell carcinoma in chronic hemodialysis patients—a 1994 questionnaire study. *Journal of Japanese Society for Dialysis Therapy*, **29**, 109–16. (Japanese).

Ishikawa, I., and Kovacs, G. (1993). High incidence of papillary renal cell tumours in patients on chronic haemodialysis. *Histopathology*, **22**, 135–9.

Ishikawa, I., and Shinoda, A. (1983). Renal adenocarcinoma with or without acquired cysts in chronic hemodialysis patients. *Clinical Nephrology*, **20**, 321–2.

Ishikawa, I., Saito, Y., Onouchi, Z., *et al.* (1980). Development of acquired cystic disease and adenocarcinoma of the kidney in glomerulonephritic chronic hemodialysis patients. *Clinical Nephrology*, **14**, 1–6.

Ishikawa, I., Yuri, T., Kitada, H., and Shinoda, A. (1983). Regression of acquired cystic disease of the kidney after successful renal transplantation. *American Journal of Nephrology*, **3**, 310–14.

Ishikawa, I., Onouchi, Z., Saito, Y., *et al.* (1985). Sex differences in acquired cystic disease of the kidney on long-term dialysis. *Nephron*, **39**, 336–40.

Ishikawa, I., Shikura, N., Horiguchi, T., *et al.* (1988). Size distribution of acquired cysts in chronic hemodialysis patients. *Journal of Kanazawa Medical University*, **13**, 171–5.

Ishikawa, I., Horiguchi, T., and Shikura, N. (1989*a*). Lectin peroxidase conjugate reactivity in acquired cystic disease of the kidney. *Nephron*, **51**, 211–14.

Ishikawa, I., Saito, Y., Shikura, N., *et al.* (1989*b*). Excretion of hippuran into acquired renal cysts in chronic hemodialysis patient. *Nephron*, **52**, 110–11.

Ishikawa, I., Shikura, N., Kitada, H., Yuri, T., Shinoda, A., and Nakazawa, T. (1989*c*). Severity of acquired renal cysts in native kidneys and renal allograft with long-standing poor function. *American Journal of Kidney Diseases*, **14**, 18–24.

Ishikawa, I., Saito, Y., Shikura, N., Kitada, H., Shinoda, A., and Suzuki, S. (1990). Ten-year prospective study on the development of renal cell carcinoma in dialysis patients. *American Journal of Kidney Diseases*, **16**, 452–8.

Ishikawa, I., Shikura, N., Nagahara, M., Shinoda, A., and Saito, Y. (1991*a*). Comparison of severity of acquired renal cysts between CAPD and hemodialysis. *Advances in Peritoneal Dialysis*, **7**, 91–5.

Ishikawa, I., Shikura, N., and Sinoda, A. (1991*b*). Cystic transformation in native kidneys in renal allograft recipients with long-standing good function. *American Journal of Nephrology*, **11**, 217–23.

Ishikawa, I., Shikura, N., and Ozaki, M. (1993). Papillary renal cell carcinoma with numeric changes of chromosomes in a long-term hemodialysis patient: a karyotype analysis. *American Journal of Kidney Diseases*, **21**, 553–6.

Ishikawa, I., Ozaki, M., Tominaga, Y., and Nakamura, Y. (1996*a*). Cytogenetic abnormalities in renal cell carcinomas associated with uremic acquired renal cystic disease. *Journal of Kanazawa Medical University*, **21**, 76–81.

Ishikawa, I., Yamaya, H., Nakamura, M. *et al.* (1996*b*). Erythropoietin does not affect the development and progression of acquired renal cystic disease. *Nephrology, Dialysis, Transplantation*, **11**, A262. (Abstract).

Ishikawa, I., Saito, Y., Nakamura, M., *et al.* (1997). Fifteen-year follow-up of acquired renal cystic disease—a gender difference. *Nephron*, **75**, 315–20.

Ito, F., Horita, S., Yanagisawa, H., *et al.* (1993). Bellini's duct tumor associated with end stage renal disease: a case diagnosed by lectin immunohistochemistry. *Acta Urologica Japonica*, **39**, 735–8.

Kessler, M., Testevuide, P., Aymard, B., and Huu, T. C. (1991). Acquired renal cystic disease mimicking adult polycystic kidney disease in a patient undergoing long-term hemodialysis. *American Journal of Nephrology*, **11**, 513–17.

Klotz, L. H., Kulkarni, C., and Mills, G. (1991). End stage renal disease serum contains a specific renal cell growth factor. *Journal of Urology*, **145**, 156–60.

Kovacs, G. (1993). Molecular differential pathology of renal cell tumours. *Histopathology*, **22**, 1–8.

Kovacs, G. (1995). High frequency of papillary renal-cell tumours in end-stage kidneys—is there a molecular genetic explanation? *Nephrology, Dialysis, Transplantation*, **10**, 593–6.

Levine, E. (1992). Renal cell carcinoma in uremic acquired renal cystic disease: incidence, detection, and management. *Urologic Radiology*, **13**, 203–10.

Levine, E., Grantham, J. J., Slusher, S. L., Greathouse, J. L., and Krohn, B. P. (1984). CT of acquired cystic kidney disease and renal tumors in long-term dialysis patients. *American Journal of Roentgenology*, **142**, 125–31.

Levine, E., Grantham, J. J., and MacDougall, M. L. (1987). Spontaneous subcapsular and perinephric hemorrhage in end-stage kidney disease: clinical and CT findings. *American Journal of Roentgenology*, **148**, 755–8.

Levine, E., Slusher, S. L., Grantham, J. J., and Wetzel, L. H. (1991). Natural history of acquired renal cystic disease in dialysis patients: a prospective longitudinal CT study. *American Journal of Roentgenology*, **156**, 501–6.

Lien, Y-H.H., Hunt, K. R., Siskind, M. S., and Zukoski, C. (1993). Association of cyclosporin A with acquired cystic disease of the native kidneys in renal transplant recipients. *Kidney International*, **44**, 613–6.

MacDougall, M. L., Welling, L. W., and Wiegmann, T. B. (1987). Renal adenocarcinoma and acquired cystic disease in chronic hemodialysis patients. *American Journal of Kidney Diseases*, **9**, 166–71.

MacDougall, M. L., Welling, L. W., and Wiegmann, T. B. (1990). Prediction of carcinoma in acquired cystic disease as a function of kidney weight. *Journal of the American Society of Nephrology*, **1**, 828–31.

Makita, Y., Inenaga, T., Kinjo, M. Komatsu, K., Onoyama, K., and Fujishima, M. (1991). Renal oncocytoma developed in a long-term hemodialysis patient. *Nephron*, **57**, 355–7.

Marco-Franco, J. E., Torres, V. E., Nixon, D. E., *et al.* (1991). Oxalate, silicon and vanadium in acquired cystic kidney disease. *Clinical Nephrology*, **35**, 52–8.

Maruyama, S., Gejyo, F., Arakawa, M. (1991). A case of erythropoietin producing renal cell carcinoma with hemodialysis. *Japanese Journal of Nephrology*, **33**, 1205. (Japanese abstract).

Matson, M. A., and Cohen, E. P. (1990). Acquired cystic kidney disease: occurrence, prevalence, and renal cancers. *Medicine*, **69**, 217–26.

Matsumoto, M., Sakamoto, K., Kamura, K., *et al.* (1995). A case of renal cell carcinoma of the left native kidney following renal transplantation. *Ishoku*, **30**, 605–10. (Japanese).

Mickisch, O., Bommer, J., Bachmann, S., Waldherr, R., Mann, J. F. E., and Ritz, E. (1984). Multicystic transformation of kidneys in chronic renal failure. *Nephron*, **38**, 93–9.

Miller, L. R., Soffer, O., Nassar, V. H., and Kutner, M. H. (1989). Acquired renal cystic disease in end-stage renal disease: an autopsy study of 155 cases. *American Journal of Nephrology*, **9**, 322–8.

Moskowitz, D. W., Bonar, S. L., Liu, W., Sirgi, C. F., Marcus, M. D., and Clayman, R. V. (1995). Epidermal growth factor precursor is present in a variety of human renal cyst fluids. *Journal of Urology*, **153**, 578–83.

Nadasdy, T., Laszik, Z., Lajoie, G., Blick, K. E., Wheeler, D. E., and Silva, F. G. (1995). Proliferative activity of cyst epithelium in human renal cystic diseases. *Journal of the American Society of Nephrology*, **5**, 1462–8.

Narasimhan, N., Golper, T. A., Wolfson, M., Rahatzad, M., and Bennett, W. M. (1986). Clinical characteristics and diagnostic considerations in acquired renal cystic disease. *Kidney International*, **30**, 748–52.

Oliveras, A., Puig, J. M., Lloveras, J., *et al.* (1993). Risks of acquired renal cystic disease in long-term renal transplant recipients: report of one case and general review. *Clinical Transplantation*, **7**, 578–81.

Penn, I. (1987). Cancers following cyclosporine therapy. *Transplantation*, **43**, 32–5.

Port, F. K., Ragheb, N. E., Schwartz, A. G., and Hawthorne, V. M. (1989). Neoplasms in dialysis patients: a population-based study. *American Journal of Kidney Diseases*, **14**, 119–23.

Sarasin, F. P., Wong, J. B., Levey, A. S., and Meyer, K. B. (1995). Screening for acquired cystic kidney disease: a decision analytic perspective. *Kidney International*, **48**, 207–19.

Shikura, N., Ishikawa, I., Ishii, H., *et al.* (1991). Double cancer in dialysis patients. *Journal of Japanese Society for Dialysis Therapy*, **24**, 678. (Japanese abstract).

Suvarna, S. K., Ahuja, M., and Brown, C. B. (1994). Sarcomatoid renal cell carcinoma arising in hemodialysis-associated acquired cystic kidney disease presenting with disseminated bone marrow infiltration. *American Journal of Kidney Diseases*, **24**, 581–5.

Takahashi, S., Shirai, T., Ogawa, K., *et al.* (1993). Renal cell adenomas and carcinomas in hemodialysis patients: relationship between hemodialysis period and development of lesions. *Acta Pathologica Japonica*, **43**, 674–82.

Takase, K., Takahashi, S., Tazawa, S., Terasawa, Y., and Sakamoto, K. (1994). Renal cell carcinoma associated with chronic renal failure: evaluation with sonographic angiography. *Radiology*, **192**, 787–92.

Terasawa, Y., Suzuki, Y., Morita, M., Kato, M., Suzuki, K., and Sekino, H. (1994). Ultrasonic diagnosis of renal cell carcinoma in hemodialysis patients. *Journal of Urology*, **152**, 846–51.

Terens, W. L., Gluck, R., Golimbu, M., and Rofsky, N. M. (1992). Use of gadolinium–DTPA-enhanced MRI to characterize renal mass in patient with renal insufficiency. *Urology*, **40**, 152–4.

Thoenes, W., Storkel, S., Rumpelt, H. J., and Moll, R. (1990). Cytomorphological typing of renal cell carcinoma—a new approach. *European Urology*, **18** (Suppl. 2), 6–9.

Tosaka, A., Ohya, K., Yamada, K., *et al.* (1990). Incidence and properties of renal masses and asymptomatic renal cell carcinoma detected by abdominal ultrasonography. *Journal of Urology*, **144**, 1097–9.

Vandeursen, H., vanDamme, B., Baert, J., and Baert, L. (1991). Acquired cystic disease of the kidney analyzed by microdissection. *Journal of Urology*, **146**, 1168–72.

Wilson, P. D., Sherwood, A. C., Palla, K., Du, J., Watson, R., and Norman, J. T. (1991). Reversed polarity of Na$^+$–K$^+$-ATPase: mislocation to apical plasma membranes in polycystic kidney disease epithelia. *American Journal of Physiology*, **260**, F420–F430.

Yoshida, M. A., Shishikura, A., Oshima, H., and Ikeuchi, T. (1993). Cytogenetic analyses of renal cell carcinoma cells from a patient with chronic renal failure, acquired cystic disease of the kidney and a constitutional chromosome translocation. In *Proceedings of the Japanese Cancer Association*, 52nd *Annual Meeting*, p. 208. Japanese Cancer Association, Sendai. (Abstract.)

8

Psychological adaptation and quality of life of the patient with end-stage renal disease

Fredric O. Finkelstein and Susan H. Finkelstein

Introduction

Successful psychosocial adaptation to dialysis is the key to long-term survival. This chapter sets out to review the various psychological and social problems that dialysis patients have to face.

The assessment of the psychological adaptation of the patient with end-stage renal disease (ESRD) has intrigued investigators for many years. In the initial years of ESRD therapy, researchers focused their attention on the physical and psychological limitations and the difficulties and restrictions imposed on patients by their illness and treatment modality (Abram, 1974; Levy, 1994). The increased mortality of patients with ESRD, the demands placed on these patients by their therapy, and the myriad physical and social problems that engulf them because of their illness have been repeatedly emphasized. Developing effective tools and strategies of psychosocial assessment and intervention has perhaps become more important as the incidence and prevalence of end-stage renal failure has increased and the mean age of the ESRD population has increased throughout the world. More recently, however, efforts to understand better the experience of the dialysis patient have focused researchers' attention on the quality of life experienced by these patients (Gokal, 1993; Powe *et al.*, 1996; Salek, 1996; Steele *et al.*, 1996*a*). The assessment of quality of life has presented problems and raised basic philosophical issues for investigators (Gill and Feinstein, 1994; Nissenson, 1994; Anonymous, 1995; Fallowfield, 1996). Just how should quality of life be measured? What in fact is important in assessing a patient's quality of life? It is perhaps surprising that preliminary work has suggested that when dialysis patients are asked about their quality of life, they frequently perceive their quality of life as being as good if not better than members of the general population (Evans *et al.*, 1985, 1990; Steele *et al.*, 1996*a*).

Specific areas of psychological and psychosocial difficulties experienced by the patient with ESRD have been studied by several investigators. Although these areas have often been studied in isolation, their inter-relationship is obviously important. Furthermore, the relationship among these variables and the medical condition and therapy of the patient must be considered. The medical status of the patient may affect the criteria used to assess their psychological status. For example, symptoms of uremia may overlap with symptoms of depression. The presence of anemia and hyperparathyroidism may affect the assessment of several psychosocial variables. Side-effects of medication, particularly antihypertensive medication, may affect the assessment of psychological distress. And, the patient's sense of well-being may be positively affected by the adequacy of the dialysis therapy or negatively affected by the intensity of the dialysis regimen.

The areas of psychosocial difficulties experienced by the patient with ESRD can be conveniently thought of in two general domains: areas of intrapsychic distress and areas of interpersonal stress. Areas of intrapsychic distress include depression, anxiety, problems of self-esteem and body image, organic dysfunction, and underlying psychosocial illness. Interpersonal stressors include family dysfunction, marital discord, sexual difficulties, and employment and rehabilitation. It is important to keep in mind that the overall goal of understanding these areas of stress for the medical team providing care to the ESRD patient is to understand the difficulties of the patient better, to intervene more effectively with patient care, to maximize the patient's overall quality of life, and to facilitate the medical management of the patient.

Areas of intrapsychic distress

Depression

Depression is generally regarded as the most common psychological problem encountered in patients with ESRD (Levy, 1994). However, the incidence of depressive disorders in ESRD patients is reported to be quite variable, with some investigators reporting an incidence of up to 60% and others reporting an incidence as low as 5% (De-Nour, 1994). Wolcott *et al.* (1988) have suggested that 20–30% of dialysis patients have clinically significant affective disorders. Bonney *et al.* (1978), in a study of a large cohort of hemodialysis patients, have reported that ESRD patients have similar depression scores on self-administered questionnaires as patients seeking help at an outpatient psychiatric clinic. The problems with diagnosing depression in ESRD patients using standardized questionnaires have recently been reviewed by De-Nour (1994). This author has emphasized that the incidence may vary not only because of the patient mix (age of patients and the presence of comorbid disease) but also because of the instrument used to assess the depressive symptomatology. For example, the Beck Depression Inventory (BDI) often indicates higher degrees of depression than the Multiple Affect Adjective Check List (MAACL) because of the presence of numerous 'physical' items on the BDI.

Since patients with physical illness may feel sad and anhedonic, it is important to specify what in fact is meant by depression. The syndrome of clinical depression consists of depressive affect (feelings of sadness, being downhearted and blue, hopelessness, helplessness, guilt, pessimism, etc.), and is accompanied by changes in sleep, appetite, and libido. The evaluation of depression must include a systematic assessment of the unique physical and psychosocial factors that characterize each individual. While symptoms of depression can be related to specific details of the patient's medical condition, they can also develop as a result of loss. Individuals with ESRD experience many losses, ranging from losses of their normal physical function, to changes in their daily structure, to changes in their marital and occupational roles. The specific concerns which depressed people express may be a function of their life-stage situation and the demands placed on them, and determined by where they may be in their life. For example, the depressed young adult worries about the choice of career and partner; the depressed person in middle age worries about adjusting to marriage after the children have left the home, or about problems with work or career; and the depressed, older person worries about health, declining financial resources, the death of friends, family members, and spouse, and one's own mortality. People who are not depressed share these same concerns but seem less severely affected by them. The demand on the individual's capacity for adaptation and adjustment to these psycho-social changes inevitably impacts on how he/she responds to the dialysis regimen.

The details and specifics of the overall medical management of the ESRD patient will affect the assessment of the presence of depressive symptomatology. Thus, the extremely high incidence of depression noted in the early years of renal replacement therapy (the 1960s and 1970s) may not be applicable to current treatment modalities. For example, the treatment of anemia with recombinant erythropoietin can result in an improvement in depressive symptomatology when hematocrit levels are increased to 32–38% (Evans *et al.*, 1990; Levin, 1992). Will further increases in hematocrit, with the more judicious use of recombinant erythropoietin, result in a still further decrease in depressive symptomatology? In addition, recent work has focused attention on the importance of maintaining adequate doses of dialysis therapy, both for hemodialysis as well as a continuous ambulatory peritoneal dialysis (CAPD). Optimal doses of dialysis for both modalities are still not yet defined, but many investigators feel that the provision of adequate doses of dialysis may not only lessen mortality rates but may also improve the patients' sense of psychological well-being, lessen the frequency of physical symptoms, and thus decrease the incidence of depressive symptomatology. For example, the results of the National Cooperative Dialysis Study suggested that the patients randomized to treatment modalities designed to maintain low blood urea nitrogen levels had significantly lower depression scores on the Minnesota Multiphasic Personality Inventory than patients randomized to maintain high blood urea nitrogen levels (Maher *et al.*, 1983).

A discussion of depression must also include suicidality and homicidality. Depressed patients may feel that they are a terrible burden and that others would be better off if they were dead. They might wish they would go to sleep and never wake up. In addition to passive suicidal ideation, more severely depressed patients may be preoccupied with a specific plan about how they might take their own lives (e.g. they may consider stopping dialysis or overdosing on their medication). Some patients may lash out and blame others for their condition and ruminate about how they will retaliate. Suicidal ideation, whether passive or active, as well as homicidal ideation are not uncommonly encountered in dialysis patients. Often these feelings are casually or humorously tossed out. In whatever manner they are presented, it is essential that they be taken very seriously. It is important to listen to what the patient is thinking and feeling and to explore the specifics of his ideations, plans, and intentions. It is also important to mobilize a support system of family, friends, significant others, and carers, to make a plan for the safety of a patient at risk for suicide or homicide.

The importance of elective discontinuation of dialysis as a cause of mortality in ESRD patients has been emphasized by some investigators (Neu and Kjellstrand, 1986; Shulman *et al.*, 1989; De-Nour, 1994). For example, Neu and Kjellstrand (1986) reported that 9% of their patients discontinued dialysis, accounting for 22% of the deaths in their patient population. Other investigators report lower rates of elective withdrawal from dialysis as a cause of death in their ESRD treatment group (Shulman *et al.*, 1989). Discontinuation of dialysis, or a desire to do so, by long-term dialysis patients when encountering yet another complication is an important cause of death in these patients (Chapter 1). It should also be stressed that suicidality and its resulting acting-out behavior may well contribute to a substantially higher percentage of deaths in dialysis patients than is generally appreciated from the reports of elective withdrawal from dialysis. For example, dietary indiscretions (such as excess fluid intake and potassium ingestion) and poor compliance with the dialysis treatment prescription can be perhaps understood as expressions of a patient's mood and psychological condition.

The relationship between depression and patient survival on dialysis has recently been reviewed in detail by Kimmel *et al.* (1993). These authors point out that the results of the few studies that are available provide conflicting data. They note that depression can affect certain variables, such as immunological functioning, nutritional status, and patient compliance, that may well impact on the survival of dialysis patients. But a convincing demonstration of a relationship between survival and depression has thus far not been clearly demonstrated.

Effective treatment of depression in dialysis patients involves early and proactive assessment and diagnosis, psychosocial counseling, and psychopharmacologic intervention as needed. The use of antidepressant medication in patients with renal failure presents challenging problems, since the appropriate dosing of these drugs in patients without renal function is not clear and the side-effects of these medications often overlap with the difficulties experienced by the patients. Thus, tricyclic antidepressants can cause orthostatic hypotension, tachycardias, cardiac conduction disturbances, dryness of the mouth, bowel disturbances, and central nervous system dysfunction. The selective serotonin uptake inhibitors can cause headache, tremor, gastrointestinal problems such as nausea and diarrhea, agitation and nervousness, and anorgasmia in both males and females. Monoamine oxidase inhibitors can cause significant problems with hypotension. Thus they must be used with extreme caution in dialysis patients (Levy, 1994). Although many of these drugs are primarily metabolized by the liver, the metabolites are often excreted, at least in part, by the kidney, making precise dosing adjustments in patients with renal failure somewhat problematical. There are in fact few studies in the literature that specifically examine the effectiveness of antidepressant medication in dialysis patients. Kennedy *et al.* (1989), examining the effect of tricyclic medication in a small cohort of dialysis patients suffering from major depression, reported an amelioration of depressive symptomatology in the majority of patients. These authors noted that a lower dosage was used in their patients than in patients with normal renal function. They suggested that this may reflect the patients' increased sensitivity to the adverse and possibly the thera-peutic effects of the drugs.

Lithium carbonate can be used in dialysis patients, when clinically indicated, despite the fact that the drug is entirely excreted by the kidney and is removed by both peritoneal and hemodialysis (Levy, 1994). Careful attention to dosing regimens is clearly necessary.

Anxiety

Dialysis patients are exposed to a variety of stresses—stresses that result from their illness, treatment, comorbid disease, and social interactions. Thus, it is not surpris-ing that ESRD patients have symptoms and complaints that reflect the effects of these stresses. It is not uncommon for dialysis patients to experience symptoms of anxiety. Scores for ESRD patients on various tools to assess anxiety are higher than for control patients (Bonney *et al.*, 1978; Steele *et al.*, 1996a). Wolcott *et al.* (1988) have suggested that 50–70% of dialysis patients report moderate to severe degrees of stress related to a variety of factors, including health status, social relationships and function, financial status, and vocational activity. Generalized anxiety, anticipatory anxiety, even performance anxiety are not unusual when dialysis treatment begins. Changes in the treatment regimen and/or the condition of the patient can also result in not-unexpected symptoms of anxiety. Long-term patients can become anxious about vascular access failure and the emergence of new complications.

Assessing the anxiety level of the individual patient is important since it may pro-vide clues to the carer about the level of stress and discomfort experienced by the patient. It is well documented that anxiety and stress may affect various aspects of the medical care of patients (Ruberman *et al.*, 1984; Kiecolt-Glaser *et al.*, 1995; Juer-gensen *et al.*, 1996). For example, anxiety levels, as assessed by the Patient Related Anxiety Scale in a cohort of CAPD patients, significantly correlated with the inci-dence of peritonitis (Juergensen *et al.*, 1996). Thus, the anxiety level may serve as a bar-ometer of the overall difficulties and stresses imposed on the patient.

When symptoms of anxiety are severe, persistent and intense, interfere with a patient's medical management, and/or interfere with a patient's overall adjustment to his illness and/or daily living, then therapeutic interventions become necessary. Therapy should initially consist of the appropriate psychosocial intervention, which can include brief individual treatment, cognitive, behavioral therapy focusing on stress reduction techniques, or couples/family counseling. Administration of short-acting benzodiazepine derivatives, such as lorazepan or alprazolam, may be of benefit in conjunction with counseling. Benzodiazepine drugs which have pharmacologically active metabolites, such as chlordiazepoxide amd diazepam, should be avoided since accumulation of these metabolites can result in significant toxicity (Levy, 1994).

Self-esteem and body image

Each individual has a public persona and a private self. The sense of inner self is based on one's personal history, especially the reflection and integration of how the nurturing adults responded in childhood. A childhood pattern of experiencing shaming responses (e.g. 'You stupid, clumsy oaf', in response to a spilled glass of milk) can result in feelings that one is defective and hopelessly beyond repair. In contrast, a pattern of positive, affirming responses (e.g. 'A little spilled milk is easy to clean up, let's do it together') helps to build self-confidence and the ability to be self-affirming. One's self concept is a critical factor in how an individual is able to manage the personal challenges and demands imposed by a chronic illness. If one's self-esteem is largely dependent on how others view oneself (e.g. 'I'm a successful business man', 'I'm an impeccable homemaker', 'I'm a fabulous athlete', etc.), the erosion of these functions and images as one is coping with the demands of a chronic treatment regimen, such as CAPD or hemodialysis, can result in a variety of emotional reactions, such as apathy, withdrawal, and irritability, or symptoms of anxiety and depression. The importance of the issue of the patient's self-esteem for the treatment team cannot be overlooked. Since all of us struggle with issues of self-esteem, being sensitive to these issues in dealing with the ESRD patient enables the treatment team to support and mobilize the patient's inner resources.

Every individual has a unique relationship with his or her own body. One's body image, like self-esteem, is more or less positive depending upon early childhood and personal experiences. In today's world, the media has created idealized images of beauty that we all compare ourselves to. Thinness is equated with goodness; fattness with slovenliness and stupidity. Plastic surgeons are kept busy helping individuals achieve a more ideal appearance. It is important, therefore, to be sensitive to how the dialysis patient is experiencing changes in his or her body. The decrease or cessation of urination, fluid and dietary restrictions, abdominal fullness, weight gain or loss, and the presence of a permanent catheter or fistula are assaults on the body and impact on one's body image. Acknowledging these effects and being sensitive to how patients are dealing with these changes supports their adjustment and maximizes their ability to successfully integrate these changes.

Organic dysfunction

Organic central nervous system dysfunction is commonly encountered in the ESRD patient and can be detected by standard psychological and neuropsychiatric tests. Thus, patients with renal failure have poorer performances than normal individuals on a variety of tests, including the Trailmaking Test, the Continuous Memory Test, and the Choice Reaction Test (Fraser and Arieff, 1988). In addition, these patients may demonstrate organic-like loss of intellectual function, particularly information processing. But, verbal learning, as measured by the Walton–Black Modified Word Learning Test, and performance learning, as measured by the Block Design Learning Test, may be normal in patients with renal failure (Fraser and Arieff, 1988).

The presence of organic dysfunction certainly impacts on the capacity and flexibility of the patient to cope with the various problems imposed on him by his illness and treatment. As the age of the dialysis population advances and the level of comorbid disease increases in severity, consideration of the impact of organic dysfunction will become more important in understanding the psychosocial adaptation of the

ESRD patient. Confusion, disorientation, short-term memory difficulty, problems with concentration, and other cognitive disturbances can be the result of a variety of factors. They may represent signs of or result from senility and dementia, a neuro-logical event, or clinical depression. In addition, a critical issue to consider in attempting to understand this organic dysfunction is the relationship between the medical management of the ESRD patient and the degree of organic dysfunction. For example, the treatment of anemia with recombinant erythropoietin has been shown to improve cognitive functioning in a large cohort of ESRD patients (Marsh *et al.*, 1991). Recently, increased attention has been paid to the development of more detailed standards for assessing the adequacy of dialysis delivered to both CAPD and hemodialysis patients. More careful attention will, therefore, need to be focused on the relationship between dialysis dose and measurements of organic brain dys-function and the neuropsychological status. These issues certainly require further investigation.

Underlying psychosocial illness

The assessment of the current psychosocial problems of the dialysis patient requires a detailed exploration of the pre-illness psychological and social adjustment of the in-dividual. Information about developmental patterns (including the attainment of milestones), cognitive and social patterns of family coping (especially conflict resolu-tion and problem solving), and resolution of issues of separation and emancipation is essential to the understanding of the current clinical picture of each patient. It is also important to elicit information concerning family history of significant psychiatric illness, such as psychotic, depressive, and anxiety disorders, as well as data about pre-vious episodes of psychiatric problems in the patient. Knowledge of the patient's psy-chosocial adjustment prior to the onset of dialysis, including experiences with prior psychiatric treatment and the results of therapy, will allow the clinical team to struc-ture and present the dialysis regimen and associated supportive services to best meet the specific and unique needs of the individual patient and his family.

Areas of interpersonal stress

Family problems

To understand the patients' adjustment to chronic dialysis therapy more fully, it is necessary to view patients in the context of their family. Family systems' theory assumes that the family is the single most powerful emotional system to which we belong and that the family is critical in shaping our experience and us as individuals. The family determines our belief system; it affects how we explain to ourselves what is happening (e.g. 'I'm being punished', 'It's God's will', 'I won't take this lying down'). The family determines our responses to and our ability to communicate with persons outside the family. It may thus determine a patient's response to the medical team, influencing attitudes that range from 'I'm in your hands', to 'I want to know everything you're doing and why'. Furthermore, the family can affect the patient's ability to give and receive information—crucial aspects of patient interaction with the health-care team. Family boundaries affect how an individual interacts with others. These boundaries have been classified as ranging on a continuum from rigid and impermeable (every man is out for himself), to enmeshed and permeable (it is difficult to tell where one person leaves off and the other begins), to intact (where autonomy is possible, and respectful negotiation, and giving and receiving of feedback characterize communication). Thus, families, like individuals, can be viewed as spanning a spectrum from healthy and high functioning, through rigid and neurotic, to chaotic and dysfunctional. Understanding the patient in the context of the family system allows the formulation of realistic expectations and appropriate treatment strategies to guide the treatment team's approach more effectively to the successful management of the individual.

Family function then must be seen as more than the sum of its parts. The structure, organization, and transactional patterns (how members typically interact with one another) of the family are important variables in determining the behavior of individual family members. In fact, according to family system's theory, understanding these variables may be more important than understanding intrapsychic dynamics in designing treatment strategies for individual patients.

Few investigators have directly studied the impact of family dynamics on the outcome of therapy for patients with ESRD. In a study of 23 patients maintained on in-center hemodialysis, Steidl *et al.* (1980) observed a correlation between overall family functioning and the staff's assessment of the patients' adjustment to their illness and compliance with their treatment regimen. It might be expected that the impact of family dynamics would be most evident in patients maintained on home dialysis, since these dynamics can affect the patient's ability to give and receive information, solve problems, and lucidly communicate with the medical team and family members providing supportive care for the patient. This in fact was studied by Carey *et al.* (1990) in an interesting review examining the causes for patient drop-out from CAPD and transfer to hemodialysis. In this study, families of CAPD patients were rated using the Beavers–Timberlawn Family Evaluation Scale. These investigators observed that psychosocial factors were primarily responsible for patient transfer from CAPD to hemodialysis in 24% of patients transferring and that peritonitis was responsible in 49% of patients. However, in patients who were members of poorly functioning families, 55% of transfers were due to psychosocial factors, while in patients who were members of highly functioning families only 12.5% of transfers were due to psychosocial factors. Furthermore, in patients over 60 years of age, 67% of patient transfers were due to psychosocial factors in patients from poorly functioning families, while only 5% of transfers were due to these factors in patients from highly functioning families. Thus, family dynamics appeared to influence the rate of transfer of patients with ESRD maintained on CAPD to hemodialysis, particularly for those patients over 60 years of age.

Marital problems

Just as it is important to understand the impact of the family dynamics on the adjustment of the dialysis patient, it is also important to understand the effects of the chronic illness and treatment regimen on the spouse, who inevitably shares the stress and burden of the illness often without the benefit of adequate attention and support, and the effects on the marital relationship itself. In fact, some investigators have suggested that the patients' ability to cope with the stresses of their illness may be more dependent on the nature and flexibility of their marital interactions than on the nature of their individual psyches (Streltzer *et al.*, 1978). The ways in which patients' chronic illness and dialysis treatments stress a marriage are often not fully explored by carers. Some symptoms of depression, anxiety, and organicity may well be present in the married dialysis patient. How these symptoms, as well as the treatment regimen itself, affect the spouse and the marital relationship are critically important. How couples view, share, and communicate about their situation can directly affect their ability to cope with the demands of their changing roles and functions. Marital discord usually results from problems in communication, difficulties with conflict resolution, and unresolved issues of autonomy and intimacy. If couples are experiencing prolonged and intense difficulties in these areas, marital counseling may be indicated, especially since marital discord can add to the stress of the dialysis patient. Additionally, with all couples, being able to successfully engage the spouse or partner as a valued member of the treatment team can help to support the couple and modulate the impact of the demands of chronic illness and its unrelenting treatment regimen.

Only a few studies have attempted to assess the marital relationships of dialysis patients. In a detailed study of marital relationships of medically stable hemodialysis patients, 53% of couples were noted to exhibit moderate to severe degrees of marital discord (Finkelstein *et al.*, 1976). The extent of discord in these couples was comparable to that of couples seeking marital counseling in an outpatient psychiatric clinic. However, it was striking that despite the presence of multiple areas of conflict in dialysis couples, the vast majority globally viewed their marriages as having few or no problems. One reason for this discrepancy may well be that denial plays a prominent role in the psychological defenses of the dialysis patient (Short and Wilson, 1969; Reichsman and Levy, 1972). An alternative explanation might be that the shared burdens of dialysis in these couples eclipse those problems that in physically healthy couples often lead to overt disruption. In any case, the fact that these couples do not seriously view these problems in their global marital assessment does not obviate their importance and does not mean that therapeutic interventions designed to confront and deal with these problems will not be of benefit. Clearly, intervention must be undertaken with care, however, since it is not meant to disrupt and disorganize basic adaptive defenses but rather to improve the overall care of the patient.

Sexual dysfunction

Another stress on the dialysis couple that is frequently reported concerns sexual dysfunction. Patients with ESRD maintained on chronic dialysis have a high prevalence of sexual dysfunction. The extent of sexual dysfunction is similar for patients treated with chronic peritoneal dialysis and chronic hemodialysis (Juergensen *et al.*, 1996). About 60–65% of dialysis patients report that they never have intercourse, 33% report an inability to have an orgasm, and 60% report difficulty getting or maintaining an erection or sexual excitement. Dialysis patients engage in intercourse less often and report a higher incidence of specific symptoms of sexual dysfunction after developing ESRD (Levy, 1994).

It is important to note that the sexual difficulties experienced by the dialysis patients are perceived by them as an area of difficulty (Finkelstein *et al.*, 1976; Steele *et al.*, 1996*b*). Thus, about half of the dialysis patients would like to have intercourse more frequently. Furthermore, when patients evaluate their degree of satisfaction with their sexual activity, those 60–65% of dialysis patients never having intercourse (Steele *et al.*, 1996*b*) report a low level of satisfaction, significantly lower in fact than those patients having intercourse .

The relationship between ESRD patients' sexual dysfunction and their overall psychosocial adaptation is of considerable interest. Patients never having intercourse have significantly higher scores on standard measures of depression and anxiety than patients having intercourse at least twice per month (Steele *et al.*, 1996*b*). Steele *et al.* (1996*b*) explored the relationship between patients' assessment of their quality of life and their level of sexual functioning. Using a global patient assessment of quality of life, these investigators described, perhaps not surprisingly, an association between the assessment of quality of life and the frequency of sexual intercourse. Those patients never having intercourse reported a significantly lower assessment of their overall quality of life than those patients having intercourse at least twice a month. But issues of cause and effect are complex. Thus, the roles that depression and anxiety play in contributing to the sexual dysfunction of the ESRD patient have not been fully evaluated. And, the role that sexual activity plays in contributing to the patients' depression and anxiety and patients' overall assessment of their quality of life has not been clearly elucidated.

The factors responsible for the sexual dysfunction of the ESRD patient are complex and multifactorial, involving a variety of medical and psychological issues that are often inter-related.

Many of the psychological issues have been discussed in the above sections. Thus, depressive symptomatology is often associated with decreased sexual functioning. Patients who are experiencing sexual dysfunction for whatever reason may withdraw from sexual activity because of their 'fear of failure' to achieve orgasm and to give adequate pleasure to their sexual partner. This performance anxiety can further compromise sexual functioning. Marital discord, commonly encountered in dialysis patients' marriages (as noted above), closely correlates with the level of sexual functioning (Finkelstein *et al.*, 1976). And, when dialysis patients and their spouses are asked to identify their marital problems, sexual difficulties are cited frequently and noted as a problem area by 60% of these couples (Finkelstein *et al.*, 1976). In addition, changes in body image and self-esteem can affect sexual interest and desire.

From a medical standpoint, a variety of factors have been implicated as contributing to the sexual dysfunction of the ESRD patient. Medication may affect the level of sexual functioning. This is particularly true of various antihypertensive medications (e.g. centrally acting agents, beta-blocking agents) that may result in not only loss of libido but also in specific symptoms of sexual dysfunction.

Investigations into hypothalamic, pituitary, gonadal, and parathyroid functioning have indicated a variety of abnormalities that may contribute to sexual dysfunction. In male dialysis patients, several studies have suggested that testicular dysfunction is common, often resulting in low sperm counts and testosterone levels (Holdsworth *et al.*, 1977; Lim, 1995). Follicle-stimulating hormone (FSH) and luteinizing hormone (LH) levels are frequently, but not always, elevated (Lim, 1995). However, the degree of elevation does not always seem appropriate for the degree of depression of the testosterone level. Pituitary hormone responsiveness to luteinizing-releasing hormone (LRH), however, is usually intact, although abnormal responses are noted in some patients (Schalch *et al.*, 1975). Thus, these data suggest that pituitary response to LRH is usually intact, but that the feedback response to reduced testosterone levels at the level of the pituitary gland may, at least in some patients, be deficient.

Prolactin levels range from normal to markedly elevated (Foulks and Cushner, 1986; Lim, 1995). A causal relationship has been suggested between prolactin levels and sexual dysfunction in both male and female patients. The elevated prolactin levels can contribute to sexual dysfunction by limiting FSH and LH responses and impairing gonadal function as well as by directly inhibiting libido. However, the actual contribution of the abnormal prolactin secretion to the sexual dysfunction of the ESRD patient remains uncertain (Foulks and Cushner, 1986). Elevated prolactin levels can be lowered by treatment with dopamine agonists, e.g bromocriptine, which acts on the pituitary lactotroph to inhibit prolactin synthesis and release. However, lowering prolactin levels with such drugs may not always improve libido, spermatogenesis, and/or testosterone production in patients with renal failure (Gomez *et al.*, 1980, Finkelstein and Finkelstein, 1993).

Zinc deficiency has been implicated by some investigators as contributing to the testicular dysfunction of male dialysis patients (Mahajan *et al.*, 1982). Thus, an association has been reported between zinc deficiency and impaired testicular function. Therapy with oral zinc replacement has been reported to result in an improvement in sperm counts and testosterone levels and fall in FSH and LH levels. These physiological changes may contribute to an improvement in libido, enhanced sexual performance, and decreased impotence. However, other investigators have not been impressed with the clinical response of ESRD patients to oral zinc replacement therapy (Finkelstein and Finkelstein, 1993).

Hyperparathyroidism, a commonly encountered abnormality in ESRD patients, has also been implicated as a cause of the sexual dysfunction of the male dialysis patient (Massry *et al.*, 1977). Studies have suggested that increased levels of parathyroid hormone may specifically interfere with some of the physiological aspects of male sexual functioning. However, other investigators have been unable to confirm an association between hyperparathyroidism in the ESRD patient and the degree of sexual dysfunction (Finkelstein and Finkelstein, 1993).

Additional physiological problems that can contribute to the sexual dysfunction of the dialysis patient include autonomic neuropathy and peripheral vascular disease. Both of these problems occur significantly more commonly in the diabetic patient and can contribute to the development of erectile dysfunction. Physiological derangements that result in erectile dysfunction in male patients have been examined using a variety of relatively new techniques (Whitehead *et al.*, 1990). These studies have been designed to sort out the relative contributions of afferent and efferent neurological abnormalities and arteriolar and venous dysfunction to the erectile problems of the male patient. Penile biothesiometry, sacral evoked-potential testing, bulbocavernous electromyography, and dorsal nerve, somatosensory evoked-potential testing are designed to examine various components of the neurological axis involved in achieving an erection. The penile brachial index (the ratio between the systolic penile blood pressure and systolic brachial blood pressure) is a widely used non-invasive test to examine arteriogenic impotence. Additional, invasive studies that can be used to assess arterial or venous abnormalities preventing successful achievement and maintenance of an erection include penile injection with vasodilators, pulse duplex sonography with corpora cavernosa papaverine injection, and pelvic angiography with internal pudendal arteriography. At the present time, few of these complex investigations have been used to study a large cohort of ESRD patients. However, they may well be useful in examining the cause of erectile dysfunction in an individual patient and thus perhaps designing an optimal treatment modality.

The endocrine abnormalities encountered in the female dialysis patient are similar to those found in the male. Absence of menstruation or irregular menstrual cycles are commonly noted in the premenopausal female dialysis patient. These problems may reflect abnormalities in ovarian function and pituitary control of ovarian hormone release (Ramirez *et al.*, 1994). Appropriate FSH and LH responses to LRH suggest normal pituitary responses to hypothalamic stimuli. However, low estradiol and progesterone levels at critical points during the menstrual cycle without corresponding increases in FSH and LH suggest a defective pituitary–ovarian feedback loop.

The contribution of the elevation of the prolactin levels to the abnormalities in estrogen, progesterone, FSH, and LH secretion is unclear. The known association of high prolactin levels with amenorrhea in female patients without renal disease and the response of the menstrual abnormalities to therapy with dopamine agonists raises the question of the possible therapeutic benefit of these agents in female patients with ESRD. However, this has not yet been systematically studied.

Recent work has emphasized the importance of testosterone in maintaining female libido. Treatment of estrogen-deficient women with estrogen therapy alone may not return female libido to normal, but combinations of estrogen and testosterone may result in a better clinical response. The role of testosterone in maintaining female libido in the patient with ESRD has not been explored.

Whatever the etiology of a patient's diminished sexual interest and activity, it is important to openly discuss and explore the specifics of each person's situation. Obstacles exist to accomplishing this. Discussions about sexual activity often elicit discomfort in both the staff and the patient. It is, therefore, important to heighten the staff's consciousness of the importance of investigating this arena. Facilitating a discussion of sexual difficulties requires active effort to overcome inhibitions and resistance that often contribute to keeping this area closed for discussion. Patients are not likely to feel free and comfortable revealing and sharing their sexual feelings without a clear message from the staff that this is a standard, normal operating procedure.

Employment and rehabilitation

The aim of rehabilitation for the patient with renal failure is to improve the patient's physical and mental functioning and to maximize his quality of life (Blagg and Fitts, 1994). Achievement of this goal requires that the staff make a realistic appraisal of the patient's capacities and that the degree of rehabilitation be monitored with standardized measures and timely and effective interventions (Blagg and Fitts, 1994). The process of rehabilitation thus involves assessing the patient's goals and desires, understanding his physical and mental capacities, appraising the resources available to provide support, and optimizing his medical care.

That dialysis patients are limited in their vocational capacity is well documented (Fragola *et al.*, 1983; Levy, 1994). About three-quarters of dialysis patients are unemployed. About two-thirds do not return to the employment they had engaged in prior to the onset of renal failure (Fragola *et al.*, 1983; Levy, 1994). However, the reasons for the low employment rates are not clear, and probably reflect a complex interaction amongst disability insurance plans, government policy regarding disability payments, labor market conditions, comorbid disease, psychosocial aspects of the individual, family and martial relationships, and the dialysis treatment regimen. The varying contributions of these factors to the low employment rates in dialysis patients has not been fully elucidated. However, active intervention with psychosocial assessment, education, counseling, and support can maximize patients' employment capabilities. For example, such intervention in the 6 months prior to the onset of dialysis resulted in 74% of patients maintaining employment after dialysis started (Rasgon *et al.*, 1996).

The physical limitations and disability of the dialysis patient have been well documented by various authors (Bonney *et al.*, 1978; Fragola *et al.*, 1983; Levy, 1994). Most investigators agree that these difficulties occur for a variety of reasons, including the effects of the renal failure itself, comorbid disease, the treatment regimen, and the psychosocial problems of the dialysis patient. It is important for carers to attempt to assess the varying contributions of these factors to the limitations of the dialysis patient so that therapeutic interventions can be designed to maximize the rehabilitation of the patient.

Quality of life

During the last decade, there has been a burgeoning interest in the concept of quality of life assessment as an outcome measure of therapeutic interventions for medical diseases. However, what in fact constitutes quality of life has been subject to a wide variety of opinions. Thus measuring quality of life has presented a confusing and perplexing problem.

Why has there been this recent interest in the notion of quality of life? Various investigators and authors have come to realize that the ultimate goal of treatment for patients with a chronic illness, such as renal failure, is ultimately to improve and maximize the patient's quality of life (Schrier *et al.*, 1995; Cohn, 1996; Steele *et al.*, 1996a). For any medical intervention in these patients, investigations must address and evaluate the impact of that intervention on the patients' quality of life. This requires that researchers not just focus attention on specific physical and psychological outcome measures, but that they also consider the patients' own sense of well-being (Gill and Feinstein, 1994). However, how to measure and define this sense of well-being precisely has perplexed investigators not just for patients with chronic renal disease but for all patients with a chronic illness. Physicians too often rely on specific and objective measurements of physical and psychological functioning and often ignore or disregard the patients' subjective symptoms and overall perception of their quality of life (O'Boyle *et al.*, 1992; Gill and Feinstein, 1994; Cohn, 1996; Steele *et al.*, 1996*a*).

Recently, Gill and Feinstein (1994) published an in-depth review evaluating the quality of life measurements that had been used in the medical literature. These authors concluded that quality of life measurements are too often aimed at the wrong target and are usually focused on various aspects of the patients' health status. Quality of life, they argue, is inherently an attribute and perception of the patient. The incorporation of the patients' values and preferences must be utilized to distinguish true quality of life measurements from those that simply assess health status. These authors conclude by offering three suggestions for investigators concerning the design of quality of life measurements. First, they stress the use of global ratings which can reflect individual values and unique patient preferences. Second, they underscore the utility of permitting patients to rate the severity and importance of various items. Third, they emphasize the need to permit supplemental items to be selected by the patient so that items that are uniquely important to an individual patient can find expression.

Other recent reviews of quality of life assessments have stressed the need to define appropriate domains of interest for specific targeted patient populations (Kimmel *et al.*, 1995; Powe *et al.*, 1996; Testa and Simonson, 1996). The instrument used must take into account the specific characteristics of the patient group being studied. In addition it must have an internal reliability and validity to establish its meaning, as well as a responsiveness and sensitivity to allow relevant changes to be detected.

How has quality of life been examined in the patient with ESRD? There remains considerable controversy about not only the optimal way of assessing but also the actual meaning of the notion of quality of life for dialysis patients. Some investigators have continued to stress primarily objective measures of functional status (Schrier *et al.*, 1995). Others recognize the importance of unique patient assessments of what, for each individual, constitutes significant contributors to their quality of life (Steele *et al.*, 1996*a*). It is becoming more widely recognized, however, that there is a need for some standardization and some general agreement as to how quality of life should be measured to permit clinical trials to incorporate the concept into their outcome measures in a meaningful and generally applicable fashion (Nissenson, 1994; Schrier *et al.*, 1995; Salek, 1996). If nephrologists are going to attempt to define the optimal renal replacement therapy and define what is optimal dialysis dosing, then the notion of what constitutes and how to measure quality of life must be more generally accepted and should accompany the reporting of standard measures of mortality, hospitalization, and patient rehabilitation.

Recent work from several investigators (Wolcott *et al.*, 1988; Laupacis *et al.*, 1994;

Nissenson, 1994; Kallich *et al.*, 1995; Kimmel *et al.*, 1995; Wilson and Cleany, 1995) has attempted to consolidate the notion of quality of life measurement into specific domains. These include physical health, mental health, social health, and general health. Wolcott *et al.* (1988) have emphasized the independence of these domains, and suggest that studies of adaptation of the ESRD patient must assess all these areas individually. Kimmel *et al.* (1995) have also stressed the importance of focusing attention on a variety of domains to assess quality of life. The Rand Corporation has developed a generic quality of life assessment tool targeting these four general areas (The Rand-36 Item Health Survey, known as the SF-36), to assess quality of life in the general population and in patients with a variety of medical disorders (Kallich *et al.*, 1995). This instrument has been gaining widespread use in the United States of America and elsewhere. However, it is limited by its generic focus and is not designed to examine critically the particular needs and issues of patients with ESRD. Thus, investigators from Rand have subsequently expanded this core questionnaire—after conducting in-depth focus group discussions with both dialysis patients and dialysis unit staff members—to include a variety of questions specifically targeting the effects of chronic renal disease and dialysis therapy on the patients' perception of their quality of life (Kallich *et al.*, 1995). Other investigators have adopted a similar approach by carefully discussing the notion of quality of life with ESRD patients and their carers (Laupacis *et al.*, 1994; Powe *et al.*, 1996).

Yet other investigators have focused attention primarily on the patient's own perception of his quality of life, suggesting that this may in fact be more important than objective measurements of the level of functioning (O'Boyle *et al.*, 1992; Steele *et al.*, 1996). Thus, it has been observed that dialysis patients often rate their overall quality of life as equal to or even higher than members of the general population, despite the obvious restrictions placed on the patients by their illness and treatment (Evans *et al.*, 1985, 1990; Blagg and Fitts, 1994; Steele *et al.*, 1996*a*). This observation applies to the older dialysis patients (over 70 years of age) as well as the younger patients (Nissensin, 1996; Westlie *et al.*, 1984). Some authors have argued that this may represent patient denial or distortion of reality (Cramond *et al.*, 1967; Short and Wilson, 1969). But this indeed seems unlikely given the dialysis patients' willingness to report a host of medical and psychological symptoms on self-administered questionnaires as well as direct patient interviews. More likely, the explanation for this perhaps surprising finding lies in the complex interactions among objective problems, the subjective experience of these problems, and the patients' own assessment and personal interpretation of these subjective experiences.

Recently, therefore, several investigators have asked patients to rate their own quality of life. Steele *et al.* (1996*a*) Juergensen *et al.* (1996), and Wuerth *et al.* (1997) asked patients to rate their overall quality of life as well as to rate an 18-item questionnaire covering a variety of domains such as energy level, family relationships, sexual function, living conditions, health and work status, etc. using a 10-point scale from a score of 1 ('as bad as it could possibly be') to a score of 10 ('as good as it could possibly be'). In addition, patients were asked to select the five areas that are most important in determining their overall quality of life, either using domains from the 18-item questionnaire or selecting their own unique domains. These researchers observed a significant correlation between the patients' overall perception of their quality of life and the dose of dialysis provided (as measured by Kt/V urea), depression scores (as measured by the BDI), and anxiety scores (as measured by the Patient Related Anxiety Scale). After adjustment for interacting variables, depression retained the strongest correlation with patient-assessed overall quality of life. These investigators observed several other significant findings. First, there was a very high correlation between the sum of the scores on the individual items on their questionnaire and the overall patient assessment of quality of life. Second, there was a weak correlation between the staffs' assessment of the patients' quality of life and the patients' assessment of their own quality of life, supporting the notion that patients and clinicians often differ in their evaluation of quality of life (Evans *et al.*, 1985; McGee *et al.*, 1991; Von Korff *et al.*, 1992; Meers *et al.*, 1995). Third, patients were particular in selecting the five areas that they felt were the most important domains in determining their quality of life. The most frequently selected domains included family relationships, social supports other than family, issues of autonomy and independence, structured daily activities, and overall physical condition.

With regard to long-term dialysis patients, one aspect of quality of life assessment that has been conspicuously absent thus far from the literature is the longitudinal assessment over time of the patients' perception of their quality of life and their adaptation to ESRD therapy (Wolcott *et al.*, 1988; Steele *et al.*, 1996a). The importance of these observations, which are now just beginning to be undertaken (Powe *et al.*, 1996), cannot be overemphasized. They, hopefully, will provide a clearer insight into the relationships, of various psychological and social adaptations, the patients' perception of their quality of life, and overall morbidity and mortality. Furthermore, they may enable the medical team caring for the ESRD patient to define those characteristics that are predictive of a poor response to treatment, permitting early and selective interventions to be performed. An example would be the findings of Jurgensen *et al.* (1996), who observed that in a cohort of patients maintained on CAPD, those patients with a higher incidence of peritonitis had a significantly lower self-rating of their quality of life than those not developing peritonitis.

Summary and conclusions

The goal of the therapy of patients with ESRD, as for any patient with a chronic disease, is to provide optimal medical treatment, provide adequate supportive care, and maximize patient rehabilitation and quality of life. Achievement of these goals requires that a detailed assessment of the patient's psychosocial status be undertaken by the patient's care team using a systematic approach, with attention focused on the areas of intrapsychic and interpersonal stress experienced by the patient. It is critically important to understand these areas of stress in the context of each patient's experience of his illness. The interaction of these areas with the medical condition, treatment regimen, and amount of dialysis delivered must be considered and reviewed on an ongoing basis. It must be kept in mind that a variety of medical factors can influence the psychosocial status of the patient and that the psychosocial status of the patient can affect various aspects of the medical condition of the patient.

Assessment of the quality of life experienced by the patient requires a systematic and standardized approach. This assessment must include not only objective measures of various domains of adjustment, but also the subjective experience of the patient, giving him the leeway to provide insight into those domains which for him are uniquely important.

A strategy of intervention should be considered for those patients who themselves report or who are felt by the medical team, family members, or partners to have persistent and/or troublesome psychosocial symptoms or a change in psychosocial functioning. Moreover, intervention should be considered when the medical team feels that psychosocial factors are interfering with the adequate delivery of health care to the patient.

Further studies are needed to clarify the following issues: (a) the optimal way to assess quality for life for the ESRD patient: (b) the relationship between the dose of dialysis and the quality of life and psychosocial status of the patient; (c) the relationship between the psychosocial status of the patient and specific areas of his medical condition; and (d) the longitudinal assessment of the quality of life, psychosocial status, medical condition, and dialysis dose in a large cohort of ESRD patients and the relationship amongst these variables over time.

References

Abram, H. S. (1974). Psychiatric reflections on adaptation to repetitive dialysis. *Kidney International*, **6**, 67–72.

Anonymous. (1995). Quality of life and clinical trials. *Lancet*, **346**, 1–2.

Blagg, C. and Fitts, S. S. (1994). Dialysis, old age and rehabilitation. *Journal of the American Medical Association*, **271**, 67–8.

Bonney, S., Finkelstein, F. O., Lytton, B., Schiff, M., and Steele, T. E. (1978). Treatment of end-stage renal disease in a defined geographic area. *Archives of Internal Medicine*, **138**, 1510–13.

Carey, H., Finkelstein, S., Santacroce, S., *et al.* (1990). The impact of psychosocial factors and age on CAPD dropout. *Advances in Peritoneal Dialysis*, **6**, 26–8.

Cohn, J. N. (1996). The management of chronic heart failure. *New England Journal of Medicine*, **335**, 490–8.

Cramond, W. A., Knight, P. R., and Lawrence, J. R. (1967). The psychiatric contribution to a renal unit undertaking chronic hemodialysis and homotransplantation. *British Journal of Psychiatry*, **113**, 1201–12.

De-Nour, A. K. (1994). Psychological, social, and vocational impact of renal failure: a review. In *Quality of life following renal failure* (ed. H. McGee and C. Bradley) pp. 33–42. Harwood Academic, Chur.

Evans, R. W., Manninen, D. L., Garrison, L. P., *et al.* (1985). The quality of life of patients with end stage renal disease. *New England Journal of Medicine*, **312**, 553–9.

Evans, R. W., Rader, B., Manninen, D. L., *et al.* (1990). The quality of life of hemodialysis recipients treated with recombinant erythropoietin. *Journal of the American Medical Association*, **263**, 825–30.

Fallowfield, L. (1996). Quality of life data. *Lancet*, **348**, 421.

Finkelstein, S. H., and Finkelstein, F. O. (1993). Evaluation of sexual dysfunction. *In Dialysis therapy* (2nd edn) (ed. A. R. Nissenson and R. N. Fine) pp. 270–3. Hanley and Belfus, Philadelphia.

Finkelstein, F. O., Finkelstein, S. H., and Steele, T. E. (1976). Assessment of marital relationships of hemodialysis patients. *American Journal of Medical Sciences*, **271**, 21–8.

Foulks, C. J., and Cushner, H. M. (1986). Sexual dysfunction in male dialysis patients: pathogenesis, evaluation and therapy. *American Journal of Kidney Diseases*, **8**, 211–22.

Fragola, J. A., Grube, S., Von Bloch, L., and Bourke, E. (1983). Multicentre study of physical activity and employment status of continuous ambulatory peritoneal dialysis patients in the United States. *Proceedings of European Dialysis and Transplant Association*, **20**, 243–9.

Fraser, C. L., and Arieff, A. I. (1988). Nervous system complications in uremia. *Annals of Internal Medicine*, **109**, 143–53.

Gill, T. M., and Feinstein, A. R. (1994). A critical appraisal of the quality of life measurements. *Journal of the American Medical Association*, **272**, 619–26.

Gokal, R. (1993). Quality of life in patients undergoing renal replacement therapy. *Kidney International*, **43** (Suppl. 40), S23–S27.

Gomez, F., de la Cueva, R., and Wauters, J. P. (1980). Endocrine abnormalities in patients undergoing long term hemodialysis: the role for prolactin. *American Journal of Medicine*, **68**, 522–30.

Holdsworth, S., Atkins, R. C., and deKretser, D. M. (1977). The pituitary–testicular axis in men with chronic renal failure. *New England Journal of Medicine*, **296**, 1245–9.

Juergensen, P. H., Juergensen, D. M., Wuerth, D. B., *et al.* (1996). Psychosocial factors and incidence of peritonitis. *Advances in Peritoneal Dialysis*, **12**, 196–8.

Kallich, J. D., Hays, R. D., Mapes, D. L., Coons, S. J., and Carter, W. B. (1995). The RAND kidney disease and quality of life instrument. *Nephrology News and Issues*, September, 29–36.

Kennedy, S. H., Craven, J. L., and Roin, G. M. (1989). Major depression in renal dialysis patients: an open trial of antidepressant therapy. *Journal of Clinical Psychiatry*, **50**, 60–3.

Kiecolt-Glaser, J., Marucha, P. T., Malarkey, A. M., and Glaser, R. (1995). Slowing of wound healing by psychological stress. *Lancet*, **346**, 1194–6.

Kimmel, P. L., Weihs, K., and Peterson, R. A. (1993). Survival in hemodialysis patients: role of depression. *Journal of the American Society of Nephrology*, **4**, 12–27.

Kimmel, P. L., Peterson, R. A., Weihs K. L., *et al.* (1995). Aspects of quality of life in hemodialysis patients. *Journal of the American Society of Nephrology*, **6**, 1418–26.

Laupacis, A., Muirhead, N., Keown, P., and Wong, C. (1994). A disease specific questionnaire for assessing quality of life in patients on hemodialysis. *Nephron*, **60**, 302–6.

Levin, N. W. (1992). Quality of life and hematocrit level. *American Journal of Kidney Diseases*, **20** (Suppl. 1), S16–S20.

Levy, N. B. (1994). Psychology and rehabilitation. In *Handbook of dialysis* (2nd edn) (ed. J. T. Daugirdas and T. S. Ing), pp. 369–73. Little Brown, Boston.

Lim, V. S. (1995). Peritoneal dialysis and endocrinology. *Peritoneal Dialysis International*, **16** (Suppl. 1), S257–S259.

McGee, H. M., O'Boyle, C. A., Hickey, A., O'Malley, K., and Joyce, C. R. B. (1991). Assessing the quality of life of the individual: the SEIQoL with a healthy and a gastrointestinal unit population. *Psychological Medicine*, **21**, 749–59.

Mahajan, S. K., Abbasi, A. A., and Prasad, A. S. (1982). Effect of oral zinc therapy on gonadal function in hemodialysis patients. *Annals of Internal Medicine*, **97**, 357–61.

Maher, B. A., Lamping, D. L., Dickinson, C. A., Murawski, B. J., Olivier, D. C., and Santiago, G. C. (1983). Psychosocial aspects of chronic hemodialysis: the National Cooperative Dialysis Study. *Kidney International*, **23** (Suppl. 13), S50–S57.

Marsh, J. T., Brown, W. S., Wolcott, D. *et al.* (1991). rHuEPO treatment improves brain and cognitive function of anemic dialysis patients. *Kidney International*, **39**, 155–63.

Massry, S. G., Goldstein, D. A., and Procci, W. R., (1977). Impotence in patients with uremia: a possible role for parathyroid hormone. *Nephron*, **19**, 305–11.

Meers, C., Hopman, W., Singer, M. A., MacKenzie, T. A., Morton, A. R., and McMurray, M. (1995). A comparison of patient, nurse and physician assessment of health-related quality of life in end-stage renal disease. *Dialysis and Transplantation*, **24**, 120–4.

Neu, S., and Kjellstrand, C. M. (1986). Stopping long term hemodialysis. *New England Journal of Medicine*, **314**, 14–20.

Nissenson, A. R. (1994). Measuring, managing, and improving quality in the end-stage renal disease treatment setting: peritoneal dialysis. *American Journal of Kidney Diseases*, **24**, 368–75.

Nissenson, A. R. (1996). Quality of life in elderly and diabetic patients in peritoneal dialysis. *Peritoneal Dialysis International*, **16** (Suppl. 1), S406–S409.

O'Boyle, C. A., McGee, H., Hickey, A., O'Malley, K. O., and Joyce, C. R. B. (1992). Individual quality of life in patients undergoing hip replacement. *Lancet*, **339**, 1088–91.

Powe, N. R., Klag, M. J., Sadler, J. H., *et al.* (1996). Choices for healthy outcomes in caring for end stage renal disease. *Seminars in Dialysis*, **9**, 9–11.

Ramirez, G. (1994). Abnormalities in the hypothalamic–hypophyseal axes in patients with chronic renal failure. *Seminars in Dialysis*, **7**, 138–46.

Rasgon, S. A., Chemleski, B. L., Ho, S., *et al.* (1996). Benefits of a multidisciplinary predialysis program in maintaining employment among patients on home dialysis. *Advances in Peritoneal Dialysis*, **12**, 132–5.

Reichsman, F., and Levy, N. B. (1972). Problem in adaptation to maintenance hemodialysis: a four year study of twenty-five patients. *Archives of Internal Medicine*, **130**, 859–65.

Ruberman, W., Weinblatt, E., Goldberg, J. D., and Chaudhary, B. S. (1984). Psychosocial influences on mortality after myocardial infarction. *New England Journal of Medicine*, **311**, 552–9.

Salek, S. (1996). Quality of life assessment in patients on peritoneal dialysis: a review of the state of the art. *Peritoneal Dialysis International*, **16** (Suppl. 1), S398–S401.

Schlach, D. S., Gonzalez-Barcena, D., and Kastin, A. J. (1975). Plasma gonadotropins after administration of LH-releasing hormone in patients with renal or hepatic failure. *Journal of Clinical Endocrinology and Metabolism*, **41**, 921–5.

Schrier, R. W., Burrows-Hudson, S., Diamond, L., *et al.* (1995). Measuring, managing, and improving quality in the end-stage renal disease treatment setting: committee statement. *American Journal of Kidney Diseases*, **24**, 383–8.

Short, M. J., and Wilson, W. P. (1969). Roles of denial in chronic hemodialysis. *Archives of General Psychiatry*, **20**, 433–7.

Shulman, R., Price, J. D., and Shinelli, J. (1989). Biopsychosocial aspects of long term survival on end stage renal failure therapy. *Psychological Medicine*, **19**, 945–54.

Steele, T. E., Baltimore, D., Finkelstein, S. H., Juergensen, P., Kliger, A. S., and Finkelstein, F. O. (1996*a*). Quality of life in peritoneal dialysis patients. *Journal of Nervous and Mental Disease*, **184**, 368–74.

Steele, T. E., Wuerth, D., Finkelstein, S., *et al.* (1996*b*). Sexual experience of the chronic peritoneal dialysis patient. *Journal of the American Society of Nephrology*, **7**, 1165–8.

Steidl, J. H., Finkelstein, F. O., Wexler, J. P., *et al.* (1980). Medical condition, adherence to treatment regimens, and family functioning, *Archives of General Psychiatry*, **37**, 1025–7.

Streltzer, J., Finkelstein, F., Feigenbaum, H., Kitsen, J., and Cohn, G. L. (1976). The spouse's role in home hemodialysis. *Archives of General Psychiatry*, **33**, 55–8.

Testa, M. A., and Simonson, D. C. (1996). Assessment of quality of life outcomes. *New England Journal of Medicine*, **334**, 835–40.

Von Korff, M., Omel, J., Katon, W., and Lin, E. H. B. (1992). Disability and depression among high utilizers of health care. *Archives of General Psychiatry*, **49**, 91–100.

Westlie, L., Umen, A., Nestrud, S., and Kjellstrand, C. M. (1984). Mortality, morbidity, and life satisfaction in the very old dialysis patient. *Transactions of the American Society of Artificial Internal Organs*, **30**, 21–30.

Whitehead, E. D., Klyde, B. J., Zussman, S., and Salkin, P. (1990). Diagnostic evaluation of impotence. *Postgraduate Medicine*, **88**, 123–35.

Wilson, I. B., and Cleary, P. D. (1995). Linking clinical variables with health related quality of life. *Journal of the American Medical Association*, **273**, 59–65.

Wolcott, D. L., Nissenson, A. R., and Landsverk, J. (1988). Quality of life in chronic dialysis patients. *General Hospital Psychiatry*, **10**, 267–77.

Wuerth, D., Finkelstein, S., Juergensen, D., *et al.* (1997). Quality of life assessment in chronic peritoneal dialysis patients. *Advances in Peritoneal Dialysis*, **13**, 125–27.

PART III
Survival

9

Nutrition as a factor in survival

David Reaich

Introduction

The presence of protein–calorie malnutrition is well recognized in maintenance hemodialysis (HD) patients. The nutritional deficiencies are multifactorial, with both inadequate intake and increased catabolism contributing. There is increasing evidence that malnutrition in HD has a negative impact on morbidity and mortality. Long-term survival of the HD patient is therefore likely to be influenced by nutritional status. The optimum management of the HD patient must therefore include an appropriate assessment of his/her nutritional status and interventions to prevent the development of malnutrition, or correct it, should it arise.

Nutritional status of patients on maintenance HD

The assessment of nutritional status in HD patients is based on clinical evaluation; dietary history; measurement of serum proteins such as albumin, prealbumin, transferrin, and insulin–like growth factor-1 (IGF-1); and anthropometry. Serum albumin in particular is often used as an index of protein nutrition. However, it has a half–life of more than 10 days and therefore responds slowly to changes in visceral protein stores. Serum albumin concentration also falls as part of the acute-phase response. Therefore hypoalbuminemia may reflect coexisting illness rather than the nutritional status. There is also a dichotomy in that serum albumin may well be normal despite significant anthropometric abnormalities (Bansal *et al.*, 1980; Jacob *et al.*, 1990). If serum albumin is being used as a nutritional marker, the development of hypo-albuminemia should be considered as a late response and indicative of significant nutritional deficiency. As far as other serum proteins are concerned, serum IGF-1 levels may be a better nutritional indicator than albumin in the HD patient, as they have been shown to correlate well with changes in triceps skinfold thickness (Jacob *et al.*, 1990). Furthermore, longitudinal changes in serum IGF-1 concentrations can prospectively predict changes in serum albumin concentration (Parker *et al.*, 1996). It is clear that no single measurement provides a reliable indicator of the nutritional state. Instead a combination of serial measurements of body weight, anthropo-metrics, and serum proteins should be used to indicate changes in a patient's nutritional status.

More precise methods are available, including the measurement of total body nitrogen by *in-vivo* neutron activation (Allman *et al.*, 1990; Rayner *et al.*, 1991), and body composition analysis using dual-energy, X-ray absorptiometry (DEXA) (Roubenoff *et al.*, 1993). These methods involve expensive equipment that is not readily available on a routine basis, and thus they remain essentially experimental. Other assessment methods unsuitable for routine use include intramuscular amino-acid (Bergström *et al.*, 1990) and protein/nucleic acid determination (Guarnieri *et al.*, 1983). Recently the technique of bioelectrical impedance (BIA) has been shown to estimate reliably total body water and cell mass in HD patients (Chertow *et al.* 1995) and may prove to be a simple and useful monitoring tool.

Using these various methods, there is no doubt that protein–energy malnutrition is a common problem in HD patients. Quite how common is difficult to say, as reports of the incidence of protein–calorie malnutrition vary widely, signs of malnutrition being reported in 10–70% of HD patients in different studies (Bergström and Lindholm, 1993). The incidence of malnutrition may well vary between centers—indeed it would be surprising if it did not. It is therefore of interest that Guarnieri *et al.* (1983), assessing the nutritional status of HD patients from two centers, reported a greater reduction in anthropometric values in the patients from one center. This group of patients had a lower protein and calorie intake than those patients in the other center.

The anthropometric changes commonly noted include reduced body weight, body mass index, triceps skinfold thickness, and mid-arm muscle circumference (Schoenfeld *et al.*, 1983; Jacob *et al.*, 1990). *In-vivo* neutron activation analysis (IVNAA) showed lower total body nitrogen in HD patients than age-, sex-, and height-matched controls (Allman *et al.*, 1990). In a group of 62 HD patients, IVNAA revealed a greater protein loss than was estimated by anthropometry (Rayner *et al.*, 1991), suggesting that anthropometry underestimates the degree of body protein depletion. Similarly, in a group of 22 stable HD patients, DEXA and BIA revealed reduced lean body tissue in patients in whom anthropometry failed to demonstrate any reduction in fat-free mass (Woodrow *et al.*, 1996). Muscle biopsy studies show reduced muscle protein content and cell size (Guarnieri *et al.*, 1983), and altered intracellular amino-acid profiles, with, in particular, reduced levels of intracellular valine (Bergström *et al.*, 1990).

There are no reports of regularly repeated assessments of nutritional status over time in HD patients. It is therefore difficult to comment on the effect of the length of time on HD on nutrition. Clearly the presence of comorbidity and intercurrent illnesses make this very difficult to assess. The available information is conflicting. Kaufmann *et al.* (1994) assessed nutritional status in 96 HD patients. The patients were divided according to the length of previous HD treatment into a group at first treatment and groups treated for 1–8 months, 9–69 months, and 70–207 months. The 'first treatment' group had diminished visceral protein stores, but the other groups showed no evidence of malnutrition. Serum albumin increased progressively in a group of 159 new HD patients over the first 18 months of their treatment (Parker *et al.*, 1996). In contrast, measurement of body nitrogen in 62 patients showed a negative correlation between body nitrogen and time on dialysis (i.e. body nitrogen fell as the duration of dialysis increased) (Rayner *et al.*, 1991).

Nutritional status at commencement of hemodialysis

Many individuals enter dialysis programs in a malnourished state (Kopple, 1984), reflecting the anorexia and catabolism of untreated chronic renal failure, and clearly this may affect outcome. Individuals will therefore begin their dialysis 'careers' with different baseline nutritional states. Anorexia and nausea are well-recognized symptoms of severe uremia, and from common clinical experience we know that these symptoms resolve with the introduction of adequate dialysis. We would therefore hope that the introduction of dialysis will improve the patient's nutritional status. However, it would be preferable for patients to reach end-stage renal failure well nourished. Nutritional vigilance is therefore of importance throughout the pre-dialysis period as well as after the commencement of renal replacement therapy.

Nutritional status and outcome

There are many studies supporting the hypothesis that poor nutrition influences both morbidity and mortality. However, as discussed by Bergström (1995), the USRDS Annual Report does not list cachexia and malnutrition amongst its causes of death, and in the EDTA/ERA report, only 3% of patients aged 16–64 years and 10% aged 65 and over have cachexia given as a cause of death. In contrast to this, Piccoli *et al.* (1993) in a group of dialysis patients in Northern Italy, found malnutrition to be a cause of death in 32.5% of patients aged 65 or over, and 41% of those aged over 75. The discrepancies in these figures may represent significant under-reporting of malnutrition in the registries, but may also be because malnutrition is commonly associated with (and may be secondary to) other pathologies, which are subsequently described as the cause of death.

Attempts to correlate nutrition with clinical outcome fall broadly into two groups. First, there are a number of reports in which nutritional intake is assessed and outcome measures reported. Protein intake is usually measured indirectly. One way of doing this is to use the protein catabolic rate (PCR). Use of the PCR as an index of protein intake is based on urea kinetic modeling. It is assumed that the amount of urea produced is an indicator of the net amount of protein catabolized. In patients who are in neutral nitrogen balance (i.e. they are not in a state of overall catabolism or anabolism), the amount of protein catabolized gives an estimate of the amount ingested (Gotch and Sargent, 1985). In the well-known NCDS study (Harter, 1983) a PCR of less than 0.8 g/kg body weight per day was associated with treatment failure. It was concluded that the recommended protein intake should be adequate to achieve a PCR of 0.8 g/kg body weight per day. However, the energy intake in each of the four groups studied was 23–26 kcal/kg body weight per day. This is significantly less than the recommended energy intake (see below) and may have prevented optimal utilization of the ingested protein. Thus it would seem inappropriate to draw firm conclusions regarding protein intake and clinical outcome from this study.

Other studies suggest that low protein intake may be associated with increased mortality. In a study of 120 prevalent HD patients, Acchiardo *et al.* (1983) suggested that malnutrition was the main factor in their morbidity and mortality. It is

inappropriate to draw this conclusion from the study as nutritional status was not actually assessed in the patients. However, protein intake (PCR) *was* measured, and
showed a correlation with mortality. A group of 29 patients with low PCR (mean 0.63
g/kg per day) had a mortality rate of 13.8% in 1 year. Groups with higher protein
intakes, with PCRs of 0.93, 1.02, and 1.29 g/kg per day, had mortality rates of 4, 3, and
0%, respectively. These are small groups and therefore the absolute number of deaths
is small (four in the low protein intake group). Nevertheless, the data does suggest a
relationship between protein   intake and mortality. Such a relationship must be
interpreted with caution, as it could be postulated that those patients ingesting lower
amounts of protein were doing so because of other underlying problems which
ultimately contributed to their death.

The second group of studies tried to correlate nutritional status with outcome.
Probably the best-known study of this type is the large retrospective analysis of risk
factors for mortality in HD patients by Lowrie and Lew (1990). Data from more than
12 000 HD patients in National Medical Care dialysis centers in the United States of
America were analyzed. The variables assessed included demographic data, biochemical parameters, and dialysis treatment times. Mortality data was collected over a
1-year period. A low serum albumin concentration was the strongest laboratory predictor of an increased risk of death. Taking patients with serum albumin concentrations of 40.1–45 g/l as the index group, a serum albumin in the range 35.1 to 40 g/l was
associated with a relative risk of death of 2.21. The relative risk increased to 4.86 for an
albumin level of 30.1–35 g/l and there was a greater than 7-fold increase in death in
patients with serum albumins of less than 30g/l. Assuming that serum albumin
reflects visceral protein stores, this suggests that protein malnutrition is a major risk
factor for death. Undoubtedly some patients will have had other causes contributing
to their hypoalbuminemia. Nevertheless, other biochemical parameters were also
strongly associated with death, in keeping with increased mortality secondary to undernutrition. These included an increased risk of death with both low serum creatinine and low serum cholesterol levels. The higher the serum creatinine, the lower
was the risk of death. Since the generation of creatinine is dependent on the muscle
mass, this supports the hypothesis of nutritional status being adversely affected by
reduced protein stores. The relationship between serum creatinine and mortality has
previously been reported (Degoulet *et al.*, 1982). The relationship between low serum
albumin and mortality has subsequently been confirmed not only in North American
patients (Goldwasser *et al.*, 1993; Owen *et al.*, 1993; Collins *et al.*, 1994) but also in a large
group of Japanese patients (Iseki *et al.*, 1993). In a study of Canadian patients commencing HD, patients with a serum albumin of < 30 g/l at the onset of dialysis had
an increased risk of hospitalization and infection than patients with higher serum
albumin levels (Churchill *et al.*, 1992). Therefore, there is plentiful evidence of a poor
outcome in terms of both morbidity and mortality in hypoalbuminemic patients.

Several studies of much smaller groups of patients have been reported in which
nutritional assessment has included techniques other than the measurement of
serum markers. For example, the derivation of a 'protein–calorie malnutrition index'
was described by Bilbrey and Cohen (1989). Individual scores were allocated for
anthropometry, serum protein concentrations, total lymphocyte counts, and clinical

evaluation. Addition of all scores gave the malnutrition index. Patients who scored in the moderate and severe malnutrition groups had considerably higher rates than those with little or no malnutrition. Markmann (1989) also used a scoring system based on anthropometry and biochemical markers to assess nutritional status. A group of 32 HD patients were studied. A total of five patients died over a 2-year period, all of whom were malnourished, whereas none of the patients with low scores, (indicating good nutritional status) died. Total body nitrogen has also been shown to be a prognostic marker in HD, with a low nitrogen index (i.e. measured nitrogen/ predicted normal nitrogen) being associated with an increased risk of death (Pollock *et al.*, 1995).

In conclusion, numerous studies, using various markers of malnutrition, show an increased risk of mortality with decreasing nutritional status. The very strong relationship between hypoalbuminemia and increased mortality, in repeated studies, is convincing evidence that malnourished HD patients are more likely to die than well-nourished patients. Commencing renal replacement in a poor nutritional state is associated with a poor outcome. None of the studies discussed give us hard data about the specific effects of long-term HD on nutrition. However, it seems evident that given the impact of malnutrition on mortality, assessment and maintenance of nutritional status throughout the duration of renal replacement therapy is essential to facilitate long-term patient survival.

Nutritional requirements

To maintain an individual in a well-nourished state, he or she must have an adequate intake of nutrients. An inadequate diet will result in a deficiency state. The minimal requirement for any nutrient is that amount which is necessary to prevent malnutrition. Thus, for protein this would be the amount of protein required to maintain a neutral nitrogen balance. As already discussed, the commonest form of deficiency state in HD patients is protein–calorie malnutrition. Normal young adults have average protein requirements of 0.6 g/kg body weight per day (although most adults in the western world eat significantly more protein than this). Because of normal variability, some individuals will require more than this. Thus, the minimal recommended protein intake is 0.75 g/kg per day, which is the minimal requirement of 0.6 plus two standard deviations, and therefore includes 97.5% of young adults (Young, 1993).

Protein requirements in HD patients are not well defined, but it is generally accepted that requirements in HD patients are greater than for normal subjects. The need for a greater protein intake than normal is probably multifactorial. Factors contributing to the increased protein requirement are discussed later. Based on data derived from only a few reports of nitrogen balance studies in small numbers of HD patients, the normal recommendation for protein intake in HD patients is 1.2 g/kg per day (Bergström and Lindholm, 1993).

As far as energy intake is concerned, until recently it was thought that HD patients had the same requirements as normal subjects (Slomowitz *et al.*, 1989), an intake of 35–40 kcal/kg per day generally being recommended. However, a recent report suggests that the accurate measurement of energy expenditure in a whole-room indirect calorimeter shows that resting energy expenditure is higher in HD patients than in normal subjects (Ikizler *et al.*, 1994*a*). Thus, it may be that we should be recommending higher calorie intakes than at present, although, as will be discussed, many patients do not achieve current recommended intakes.

The ability to maintain nitrogen balance is dependent upon energy intake. In normal subjects, low energy intake causes a negative nitrogen balance, whereas a high energy intake will lead to a positive nitrogen balance, despite no change in protein intake (Kishi *et al.*, 1978). It is clear that adequate caloric intake is also necessary to maintain nitrogen balance in HD patients. In a group of six HD patients, nitrogen balance was neutral or positive when energy intake was 45 kcal/kg per day. Of these, two patients had a negative nitrogen balance when the energy intake was reduced to 35 kcal/kg per day. All six patients were in negative nitrogen balance with an intake of 25 kcal/kg per day. Protein intake was maintained at a constant level throughout the study (Slomowitz *et al.*, 1989).

Pathogenesis of malnutrition in HD

The etiology of malnutrition in HD patients is multifactorial. These factors include inadequate nutritional intake, catabolic stimuli and direct effects of the hemodialysis procedure itself. These can be considered separately, although we must remember that in the individual patient they can all potentially contribute to malnutrition simultaneously.

Inadequate nutritional intake

Numerous nutritional surveys have shown an inadequate intake of both protein and energy in HD patients. For example, Guarnieri *et al.* (1983) measured mean protein intake in HD patients from one center to be 1.01 g/kg per day (compared with 1.38 g/kg per day in another center studied simultaneously by the same group). Other studies have shown mean protein intakes of less than 1 g/kg per day and energy intakes of 26–29 kcal/kg per day (Schoenfeld *et al.*, 1983; Markmann 1989; Jacob *et al.*, 1990). In a group of 29 Spanish HD patients, on HD for a mean of 68 months, there was a greater reduction in daily energy intake than daily protein intake (compared to the recommended values). Also it was of note that a greater proportion of the patients (86%) had a low caloric intake than had a low protein intake (59%) (Lorenzo *et al.*, 1995). As discussed earlier, adequate caloric intake is essential to permit the utilization of protein and to maintain nitrogen balance.

Inadequate nutritional intake in HD patients may be due to many factors. It is well recognized that anorexia, nausea, and vomiting are symptoms of 'uremia', and it is common clinical experience that these symptoms can be relieved by the commencement of dialysis. This raises the important point that patients who are inadequately dialyzed may be anorexic and therefore have inadequate nutritional intake. Clearly, therefore, the delivery of sufficient dialysis to reverse anorexia is essential. The issue of the relationship between the amount of dialysis delivered and nutritional status will be discussed more fully later. Unfortunately, the issue of inadequate intake is not simply one of 'adequate' dialysis. Many other factors contribute to the reduced intake of food in HD patients. These include psychosocial factors such as depression, loneliness, and poverty; the unpalatability of the diet because of fluid and dietary restrictions; gastropathy in diabetics, medications, and complicating or coexisting illnesses. We must not forget the importance of good dentition and oral hygiene, and the difficulties imposed on patients by poor mobility, particularly if they live alone. Many patients, particularly those who experience intradialytic cardiovascular instability, have nausea and vomiting during or after dialysis, and thus may eat less on their dialysis days. It is clear that input from all members of a multidisciplinary team may be necessary to optimize an individual patient's nutritional intake.

It is known that as renal function declines, patients spontaneously reduce their food intake. Data from the MDRD study (Kopple *et al.*, 1994) demonstrated that even at GFRs of as high as 25 ml/min, protein intake is reduced without any dietary advice. As the GFR falls, there is a further reduction in protein intake and an associated reduction in energy intake. To maintain nitrogen balance when protein intake is limited, adaptive responses must be activated. The initial major response is a reduction in amino-acid oxidation (Motil *et al.*, 1981). It has been shown that this response is intact in patients with moderately severe renal function (mean GFR = 11.56 ml/min) who are non-acidotic (Goodship *et al.*, 1990). However, patients with CRF and metabolic acidosis were unable to adapt to a low protein diet until their acidosis was corrected with sodium bicarbonate (Williams *et al.*, 1991). Thus, although patients with advanced CRF can adapt to protein restriction, metabolic acidosis will over-ride the adaptive responses. To achieve our aim of improving survival on HD, we should be aiming to have patients commence HD in a well-nourished state. Thus attention must be paid to the correction of metabolic acidosis and to ensuring adequate energy intake in the predialysis phase.

One major problem is that of the patient who presents (or is referred) to renal services at or near end-stage renal failure. Such patients are often malnourished, possibly due to a period of inadequate energy intake and uncontrolled acidosis.

Dose of dialysis and nutritional intake

In the NCDS study it was noted that patients with higher time-averaged urea concentrations had lower protein intakes (as measured by PCR) (Schoenfeld *et al.*, 1983). This suggests a relationship between the dose of dialysis and protein intake. Lindsay and Spanner (1989) investigated this further in a group of HD patients. They demonstrated a linear relationship between dose of dialysis, measured as *Kt/V*, and PCR. Attempts to increase dietary protein intake were unsuccessful unless the dose of dialysis was first increased. They also showed that the relationship between *Kt/V* and PCR was dependent upon the type of dialysis membrane. PCR increased to a greater extent with increasing *Kt/V* when a highly permeable, more biocompatible membrane (AN69S) was used than with a cellulose acetate membrane. Looking at this in another way, a specific PCR could be obtained with a lower dialysis dose when using a biocompatible membrane. In a further study, the effect of increasing *Kt/V* was assessed in a group of patients with PCR < 1 g/kg per day (Lindsay *et al.*, 1992). PCR increased significantly if *Kt/V* was increased. In a control group, whose *Kt/V* was maintained at a constant rate, there was no change in PCR. Based on this data, it has been suggested that dialysis therapy should be increased to improve protein intake in malnourished patients or when PCR is less than 1 g/kg per day. However, Panzetta (1995) reported that in 35 stable HD patients with Kt/V ranging from 0.8 to 1.51, protein intake was independent of the dose of dialysis, and concluded that if Kt/V is adequate, protein intake does not depend on the dose of dialysis delivered. Despite this, there is some evidence to suggest that an increased dose of dialysis is associated with an improvement in markers of nutrition. Acchiardo *et al.* (1994) increased the dose of dialysis delivered to 416 patients from a Kt/V of 1.09 to 1.44, and observed an increase in serum albumin of 32 ± 1 g/l to 38 ± 1 g/l. In a study by Hakim *et al.* (1994), designed to assess the effect of an increased dose of dialysis on mortality, mortality rates decreased with increased dose of dialysis, and there were significant increases in serum albumin and transferrin. It is also of note that PCR increased in this study, and that, unlike in Panzetta's study, there was a strong positive correlation between Kt/V and PCR. Thus, although there are conflicting results regarding the relationship between dose of dialysis and protein intake, these studies do suggest that increased dialysis dose can improve nutritional markers.

Catabolic factors in the HD patient

As has been discussed, HD patients have increased protein requirements compared to normal individuals. This suggests that there are factors which are increasing these patients' protein requirements, possibly by acting as a catabolic stimulus, or by preventing optimal utilization of the protein ingested. As we have seen, an inadequate energy intake will impair the patient's ability to maintain a nitrogen balance. Other factors that will be discussed are the catabolic effect of metabolic acidosis, and the effect on protein metabolism of the dialysis procedure. It is also of significance that many patients on HD are physically inactive, for a number of reasons, including fatigue, comorbid pathologies, and psychological factors. This inactivity may in itself result in a negative nitrogen balance and muscle wasting.

Metabolic acidosis

Metabolic acidosis exerts a catabolic effect in both normal human subjects and those with CRF. The first evidence of the catabolic effect of acidosis in CRF came from Papadoyannakis *et al.* (1984) who demonstrated that correction of acidosis in a group of CRF patients improved nitrogen balance. Subsequent work has demonstrated that acidosis increases the oxidation of branched-chain amino acids (BCAAs) in muscle. Plasma levels of BCAAs are low in CRF, with valine showing the greatest reduction (Alvestrand *et al.*, 1982). Low BCAAs occur even in patients fed an adequate diet. Thus, excessive BCAA catabolism is the likely cause. Rats with experimentally induced acidosis have decreased plasma levels of BCAAs, and increased rates of oxidation of leucine and valine in skeletal muscle (May *et al.*, 1987). In rats with CRF and associated acidosis, BCAA oxidation is increased in muscle (Hara *et al.*, 1987). When the acidosis is corrected with sodium bicarbonate, plasma BCAA levels and rates of oxidation in muscle are normalized. Similar results have been demonstrated in patients with CRF. In HD patients there is a strong correlation between the pre-dialysis bicarbonate concentration and the intracellular concentration of free valine measured in skeletal muscle biopsies (Bergström *et al.*, 1990). If the supply of this essential amino acid is limited, protein synthesis may be impaired. In nine HD patients, correction of acidosis over 6 months, led to an increase in the muscle con-centration of all the BCAAs (leucine, isoleucine, and valine) (Lofberg *et al.*, 1993). Direct measurement of leucine oxidation using the technique of labeled-leucine infusion, demonstrates that when metabolic acidosis is induced in normal subjects by the ingestion of ammonium chloride, leucine oxidation is increased (Reaich *et al.*, 1992). In a group of non-dialyzed CRF subjects, correction of acidosis decreased leu-cine oxidation (Reaich *et al.*, 1993). This increased oxidation of BCAAs by acidosis is secondary to the increased activity of branched-chain ketoacid dehydrogenase (the enzyme responsible for their irreversible oxidation) in muscle (England *et al.*, 1995).

As well as stimulating BCAA catabolism, metabolic acidosis increases protein degradation. Correction of acidosis in CRF patients decreases protein degradation (Reaich *et al.*, 1993). This also applies to patients on HD (Graham *et al.*, 1997) and CAPD (Graham *et al.*, 1996). Metabolic acidosis can remain a problem despite HD. A recent survey of 690 HD patients showed that 75% of the patients had predialysis plasma bicarbonate concentrations of 21 mmol/l or less (Price and Mitch, 1994). In a group of six HD patients, the predialysis plasma bicarbonate was increased from a mean of 18.5 mmol/l to 24.8 mmol/l by dialyzing against a high dialysate bicarbonate concentration (40 mmol/l) for 4 weeks. This was associated with a 28% decrease in whole-body protein degradation (Graham *et al.*, 1997). The proteolytic effect of meta-bolic acidosis is dependent upon the presence of glucocorticoids (May *et al.*, 1986) and acts by stimulating a specific proteolytic pathway, the ATP-dependent, ubiquitin-requiring pathway (Mitch *et al.*, 1994).

As discussed earlier, the presence of metabolic acidosis prevents the activation of normal adaptive responses to reduced protein intake. Thus the presence of uncor-rected metabolic acidosis in a HD patient will contribute to that individual's require-ment for a supranormal protein intake. Finally, as regards acidosis, it has recently been demonstrated that the induction of acidosis in normal subjects decreases the rate of albumin synthesis (Ballmer *et al.*, 1995). Whether the correction of acidosis in CRF increases their rate of albumin synthesis has not been studied.

Effects of HD

The hemodialysis procedure is associated with the loss of amino acids, 5–8 g of free amino acids being lost during each hemodialysis session, using low-flux dialyzers (Kopple *et al.*, 1973; Wolfson *et al.*, 1982). A further 4–5 g of peptide-bound amino acids (Kopple *et al.*, 1973) are lost. Using high-flux membranes, these losses increase by 30% (Ikizler *et al.*, 1994*b*). These amino-acid losses are associated with reductions in plasma levels of amino acids, but these changes are smaller in magnitude than would be predicted from the extent of the amino-acid loss. This implies that plasma amino acids are being replenished from intracellular stores, and calculations suggest that 25–30 g of body protein is catabolized to provide these additional amino acids. Thus, hemodialysis would seem to induce catabolism. This is supported by the finding of changes in nitrogen balance on hemodialysis days (Borah *et al.*, 1978) and of a greater urea appearance rate during hemodialysis than in the intradialytic period (Ward *et al.*, 1979; Farrell and Hone, 1980).

Studies of sham dialysis in normal subjects have shown an increased release of amino acids from the leg during dialysis with bioincompatible membranes (Gutierrez *et al.*, 1990), corresponding to the catabolism of 15–20 g of protein. Since sham dialysis causes no amino-acid loss, we can conclude that catabolism during hemodialysis is not simply secondary to the passive loss of amino acids. With more biocompatible membranes, there is no net loss of amino acids from skeletal muscle, indicating no increase in proteolysis (Gutierrez *et al.*, 1992; Ikizler *et al.*, 1994*b*). Thus we can conclude that contact between blood and a bioincompatible membrane is a catabolic stimulus, whereas biocompatible membranes, which cause less of an inflammatory reaction (Cheung, 1990), do not increase net protein catabolism. An increase in net catabolism may be due to either increased protein degradation, decreased protein synthesis, or a combination of both. Lim *et al.* (1993) demonstrated that during dialysis with Cuprophan membranes (i.e. bioincompatible), protein degradation was unaffected but there was a decrease in protein synthesis rates.

In summary, the hemodialysis procedure causes a loss of amino acids which is greater with high-flux dialyzers. Bioincompatible membranes, in sham-dialysis studies, induce net protein catabolism, and therefore may contribute to the increase in urea appearance and negative nitrogen balance seen during hemodialysis.

Prevention and treatment of malnutrition

Nutritional management involves the prevention of malnutrition if possible, its detection should it occur, and correction at as early a stage as possible. Maintenance of nutritional status throughout the predialysis phase should be a priority, hopefully ensuring that patients commence HD in as well-nourished a state as possible. Thus awareness of the spontaneous reduction in intake as GFR declines is important. Although protein restriction *per se* does not lead to malnutrition in the predialysis patient (Walser, 1993), if the diet is also deficient in calories, then the nitrogen balance will not be maintained, and so energy intake must be encouraged. Similarly, ensuring that acidosis is corrected is essential to permit appropriate adaptation to a spontaneous reduction in protein intake. When a patient reaches end-stage renal failure, reassessment of their dietary needs will be necessary. If the patient has been on a low protein diet (whether spontaneously or therapeutically), they will require re-education regarding their protein intake which will need to be increased. The need for an adequate caloric intake must be emphasized.

Despite attempts at prevention, malnutrition still occurs in HD patients. Ongoing vigilance by all members of the nephrology team should mean that any deterioration in nutritional status is recognized early. The occurrence of malnutrition in a previously stable patient should trigger a search for an underlying problem such as infection, malignancy, or other coexisting disease. Any correctable problem should be addressed. Meanwhile dietetic counseling and oral supplementation should be offered.

The role of underdialysis as a cause of anorexia and malnutrition was discussed earlier. Therefore, it is clear that an adequate dose of dialysis must be provided to prevent malnutrition. It is equally clear that our current understanding of the relationship between dialysis dose and nutritional intake is insufficient to define the optimum dose of dialysis for nutritional needs. Nevertheless, assessment of an anorexic or malnourished patient should include consideration of underdialysis as a possible cause, and the dose of dialysis should be optimized. However, it must always be remembered that anorexia in a HD patient may be due to the many other comorbid factors discussed earlier, including coexistent illnesses, psychological problems, and economic hardship.

Assessment of biochemical indices in HD patients ought to include the predialysis bicarbonate level. In view of the catabolic effects of metabolic acidosis, we should aim to maintain the predialysis bicarbonate level within normal limits, thereby decreasing protein degradation (Graham, *et al.*, 1997). Some patients may require oral sodium bicarbonate supplementation and/or high bicarbonate dialysate to achieve this.

The catabolic effect of bioincompatible dialysis membranes has already been discussed. Whether the use of bioincompatible membranes will have a long-term benefit on nutritional status and subsequent outcome is as yet undetermined. A recent publication by Parker *et al.* (1996) attempts to address the question, and there are suggestions that the use of biocompatible membranes do improve nutritional status. A group of patients just reaching ESRF were randomized to treatment with either a biocompatible or bioincompatible membrane. Those treated with the biocompatible membrane gained more weight, had an earlier and more marked rise in serum albumin, and consistently higher IGF-1 levels than those in the bioincompatible group. In contrast, the Italian Cooperative Dialysis Study Group found no difference in serum albumin and transferrin, changes in postdialysis weight, and anthropometry, in groups of stable HD patients treated with bioincompatible and biocompatible membranes for 2 years (Locatelli *et al.*, 1996). The obvious difference between these studies is that Parker *et al.* (1996) studied patients just commencing HD. These patients had lower baseline plasma albumin levels, and may well have been malnourished. All of the Italian patients were stable and had been on renal replacement therapy for at least 2 months (mean duration of dialysis prior to entry was 58 months), and had good nutritional indices. These differences suggest that in well-nourished, stable HD patients, the dialysis membrane may not have an effect on nutritional status, whereas malnourished patients may be more likely to improve (or improve more rapidly) if a biocompatible membrane is used. It would therefore seem reasonable to consider the use of a biocompatible membrane in malnourished patients.

Recognition of the limitations of dietetic counseling and oral supplementation in the correction of malnutrition (Compher *et al.*, 1991; Hakim and Levin, 1993) has led to attempts to supplement nutritional intake in other ways. One method is to use intradialytic parenteral nutrition (IDPN), consisting of an infusion of amino acids and glucose or lipids during dialysis. As hemodialysis is a catabolic stimulus, the provision of nutrients during the procedure seems a reasonable step. Clearly this method of nutritional support also has the advantages of ensuring compliance, as well as permitting the appropriate volume to be removed during dialysis. However, only a limited amount of amino acids and calories can be provided, but larger amounts can actually be provided by the regular administration of oral supplements (Wolfson, 1993).

Studies of the nutritional effect of IDPN are commonly fraught with problems such as poor control groups, small numbers of patients, and inadequate treatment times. Recent studies suggesting benefit from IDPN include a small randomized trial of 26 malnourished hemodialysis patients (Cano *et al.*, 1990), in which treatment with IDPN increased serum albumin, weight, and arm muscle cirumference. A further two retrospective studies also suggest benefit. Capelli *et al.* (1994) studied 81 malnourished patients, 50 of whom received IDPN for an average of 9 months after failing to respond to dietary counseling and oral supplements. The remaining 31, all of whom had less-marked weight loss than the treated group, did not receive IDPN. Mortality in the treated group was significantly less than in the untreated. Chertow *et al.* (1994) identified 1679 patients who had received IDPN and compared them with 22517 patients who had not (all of the patients were dialyzed in National Medical Care dialysis units). Hypoalbuminemic patients who were treated with IDPN showed increases in serum albumin and creatinine levels, and lower mortality rates than untreated hypoalbuminemic patients. Patients with normal serum albumin levels did not benefit from treatment with IDPN. Clearly these two studies suffer from the fact that they were retrospective, and unblinded. Before we are in a position to recommend IDPN in malnourished patients, long-term prospective, controlled trials are required. Meanwhile, however, it seems reasonable to use IDPN in severely malnourished HD patients in whom other methods of nutritional support have failed.

Recently there has been interest in the use of growth factors as anabolic agents in the management of malnutrition. Growth hormone and IGF-1 have significant anabolic properties, and, indeed, recombinant human growth hormone (rHGH) has been used at pharmacological doses to promote anabolism in various patient groups (Kaplan, 1993). Although rHGH has been shown to improve serum albumin, transferrin, and IGF-1 concentrations when given in combination with IDPN to malnourished HD patients (Schulman *et al.*, 1993), to date there have been no prospective controlled trials of either of these agents in HD patients. Their use therefore remains experimental, as well as prohibitively expensive.

Conclusions

Malnutrition is common in HD. The association between nutritional status and outcome has been discussed, with numerous studies suggesting an increased risk of mortality with decreasing nutritional status. The malnutrition is multifactorial, with both inadequate nutritional intake and catabolic stimuli contributing. Prevention of malnutrition should be the aim of nutritional management. To this end, regular nutritional assessment and ongoing vigilance is essential. Established malnutrition can be difficult to correct. In the prevention and treatment of malnutrition, an adequate intake of protein and energy must be ensured, and factors causing anorexia and catabolism eliminated.

References

Acchiardo, S. R., Moore, L. W., and Latour, P. A. (1983). Malnutrition as the main factor in morbidity and mortality of hemodialysis patients. *Kidney International*, **24** (Suppl. 16), 199–203.

Acchiardo, S., Fuller, J., Dyson, B., Hatten, K. W., and Ellis, K. (1994). Can we improve mortality rate in hemodialysis patients? *Journal of the American Society of Nephrology*, **5**, 430.

Allman, M. A., Allen, B. J., Stewart, P. M., *et al.* (1990). Body protein of patients undergoing haemodialysis, *European Journal of Clinical Nutrition*, **44**, 123–31.

Alvestrand, A., Furst, P., and Bergström, J. (1982). Plasma and muscle free amino acids in uremia: influence of nutrition with amino acids. *Clinical Nephrology*, **18**, 297–305.

Ballmer, P. E., McNurlan, M. A., Hulter, H. N., Anderson, S. E., Garlick, P. J., and Krapf, R. (1995). Chronic metabolic acidosis decreases albumin synthesis and induces negative nitrogen balance in humans. *Journal of Clinical Investigation*, **95**, 39–45.

Bansal, V. K., Papli, S., Pickering, S., Ing, T. S., Vertuno, L. L., and Hano, J. E. (1980). Protein-calorie malnutrition and cutaneous anergy in hemodialysis maintained patients. *American Journal of Clinical Nutrition*, **33**, 1608–11.

Bergström, J. (1995). Nutrition and mortality in hemodialysis. *Journal of the American Society of Nephrology*, **6**, 1329–41.

Bergström, J., and Lindholm, B. (1993). Nutrition and adequacy of dialysis: how do hemodialysis and CAPD compare? *Kidney International*, **43** (Suppl. 40), S39–S50.

Bergström, J., Alvestrand, A., and Furst, P. (1990). Plasma and free amino acids in maintenance hemodialysis patients without protein malnutrition. *Kidney International*, **38**, 108–14.

Bilbrey, G. L. and Cohen, T. L. (1989). Identification and treatment of protein-calorie malnutrition in chronic hemodialysis patients. *Dialysis and Transplantation*, **18**, 669–77.

Borah, M. F., Schoenfeld, P. Y., Gotch, F. A., Sargent, J. A., Wolfson, M., and Humphreys, M. H. (1978). Nitrogen balance during intermittent dialysis therapy of uremia. *Kidney International*, **14**, 491–500.

Cano, N., Labastie-Coeyrehourq, J., Lacombe, P., *et al.* (1990). Perdialytic parenteral nutrition with lipids and amino acids in malnourished hemodialysis patients. *American Journal of Clinical Nutrition*, **52**, 726–30.

Capelli, J. P., Kushner, H., Camisciola, T. C., Chen, S. M., and Torres, M. A. (1994). Effect of intradialytic parenteral nutrition on mortality rates in end-stage renal disease care. *American Journal of Kidney Diseases*, **23**, 808–16.

Chertow, G. M., Ling, J., Lew, N. L., Lazarus, J. M., and Lowrie, E. G. (1994). The association of intradialytic parenteral nutrition with survival in hemodialysis patients. *American Journal of Kidney Diseases*, **24**, 912–20.

Chertow, G. M., Lowrie, E. L., Wilmore, D. W., *et al.* (1995). Nutritional assessment with bioelectrical impedance analysis in maintenance hemodialysis patients. *Journal of the American Society of Nephrology*, **6**, 75–81.

Cheung, A. K. (1990). Biocompatibility of hemodialysis membranes. *Journal of the American Society of Nephrology*, **1**, 150–61.

Churchill, D. N., Taylor, D. W., Cook, R. J., *et al.* (1992). Canadian hemodialysis morbidity study. *American Journal of Kidney Diseases*, **19**, 214–34.

Collins, A. J., Ma, J. Z., Umen, A., and Keshaviah, P. (1994). Urea index and other predictors of hemodialysis patient survival. *American Journal of Kidney Diseases*, **23**, 272–82.

Compher, C., Mullen, J. L., and Barker, C. F. (1991). Nutritional support in renal failure. *Surgical Clinics of North America*, **71**, 597–608.

Degoulet, P., Legrain, M., Reach, I., *et al.* (1982). Mortality risk factors in patients treated by chronic haemodialysis: report of the Daiphane Collaborative Study. *Nephron*, **31**, 103–10.

England, B. K., Greiber, S., Mitch, W. E., *et al.* (1995). Rat muscle branched-chain ketoacid dehydrogenase activity and mRNAs increase with extracellular acidemia. *American Journal of Physiology*, **268**, C1395–C1400.

Farrell, P. C., and Hone, P. W. (1980). Dialysis-induced catabolism. *American Journal of Clinical Nutrition*, **33**, 1417–22.

Goldwasser, P., Mittman, M., Antignanin A., *et al.* (1993). Predictors of mortality on hemodialysis. *Journal of the American Society of Nephrology*, **3**, 1613–22.

Goodship, T. H. J., Mitch, W. E., Hoerr, R. A., Wagner, D. A., Steinman, T. I., and Young, V. R. (1990). *Journal of the American Society of Nephrology*, **1**, 66–75.

Gotch, F. A., and Sargent, J. A. (1985). A mechanistic analysis of the National Cooperative Dialysis Study (NCDS). *Kidney International*, **28**, 526–34.

Graham, K. A., Reaich, D., Channon, S. M., *et al.*, (1996). Correction of acidosis in CAPD decreases whole body protein degradation. *Kidney International*, **49**, 1396–400.

Graham, K. A., Reaich, D., Channon, S. M., Downie, S., and Goodship, T. H. J. (1997). Correction of acidosis in haemodialysis decreases whole body protein degradation. *Journal of the American Society of Nephrology* **8**, 632–37.

Guarnieri, G., Toigo, G., Situlin, R., *et al.* (1983). Muscle biopsy studies in chronically uremic patients: evidence for malnutrition. *Kidney International*, **24** (Suppl. 16), S187–S193.

Gutierrez, A., Alvestrand, A., Wahren J., and Bergstrom, J. (1990). Effect of in vivo contact between blood and dialysis membranes on protein catabolism in humans. *Kidney International*, **38**, 487–94.

Gutierrez, A., Bergström, J., and Alvestrand, A. (1992). Protein catabolism in sham dialysis: the effect of different membranes. *Clinical Nephrology*, **38**, 20–9.

Hakim, R. M., and Levin, N. (1993). Malnutrition in hemodialysis patients. *American Journal of Kidney Diseases*, **21**, 125–37.

Hakim, R. M., Breyer, J., Ismail, N., and Schulman, G. (1994). Effects of dose of dialysis on morbidity and mortality. *American Journal of Kidney Diseases*, **23**, 661–9.

Hara, Y., May, R. C., Kelly, R. A., and Mitch, W. E. (1987). Acidosis, not azotemia, stimulates branched-chain amino acid catabolism in uremic rats. *Kidney International*, **32**, 808–14.

Harter, H. R. (1983). Review of significant findings from the National Cooperative Dialysis Study and recommendations. *Kidney International*, **23** (Suppl. 13), 107–12.

Ikizler, T. A., Wingard, R. L., Sun, M., and Hakim, R. M. (1994*a*). Energy expenditure (EE) and respiratory quotient (RQ) during hemodialysis (HD) with different dialysis membranes. *Journal of the American Society of Nephrology*, **5**, 493.

Ikizler, T. A., Flakoll, P. J., Parker, R. A., and Hakim, R. M. (1994*b*). Amino acid and albumin losses during hemodialysis. *Kidney International*, **46**, 830–7.

Iseki, I., Kawazoe, N., and Fukiyama, K. (1993). Serum albumin is a strong predictor of death in chronic dialysis patients. *Kidney International*, **44**, 115–19.

Jacob, V., Le Carpentier, J. E., Salzano, S., *et al.* (1990). IGF-1, a marker of undernutrition in hemodialysis patients. *American Journal of Clinical Nutrition*, **52**, 39–44.

Kaplan, S. L. (1993). The newer uses of growth hormone in adults. *Advances in Internal Medicine*, **38**, 287–301.

Kaufmann, P., Smolle, K. H., Horina, J. H., Zach, R., and Krejs, G. J. (1994). Impact of long-term hemodialysis on nutritional status in patients with end-stage renal failure. *Clinical Investigator*, **72**, 754–61.

Kishi, K., Miytani, K., and Inoue, G. (1978). Requirement and utilization of egg protein by Japanese young men with marginal intakes of energy. *Journal of Nutrition*, **198**, 658–69.

Kopple, J. D. (1984). Causes of catabolism and wasting in acute or chronic renal failure. In *Nephrology* (ed. R. R. Robinson), pp. 1498–1514. Springer-Verlag, New York.

Kopple, J. D., Swendseid, M. E., Shinaberger, J. H., and Umezawa, C. Y. (1973). The free and bound amino acids removed by hemodialysis. *Transcripts of the American Society of Artificial Internal Organs*, 19, 309–13.

Kopple, J. D., Chumlea, W. C., Gassman, J. J., *et al.* (1994). Relationship between GFR and nutritional status: results from the MDRD study. *Journal of the American Society of Nephrology*, 5, 325.

Lim, V. S., Bier, D. M., Flanigan, M. J., and Sum-Ping, S. T. (1993). The effect of hemodialysis on protein metabolism: a leucine kinetic study. *Journal of Clinical Investigation*, 91, 2429–36.

Lindsay, R. M., and Spanner, E. (1989). A hypothesis: the protein catabolic rate is dependent upon the type and amount of treatment in dialyzed uremic patients. *American Journal of Kidney Diseases*, 132, 382–9.

Lindsay, R., Spanner, E., Heidenheim, P., *et al.* (1992). Which comes first, Kt/V or PCR— chicken or egg? *Kidney International*, 42 (Suppl. 38), S32–S37.

Locatelli, F., Mastrangelo, F., Redaelli, B., *et al.* (1996). Effects of different membranes and dialysis technologies on patient treatment tolerance and nutritional parameters. *Kidney International*, 50, 1293–302.

Lofberg, E., Wernerman, J., and Bergström, J. (1993). Branched chain amino acids in muscle increase during correction of metabolic acidosis in hemodialysis (HD) patients. *Journal of the American Society of Nephrology*, 4, 363.

Lorenzo, V., de Bonis, E., Rufino, M., *et al.* (1995). Caloric rather than protein deficiency predominates in stable chronic haemodialysis patients. *Nephrology, Dialysis, Transplantation*, 10, 1885–9.

Lowrie, E. G., and Lew, N. L. (1990). Death risk in hemodialysis patients: the predictive value of commonly measured variables and an evaluation of death rate differences between facilities. *American Journal of Kidney Diseases*, 5, 458–82.

Markmann, P. (1989). Nutritional status and mortality of patients in regular dialysis therapy. *Journal of Internal Medicine*, 226, 429–32.

May, R. C., Kelly, R. A., and Mitch, W. E. (1986). Metabolic acidosis stimulates protein degradation in rat muscle by a glucocorticoid-dependent mechanism. *Journal of Clinical Investigation*, 77, 614–21.

May, R. C., Hara, Y., Kelly, R. A., Block, K. P., Buse, M. G., and Mitch, W. E. (1987). Branched-chain amino acid metabolism in rat muscle: abnormal regulation in acidosis. *American Journal of Physiology*, 252, E712–E718.

Mitch, W. E., Medina, R., Grieber, S., *et al.* (1994). Metabolic acidosis stimulates muscle protein degradation by activating the adenosine triphosphate-dependent pathway involving ubiquitin and proteasomes. *Journal of Clinical Investigation*, 93, 2127–33.

Motil, K. J., Matthews, D. E., Bier, D. M., Burke, J. F., Munro, H. N., and Young, V. R. (1981). Whole body leucine and lysine metabolism. Response to dietary protein intake in young men. *American Journal of Physiology*, 240, E712–E721.

Owen, W. F., Lew, N. L., Liu, Y., Lowrie, E. G., and Lazarus, J. M. (1993). The urea reduction ratio and serum albumin concentration as predictors of mortality in patients undergoing hemodialysis. *New England Journal of Medicine*, 329, 1001–6.

Panzetta, G. (1995). Protein intake does not depend on the dose delivered—provided Kt/V is adequate. *Nephrology, Dialysis, Transplantation*, 10, 2286–9.

Pappadoyannakis, N. J., Stefanides, C. J., and McGeown, M. (1984). The effect of the correction of metabolic acidosis on nitrogen and protein balance of patients with chronic renal failure. *American Journal of Clinical Nutrition*, 40, 623–7.

Parker, T. F. III, Wingard, R. L., Husni, R., Ikizler, T. A., Parker, R. A., and Hakim, R. L. (1996). Effect of the membrane biocompatibility on nutritional parameters in chronic hemo- dialysis patients. *Kidney International*, **49**, 551–6.

Piccoli, G. B., Salomone, M., Bonello, F., *et al.* (1993). Dialysis choice in the elderly: cause or effect of relevant clinical problems? *Nephrology, Dialysis, Transplantation*, **8**, 1006.

Pollock, C. A., Ibels, L. S., Allen, B. A., *et al.* (1995). Total body nitrogen as a prognostic marker in maintenance dialysis. *Journal of the American Society of Nephrology*, **6**, 82–8.

Price, S. R., and Mitch, W. E. (1994). Metabolic acidosis and uremic toxicity: protein and amino acid metabolism. *Seminars in Nephrology*, **14**, 232–7.

Rayner, H. C., Stroud, D. B., Salamon, K. M., *et al.* (1991). Anthropometry underestimates body protein depletion in haemodialysis patients. *Nephron*, **59**, 33–40.

Reaich, D., Channon, S. M., Scrimgeour, C. M., and Goodship, T. H. J. (1992). Ammonium chloride-induced acidosis increases protein breakdown and amino acid oxidation in humans. *American Journal of Physiology*, **263**, E735–E739.

Reaich, D., Channon, S. M., Scrimgeour, C. M., Daley, S. E., Wilkinson, R., and Goodship, T. H. J. (1993). Correction of acidosis in humans with CRF decreases protein degradation and amino acid oxidation. *American Journal of Physiology*, **265**, E230–E235.

Roubenoff, R., Kehayias, J. J., Dawson-Hughes, B., and Heymsfield, S. B. (1993). Use of dual energy X-ray absorptiometry in body composition studies: not yet a 'gold standard'. *American Journal of Clinical Nutrition*, **58**, 589–91.

Schoenfeld, P. Y., Henry, R. R., Laird, N. M., and Roxe, D. M. (1983). Assessment of nutritional status of the National Cooperative Dialysis Study population. *Kidney International*, **23** (Suppl. 13), S80–S88.

Schulman, G., Wingard, R. L., Hutchinson, R. L., Lawrence, P., and Hakim, R. M. (1993). The effects of recombinant human growth hormone and intradialytic parenteral nutrition in malnourished hemodialysis patients. *American Journal of Kidney Diseases*, **21**, 527–34.

Slomowitz, L. A., Monteon, F. J., Grosvenor, M., Laidlaw, S. A., and Kopple, J. D. (1989). Effect of energy intake on nutritional status in maintenance hemodialysis patients. *Kidney International*, **35**, 704–11.

Walser, M. (1993). Does prolonged protein restriction preceding dialysis lead to protein mal- nutrition at the onset of dialysis? *Kidney International*, **44**, 1139–44.

Ward, R. A., Shirlow, M. J., Hayes, J. M., Chapman, G. V., and Farrell, P. C. (1979). Protein catabolism during hemodialysis. *American Journal of Clinical Nutrition*, **32**, 243–9.

Williams, B., Hattersley, J., Layward, E., and Walls, J. (1991). Metabolic acidosis and skeletal muscle adaptation to low protein diets in chronic uremia. *Kidney International*, **40**, 779–86.

Wolfson, M. (1993). The cost and bother of intradialytic parenteral nutrition are not justified by available scientific studies. *American Society of Artificial Internal Organs Journal*, **39**, 864–7.

Wolfson, M., Jones, M. R., and Kopple, J. D. (1982). Amino acid losses during hemodialysis with infusion of amino acids and glucose. *Kidney International*, **21**, 500–6.

Woodrow, G., Oldroyd, B., Turney, J. H., Tompkins, L., Brownjohn, J. M., and Smith, M. A. (1996). Whole body and regional body composition in patients with chronic renal failure. *Nephrology, Dialysis, Transplantation*, **11**, 1613–18.

Young, V. R. (1993). Nutritional requirements of normal adults. In *Nutrition and the Kidney* (ed. W. E. Mitch and S. Klahr), pp. 1–34. Little Brown, Boston.

10

Adequacy of dialysis: the key to survival

Frank Gotch and Nathan W. Levin

Introduction

The rationale for the treatment of uremia with dialysis therapy rests primarily on the premise that the uremic syndrome results from the accumulation of toxic solutes, which are normally cleared from body water by the kidney and can be successfully cleared by dialysis. It is well established that adequate dialysis therapy must normalize the extracellular fluid volume and its composition with regard to the concentrations of Na, K, Pi, Ca, HCO_3 and Mg. Consequently, the first criteria to be met for adequate dialysis are the optimal control of extracellular volume and the concentrations of these electrolytes.

Apart from the acid–base balance, volume, and electrolyte abnormalities, uremic toxicity has been presumed to result from the accumulation of organic metabolites which have a concentration-dependent toxicity. The dramatic clinical experiences in the 1950s showing the predictable reversal of uremic coma by dialysis (Teschan *et al.*, 1955; Maher *et al.*, 1961) provided the first clinical evidence to support this hypothesis. The thick cellulosic membranes used at that time strongly suggested that the toxic metabolites removed were low molecular weight materials. The bulk protein catabolite identified in dialysates was urea, which comprises 90% of waste nitrogen and had long been known to accumulate in renal failure. Other major nitrogenous constituents found in dialysates were creatinine and uric acid. Creatinine has been shown to have no correlation with clinical outcome other than as an index of nutrition (Lowrie and Lew, 1990), while uric acid is well known to have tissue toxicity at high concentration but is not used as a marker to describe the dose of dialysis. During the intervening years an enormous number of low molecular weight organic molecules have been shown to accumulate in uremic plasma (Vanholder *et al.*, 1996), but none of these have been clearly shown to exhibit specific organ system toxicities. The level of parathyroid hormone, however, may be an exception.

The first patients treated with chronic dialysis developed crippling neuropathy, this led to intense speculation regarding the molecular size of uremic toxins that must be effectively removed during dialysis (Scribner *et al.*, 1960; Scribner, 1965) and to attempts to quantify the dose of dialysis (Bass *et al.*, 1975; Sargent and Gotch, 1975). This early experience with chronic dialysis led to the middle-molecule hypothesis and world-wide efforts to identify uremic toxicity due to molecules in the molecular weight range 1000 to 2000 dalton. Despite an enormous amount of research over the past 25 years, there is no convincing evidence of toxic solutes in this molecular weight range (Vanholder *et al.*, 1996). More recently, a group of substances of molecular weight 8000–28 000 Da affecting polymorphonuclear function have been analyzed by Haag-Weber *et al.* (1994). However, no kinetic studies which could provide prescriptive guidance have been described. It is now well established that the accumulation, over 10 to 20 years of dialysis therapy, of polymerized β_2-microglobulin ($\beta 2m$) (molecular weight about 13 000), results in severe bone and soft-tissue damage (Vanholder *et al.*, 1996), and that $\beta 2m$ removal must be considered in long-term dialysis therapy. Famously good survival data have been reported in patients dialyzed in Tassin, despite the use of membranes which remove little or no $\beta 2m$ (these patients did suffer significantly from the effect of dialysis amyloidosis).

Serious peripheral neuropathy has largely disappeared during the last several decades, and, unfortunately, so has the primary clinical outcome parameter used to assess adequacy of the dialysis dose, i.e. the mortality rate achieved for a treated patient population after standardization for demographics and comorbidities. The mechanisms underlying mortality and their relationships to dialysis dose are not well understood. A recent study of cause–specific mortality concluded that a low dose appears to promote atherogenesis, infection, malnutrition, and failure to thrive through a variety of poorly defined pathophysiological mechanisms (Bloaembergen *et al.*, 1996). Consequently, the risk/dose function in dialysis therapy has been derived from statistical analyses of mortality rates in populations under therapy. The powerful effects of age and comorbid conditions, such as diabetes mellitus, myocardial dysfunction, coronary artery disease, and peripheral vascular disease, on mortality rate have been well quantified in recent years (Held *et al.*, 1996).

The dialysis dose

The dialyzer provides a clearance pathway for the removal of toxic solutes from body water, and thus dialysis therapy is an analog of pharmacological therapy. The dose and frequency of administration of a drug required to achieve a specified concentration profile and maximal clinical effect must be adequate to replace drug losses through metabolic, hepatic, renal, and other clearance pathways. In dialysis therapy, the dialysis dose constitutes a clearance pathway provided to control the concentration of toxic uremic solutes, the size of the dose being determined by the dialyzer clearance and frequency of dialyses. The dose would be most precisely defined by the clearance required to maintain the concentrations of these solutes below the levels at which clinical toxicity appears. Unfortunately, we have not achieved that level of understanding with respect to the molecular etiology of uremic toxicity. Consequently, we quantify the dose by the fractional clearance of the distribution volume of urea, which is considered a generic, low molecular weight, toxic metabolite. The fractional clearance can be quantified as the product of dialyzer clearance (K) multiplied by the treatment time (t) divided by the solute distribution volume (V), i.e. Kt/V. In addition to serving as a generic low molecular weight marker molecule, the kinetic analysis of urea mass balance can provide a precise measure of the daily protein catabolic rate: this is equivalent to the dietary protein intake in patients with a steady-state nitrogen balance, which usually exists in the absence of acute intervening illness.

Definitions of Kt/V

It is well known that there may be substantial underdelivery of the prescribed dose of dialysis (Sargent, 1990; Delmez and Windus, 1992). Consequently, the dose is best defined as the delivered (d) Kt/V, Kt/Vd, which must be calculated from an analysis of pre- and postdialysis BUNs (Co, Ct). During the early years of dialysis therapy when very, low-efficiency dialyzers were used with urea clearance (KdU) of 50–100 ml/min, urea could reasonably be considered to be distributed in a single pool equal to total body water. With the advent of high-efficiency dialyzers it has become increasingly clear that urea kinetics during rapid dialysis cannot always be adequately described by assuming single-pool kinetics. The single-pool variable volume, urea kinetic model (Gotch, 1996) assumes that urea is in concentration equilibrium throughout its volume of distribution at the end of dialysis, so that pre- and immediate post-dialysis BUNs can be used to calculate the delivered single-pool Kt/V (spKt/Vd).

Recent studies (Smye *et al.*, 1992; Daugirdas and Schneditz, 1995; Tattersal *et al.*, 1996) have shown that urea is not in concentration equilibrium at the end of dialysis with modern, efficient (i.e. high-clearance) dialysis therapy, and that there may be a substantial rebound rise in the plasma urea concentration postdialysis as equilibration occurs. A single-pool kinetic analysis will result in the overestimation of Kt/Vd due to double-pool effects with rebound. The two urea pools were long considered to be represented anatomically by extracellular and intracellular water, although more recently it has been suggested that the two compartments more likely represent organ systems with high blood flow (viscera) and low blood flow (skeletal muscle and skin) (Daugirdas and Schneditz, 1995). Since the latter organs contain the overwhelming proportion of the body's water (and therefore urea) content, reduction in flow will result in sequestration of urea with equilibration occurring postdialysis once normal blood flow has been re-established. Both these double-pool models are similar in that they contain a first-order, internal whole-body, urea transfer coefficient, which is conceptualized as either a diffusive coefficient at the cell membrane (Smye *et al.*, 1992) or a blood flow, rate-limited transfer from whole organs (Daugirdas and Schneditz (1995). The magnitude of dysequilibrium in both models is predicted to be strongly dependent on the rate of dialysis (the dialyzer urea clearance divided by the total urea distribution volume). In addition to the underestimation of dose with spKt/Vd, sp kinetic analysis will also result in an overestimation of PCR (spNPCR), since the rebound in BUN will be erroneously calculated as newly generated urea rather than simply equilibration. Correct estimates of Kt/Vd and PCR must be based on the higher equilibrated BUN value (Ct') after postdialysis equilibration which is used to calculate the equilibrated treatment and nutritional parameters, eKt/Vd and eNPCR.

Measurement of the dialysis dose

Although eKt/Vd provides the most rigorous measurement of normalized dose, it is important to note that this parameter must be calculated from spKt/Vd and that spKt/Vd is best determined from formal urea kinetic analysis using the variable volume, single-pool kinetic model (Gotch, 1996; Tattersal *et al.*, 1996). The spKt/Vd can be calculated using the simple Daugirdas formulation (Daugirdas, 1992) which will be highly reliable for the analysis of average doses in the treatment of large patient populations. It is also rigorous for individual patients *if all input parameters are correct*, but it is far less suitable for the analysis of the quality of the delivered dose in individual dialysis treatments since there is always some uncertainty about the accuracy of the treatment parameters. For example, the spKt/Vd might be 2.0 using the approximation equation, but if the Ct was drawn with the blood pump running at 400 ml/min with access recirculation, the Ct would be artifactually low. However, the volume calculated from the solution of the urea model would be very low and immediately disclose an artifact in the post-BUN measurement. The cornerstone of quality improvement is the kinetic calculation of volume (Gotch, 1996), which is used to recognize and quantify errors in dialysis delivery, provide a quantitative method to prescribe dialysis, and to calculate the total protein intake, ePCR.

The major impact of the rate of dialysis on the eKt/Vd can be seen in Fig. 10.1, where spKt/Vd is shown as a dependent variable of eKt/Vd and the treatment time. It can be seen that to deliver an eKt/Vd of 1.0, the spKt/Vd required increases from 1.08 to 1.60 as the dialysis treatment time decreases from 8 hours to 1 hour.

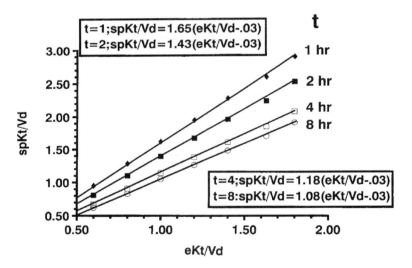

Fig. 10.1 The spKt/Vd (single-pool *kt/V* delivered) equivalent to eKt/Vd (equilibrated *kt/V* delivered) is strongly dependent on the treatment time.

Clinical outcome as a function of dose adequacy

We have recently reviewed several large clinical studies (Gotch *et al.*, 1997) relating the relative risk of mortality (RR) to the dose of dialysis, and derived a relative risk/dose function (RR/D function). The results of this analysis are shown in Fig. 10.2, where the RR is shown as a merged and normalized (nRR) function of eKt/Vd from two large databases totaling approximately 15 000 patients (Owen *et al.*, 1993; Levin *et al.*, 1995; Gotch *et al.*, 1997). Analysis of this large merged database by stepwise linear regression showed that nRR was not a continuous linear function of eKt/Vd. The curve was linear with a sharply increasing RR for eKt/Vd $\leq$ 1.03 with a breakpoint at eKt/Vd = 1.03 where the slope became 0 and nRR was constant for eKt/Vd > 1.03. The spKt/Vd values corresponding to an eKt/Vd of 1.03 would be 1.2 for 4-hour dialyses and 1.4 for 2-hour dialyses.

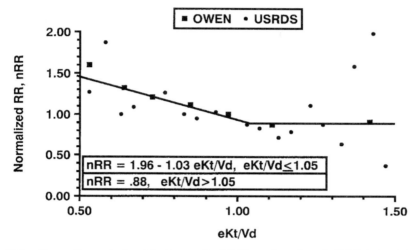

Fig. 10.2   Normalized relative risk of mortality (nRR) as a function of eKt/Vd derived from the merged Owen and USRDS data.

The doses used (Owen *et al.*, 1993; Levin *et al.*, 1995) for the construction of the RR/D function in Fig. 10.2 were not prospectively randomized, but they were relatively short-term studies and probably had a relatively small variance on the means. This is of considerable importance because many retrospective RR/D response functions have been based on mean eKt/Vd values with large standard deviations (SD) on the means (Hakim *et al.*, 1994; Parker *et al.*, 1994). With a non-linear dose response, the RR will always be overestimated relative to mean eKt/Vd levels, with large SDs covering both the steep and shallow portions of the dose-response curve.

Up to the present time the only study of clinical outcome correlated to prospectively randomized, constant doses of dialysis was the National Cooperative Dialysis Study (NCDS) (Lowrie and Laird, 1983). Analysis of the probability of failure (PF) in this study as a function of spKt/Vd clearly showed a non-linear relationship which could be fit to either an exponential or step-function change (Gotch and Sargent, 1985). We have re-examined this data after converting the dose parameter from spKt/Vd to eKt/Vd with results shown in Fig. 10.3, where the NCDS data can be seen to conform with an abrupt change to a constant *PF* of 0.10 at eKt/Vd $\geq$ 0.94. Thus the NCDS and the merged data of Owen *et al.* (1993) and the USRDS (1995) all show the change to a zero slope on clinical outcome for eKt/Vd levels greater than 1.03. These results suggest it is unlikely that survival will be increased when eKt/Vd levels are higher than approximately 1.0 to 1.1, but that mortality risk will sharply and linearly rise from 0.88 to 1.45, a 65% increase in relative risk, as eKt/Vd falls from 1.03 to 0.50. Clearly, to assure maximal survival it is necessary to provide an eKt/Vd $\geq$ 1.03 for every individual patient. It is not sufficient to maintain the average eKt/Vd for a facility at 1.03.

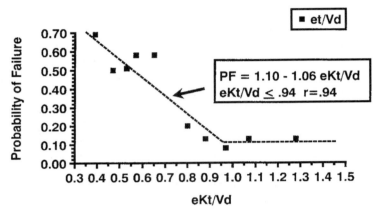

Fig. 10.3 Probability of failure of NCDS patients as a function of eKt/Vd calculated using the rate adjustment equation.

Do relatively high doses improve outcome?

A remarkably low gross mortality rate of 3.5% has been reported for 445 patients by Charra *et al.* (1992) in association with an average spKt/Vd of 1.67 and a treatment time of 8.0 hours (*see* Chapter 11). This remarkable data has been widely interpreted to indicate that an spKt/Vd of 1.7 delivered over 8 hours (which defines an eKt/Vd of 1.6) is required to achieve the maximal long-term survival of dialysis patients. Although the Tassin results are quite remarkable, very low mortality rates in the range of 2 to 3% have been reported for populations as large as 250 to 500 patients with major risk factors excluded (Shapiro and Umen, 1983; Collins and Kjellstrand, 1990) and treatment with calculated (not delivered) spKt/V doses of 1.3. The level of comorbidities in the Tassin database was very low, with a 3.5% incidence of diabetes mellitus and a mean age of 42 years. Further, the Tassin patients were not transplanted, which can be predicted to result in retention of patients with low comorbidities in the long-term survival database.

The Tassin patients also exhibited a very high incidence of normal blood pressure without a need for antihypertensive therapy. This has been attributed to the long treatment time which permits a very slow ultrafiltration rate and more optimal dry, body-weight levels (Gotch and Sargent, 1985; Scribner, 1996). However, it is of considerable importance to note that the interdialytic weight gains in Tassin patients were extremely low: 1.9 $\pm$ 0.6 kg (mean $\pm$ SD). Typical weight gains for patients in the USA are 2.5 $\pm$ 2.0 kg (Chan and Green, 1994). Assuming that the positive fluid balances are typically isotonic, it can readily be calculated that the sodium intake in Tassin patients averaged 2.5 $\pm$ 0.8 g/day (mean $\pm$ SD) compared to typical levels of

3.5 ± 2.9 g/day for USA patients. Far greater compliance with a low dietary sodium intake was achieved in the Tassin patients and is much more likely to account for the lower blood pressure than the extremely long treatment time with slow ultrafiltration. The reasons for achieving remarkably low sodium intakes with small variance are obscure but are unlikely to be due to long treatment time.

Low, gross mortality rates have been reported for unselected patient populations with short treatment times. Keshaviah and Collins reported a 12% gross mortality for 450 patients with a 30% incidence of diabetes treated with a calculated Kt/V of 1.3 (Keshaviah and Collins, 1989). In 1976, we reported the first experience with decreased treatment time guided by urea kinetic modeling (Gotch *et al.*, 1976). In that database mean t was reduced from 6 to 4.3 hours, the mean age was 56 years, incidence of diabetes was 9%, and the gross mortality rate was 13%. We reported, 17 years later, in 1993 (Uehlinger *et al.*, 1993) a mortality rate of 14% for 104 patients with a 24% incidence of diabetes and a mean age 63 years, treated with a mean eKt/Vd of 1.05 (range 0.95 to 1.4) and a mean treatment time of 2.25 h. The therapy reported in 1976 was modeled to maintain the predialysis BUN concentration constant at 80 mg/dl with monthly monitoring of NPCR and dietary counseling to maintain dietary protein intake at 1.1 ± 0.3 g/kg per day NPCR. In retrospect, this approach may have resulted in underdialysis in some patients with low NPCR despite dietary counseling. In the 1993 report, in which the gross mortality rate was similar but patients were actually older and the incidence of diabetes was substantially higher, therapy was prescribed and monitored as eKt/Vd.

In order to provide some perspective on the gross mortality rate of 14% for a group of patients with a known distribution of ages and diabetes (Uehlinger *et al.*, 1993), we can calculate the gross mortality rate expected for an identical patient cohort in a large database in which mortality rates as functions of age and diabetes are known. Registry data from EDTA, Australia, Japan, and the USA were requested and reported at the *Morbidity, Mortality and Prescription of Dialysis Symposium* in 1990 (Hull and Parker, 1990). The data reported from these registries included mortality rates as a function of age in both diabetics and non-diabetics. In all reported data sets the gross mortality rate was found to be a highly significant ($r = 0.85$ to 0.99) exponential function of age and diabetes. Consequently, the mortality rates expected in these large databases, for patient cohorts having distributions of age and diabetes identical to our patients (Uehlinger *et al.*, 1993), could be calculated from the products of the frequency distributions for age and diabetes in our patient group and the gross mortality rate functions of age and diabetes in the large databases. Data from the Japanese registry did not separate out diabetes, and the frequency of diabetes in the Tassin data was far too low to separate this comorbidity as a function of age, so these two data sets could not be normalized with respect to diabetes.

The results of such calculations are shown in Fig. 10.4, where it can be seen that the two lowest mortality rates were found with very long and very short treatment times. As noted above, the Tassin data could not be matched with respect to diabetes. Consequently, the Tassin mortality rate must be considered in the context of a very low incidence of diabetes—diabetes is widely accepted to be a major predictor of increased mortality. The curves in Fig. 10.4 do not support the concept that long treatment time is a requirement for good patient survival.

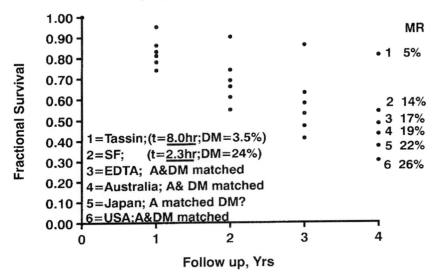

Fig. 10.4 The *lowest* normalized mortality rates (MR) were found with both the *longest* and the *shortest* treatment times.

The results of several current studies may eventually help to clarify the anomalous Tassin findings. The HEMO trial (Eknoyan *et al.*, 1996), for example, is a study of clin–

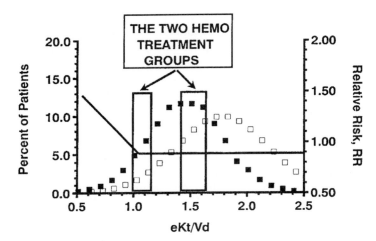

Fig. 10.5 Comparison of the two prospectively randomized eKt/Vd levels in the HEMO study to the eKt/Vd distributions in male and female patients in the population treated by Charra *et al.*

ical outcome with prospectively randomized and very tightly controlled eKt/Vd levels of 1.05 and 1.45. The domains of the two HEMO study doses, which are tightly con– trolled to 1.0–1.1 and 1.45–1.65, are depicted in Fig. 10.5 where they can be seen in sharp contrast to the broad range of eKt/Vd doses in the Tassin database. The HEMO study is designed with adequate power to determine clearly whether there is any improvement in outcome with high levels of eKt/Vd in the range of 1.5. The broad distribution of doses in the Tassin data precludes an analysis of outcome relative to $eKt/Vd > 1.0$, since the doses distribute over such a wide range of eKt/Vd.

The adequate dialysis dose

The available data indicates that an adequate dose of dialysis is provided with an eKt/V of 1.0 to 1.1. It should be emphasized that the delivered dose must be monitored at least monthly and adjusted as necessary to assure that the mean dose never falls below 1.0 in any individual patient. Prolonged periods, i.e. several months, of $eKt/Vd \geq 0.8$ was shown to result in increased mortality in NCDS group II and IV patients in a year of follow-up after the dose had been restored (Parker *et al.*, 1983). We define the mean dose as the running mean of the four most recent measurements of eKt/Vd.

Equally important is regular monthly monitoring of eNPCR and dietary counseling whenever the eNPCR falls below 1.0. Although cross-sectional analysis of the relationship of eNPCR to eKt/Vd can be spurious due to statistical artifacts (Uehlinger, 1996), in individual patients with a low eNPCR resistant to dietary counseling, an empirical trial of increased dialysis (i.e. raising eKt/Vd to 1.3 or 1.4), may be appropriate to determine if there is a dialysis-responsive impairment of protein appetite.

It is extremely important to include the optimal management of sodium and fluid balance and control of plasma Kt, Pi, HCO_3, and Ca^{2+} as important components of the quality of the delivered dialysis dose. It is very easy to achieve an eKt/Vd of 2 in small patients, but it may be at the expense of hypokalemia and a poorly controlled acid–base metabolism, resulting in an increased risk of sudden death if these solutes are not monitored and dialysate composition adjusted as needed to assure optimal pre- and postdialysis concentration profiles. The data in Fig. 10.2 suggest both high and low mortality rates in individual patient cohorts with very high eKt/Vd levels. Although the causes are unknown and may be multiple, a higher death risk may, in part, be associated with a poorer control of extracellular electrolyte composition—this is a significant risk when a 'generic' high eKt/Vd is prescribed using a high KoA dialyzer, high blood flows 0, and $t = 3–4$ hours indiscriminantly in very small patients with V of 20 l as well as in large patients. Alternatively, some of the apparent high Kt/Vs may be due to defective blood-drawing techniques.

Other factors affecting adequacy

Dialysis patients in the USA have a far higher mortality rate and a much lower life expectancy than patients in most European countries and Japan. Differences in survival have been explained by a number of factors, including alleged defects in the dialytic prescription or delivery, and some have preached the value of longer dialysis times, which reportedly result in better control of hypertension and lower rates of ultrafiltration.

While it is possible that the above argument has some merit, little direct evidence has been presented to support it. Undoubtedly, general increases in dialysis dose, measured as *Kt/V* or URR (urea reduction ratio), have resulted in improved survival. But as discussed elsewhere in this chapter, further increases are not associated with a better outcome.

We hypothesize that when adjusted for demographic and comorbidity factors, differences in survival in dialysis patients are not due exclusively to differences in the doses of dialysis, but are also related to the cardiovascular health status in the various populations from which chronic renal failure patients emerge. Differences in death rates due to ischemic cardiovascular disease are well described in an extensive WHO study of causes of death (Fig. 10.6) (Murray and Lopez, 1997). Given the 2–3-fold differences between Brazil and Finland shown in Fig. 10.6, the obvious question to test the hypothesis is the comparison of death rates in patients on dialysis in each country, adjusted for age, sex, diabetes, and dialysis dose.

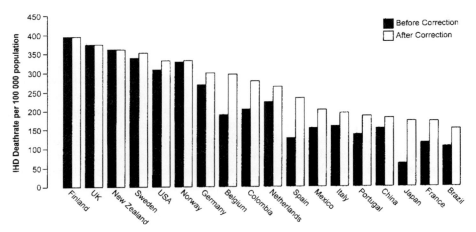

Fig. 10.6   Mortality rates by country for ischemic heart disease (IHD) before and after adjustment for miscoding. Age-standardized for men and women aged ≥ 30 years, about 1990.

Source: Murray and Lopez, 1997 with permission.

In the USA, differences in standardized mortality ratios between groups are present. According to the USRDS data, white HD patients have a much shorter life expectancy than black HD patients, and white HD patients have significantly higher rates of death due to cardiovascular causes than black patients when data are adjusted for age and diabetic status. For example, total death rates due to acute myocardial infarction, and other cardiac pathologies are 60.4 and 88.7 per 1000 patient-years among non-diabetic black and non-diabetic white HD patients, respectively. Total rates of death due to cardiac causes are 121.0 and 183.0 per 1000 patient-years among diabetic black and diabetic white HD patients ages 65 years and older, respectively (USRDS, 1994).

The USA data demonstrate that though dialysis dose might be the most obvious key to survival, many other factors affect clinical outcome and the overall adequacy of renal replacement therapy. We list several of these factors in Table 10.1. Because there is no definitive research on many of the issues we address, the relative importance of each of the points listed in the table is difficult to assess. Nonetheless, we believe that the issues we list are well founded. A comprehensive treatment plan will address these important issues according to the individual needs of each patient.

Table 10.1 What is adequate dialysis?

---

1. At least 75% of the dialysis population have a Kt/V (single pool) $\geq$ 1.2 (or eKt/V >1.0 double pool).
   –Pre- and post-blood samples drawn correctly.
   –Appropriate choice of dilayzer and blood flow rate;
   –Continuous audit of Qb (blood flow), time, and volume (V).
2. Use of high-flux biocompatible dialyzers (at present high-flux justified for $\beta2m$ removal only).
3. Infrequent hypotensive episodes, as assisted by on-line volume measurement, and/or controlled core cooling as technology advances.
4. Absence of symptoms during dialysis.
5. Access flow above 800 ml/min, preferably with regular direct measurements of access flow.
6. Dialysis time as short as possible commensurate with the delivery of prescribed dose and achievement of dry weight.
7. Participation in an exercise program with continuing evaluation (Harter, 1994).
8. Rehabilitation plans (Oberley, 1994).
9. Hematocrit 32–36% in 80% of the dialysis population, with erythropoietin administration based on kinetic principles.
10. Replete iron stores—transferrin saturation 20–30%, ferritin 100–400 mg/ml. Appropriate use of maintenance iron (usually intravenous).
11. Phosphorus < 6.0 mg/dl; calcium 9–11 mg/dl; intact PTH 2–3 times normal. Appropriate use of 1:25 DHCC (dihydrocholecalciferol).
12. Use of water better than AAMI Standard, e.g. bacteria < 20 c.f.u./ml; endotoxin < 0.25 endotoxin units/ml.
13. Dialyzer reprocessing following the AAMI recommended practise.
14. AV fistula rather than graft as initial vascular access (in conjunction with the use of jugular vein catheters during maturation of fistula).
15. Nutritional requirements: energy 30–35 kcal/kg; PCR > 1.0 g/kg.
16. Dry weight reached usually.
18. Routine psychosocial support to deal with the rigors of dialysis.
19. Regular measurements of quality of life of patients.
20. On transplant list if appropriate.
21. General health measures applied routinely, e.g. treatment of hyperlipidemia, hyperhomo-cysteinemia, diabetic control, relevant immunizations, mammography, stool occult blood screening, etc.
22. Patients receive a 'report card' containing relevant data concerning their course.
23. Patients and their families or friends are knowledgeable about their treatment, including the concept of adequacy, access care, nutrition, uremic complications.
24. All of the above are part of a comprehensive quality assurance program with continuous quality improvement.

Removal of larger molecules

Dialysis can, to an extent, replace the renal catabolic removal of larger molecules. The surrogate for this is β_2-microglobulin. Cellulosic dialyzers, including Cuprophan and regenerated cellulose and most types of cellulose acetate, do not remove β2m. High-flux membranes with high ultrafiltration coefficients (KUF) remove molecules of molecular weights up to 25000 KD the amount depending on initial sieving coeffi-cients and other factors, particularly the effects of dialyzer reprocessing.

The effects of the composition of the dialyzer membrane on chronic outcomes are not well determined. The use of biocompatible membranes may be associated with lower production rates of β2m (Hakim *et al.*, 1996*a*), and might improve outcome. Hakim, *et al.* in USRDS studies showed that in 2410 patients—adjusted for comorbid factors, geographical region and dialysate composition—mortality was 20% lower when modified cellulose or synthetic membranes were used compared to unsubsti-tuted cellulose membranes (Hakim *et al.*, 1996*b*). Unfortunately, the effects of flux were not separated from biocompatibility. Previously, Hakim and Parker found that the use of biocompatible membranes was associated with an increase in patients' weight and concentrations of serum albumin (Parker *et al.*, 1996).

In contrast to these non-randomized trials, Locatelli *et al.* (1996) compared Cupro-phan, polysulfone low-flux, polysulfone high-flux dialyzers, and hemodiafiltration in a multicenter randomized trial. The only positive result in a 2-year study was a de-crease in predialysis plasma β2m levels in high-flux dialysis and hemodiafiltration compared to the other membranes—morbidity and mortality did not differ. However, the prevalence of morbidity and mortality was universally low, hence the implications of this study for these parameters is unclear. A longer trial might have revealed sig-nificant differences in morbidity and mortality among the different patient groups.

Reprocessing high-flux membranes with Renalin® reduces, and bleach increases, the permeability of the dialyzer to β2m (Leypoldt *et al.*, 1996). An interesting aspect of the effectiveness of high-flux membranes is the extent of the removal of other larger mol-ecules which are normally catabolized by the kidney. These include homologs of β2m, light chains, and angiogenin (Haag-Weber and Horl, 1994). These substances have been associated with a decreasing functional ability of polymorphonuclear leutocytes.

Dialysate

Dialysis provides a huge exposure to water (30–48 1/h). Water contaminated with endotoxin may result in the chronic stimulation of inflammatory processes. AAMI (Association for the Advancement of Medical Instrumentation) standards permit bacterial counts of up to 200 cfu/ml (colony-forming units) and endotoxin concentra-tions of five endotoxin units in water used for the preparation of dialysates. Current methods of water reprocessing permit the production of water which contains < 0.06 endotoxin units/ml and virtually no bacteria.

Nutrition

Even when the prescribed dialysis dose is adequate, a significant proportion of dialy-sis patients suffer malnutrition, mostly due to anorexia (Kopple and Massry, 1997). While nutritional support alone is of limited value, intradialytic parenteral nutri-tional support combined with doses of recombinant growth hormone factor may be useful (Fouque, 1997). The use of biocompatible membranes may be associated with increased intake. Hypoalbuminemia, an important indicator of poor outcome, is often independent of nutritional intake and may be due to suppression of hepatic synthesis associated with states of chronic inflammation, as identified by high levels of C-reactive protein and serum amyloid A (Kaysen *et al.*, 1955). No convincing explanation has yet been given for this state.

Iron intake and erythropoietin therapy should be coordinated so that hematocrit levels reach 32–36%. Phosphorous intake should be monitored, since dialytic removal is limited by a lack of equilibration of the extracellular fluid with intracellular phosphorous. A new phosphate binder in gel form may induce better patient compliance and improve patients' phosphorus profile (Chertow *et al.*, 1997).

Oxidative stress

Several studies have found increased concentrations of the products of oxidative reactions in the sera of HD patients (Loughrey *et al.*, 1994; Haklar *et al.*, 1995). While results have been contradictory, these findings, coupled with findings that dietary and enzymatic antioxidants are depleted in HD patients (Peuchant *et al.*, 1994; Jackson *et al.*, 1995), suggest that oxidative activity is increased.

Increased activity might reflect an increase in free radicals or a decrease in the tissue's capacity to prevent oxidation. Free radicals may increase due to the inflammation and degranulation that occur as blood comes into contact with the bio-incompatible membrane. A decrease in antioxidant capacity might result from a defect in the production of the oxidizable form of the antioxidant enzyme glutathione (Yawata and Jacob, 1975) or from a dietary deficiency of antioxidant vitamins or cofactors (Peuchant *et al.*, 1994; Jackson *et al.*, 1995). Increased oxidative activity may play a role in the pathogenesis of cardiovascular disease in CRF patients.

It may also play a role in dialysis-related amyloidosis. Miyata *et al.* (Miyata *et al.*, 1996; Miyata and van Ypersele de Strihou, 1997) found that oxidation of several glucose and ascorbate derivatives can augment advanced glycation and product (AGE) production and induce the deposition of amyloid. These findings lead us to the intriguing possibility that the efficacy of high-flux membranes in reducing the incidence of severe amyloidosis may lie in their greater biocompatibility and consequent reduced production of free radicals. Though the data on these and other hypotheses concerning the role that oxygen free radicals play in the pathogenesis of disease in HD are not definitive, we believe that antioxidant supplementation will play an increasingly important role in renal replacement therapy.

Control of hypotensive episodes

Hypotension, defined as a decrease in blood pressure requiring a medical or nursing therapeutic response, occurs variably depending on a number of factors, including underlying cardiovascular disease, presence of autonomic dysfunction, rate of ultrafiltration (and therefore rate of plasma refilling), compensatory vasoconstriction, and serum sodium concentration. Relative blood volume change using a variety of sensors

Adequacy of dialysis: the key to survival

(all of which have, in common, the indirect measurement of the effects of water removal), has been a topic of much interest (Leypoldt *et al.*, 1995; Santoro *et al.*, 1996).

An adequate dialysis clearly requires the removal of fluid blood above the target dry weight. The longer the dialysis, the less likely that removal of this volume will produce symptoms. Dialysis times of less than 3 hours (which are based on the provision of an appropriate Kt/V) are more frequently associated with symptoms, particularly in the elderly.

Zocalli *et al.* (1997) examined the question of whether dialysis patients are predisposed to vasodepressor syncope by examining heart rate responses following dialysis hypotension. Tachycardia was a more frequent response than bradycardia. They suggested that bradycardia following hypotension is probably a response to hypovolemia, a special case of this being severe diastolic dysfunction in which poor ventricular filling provokes a paradoxical baroreceptor stimulation and syncope (Converse *et al.*, 1992).

Methods to reduce hypotension

During an idealized dialysis session, no changes in plasma volume would occur and there would be no danger of hypotension. However, practical considerations of time and cost dictate that we speed up the dialysis process, and hypotension is an important concern. Relatively minor changes in hemodialysis equipment and methods could be implemented to reduce the incidence of hypotensive episodes. When highly efficient, high-flux dialyzers are used, controlled ultrafiltration machines can help to prevent hypotension. Filtration rates can be decreased over the course of the hemodialysis session, so that the greatest amount of fluid is removed early in the treatment when plasma refilling is more rapid from an expanded extracellular fluid volume.

Dialysates with greater sodium concentrations will cause small increases in osmotic pressure, enhance plasma refilling, and possibly shift fluids from the intracellular compartment. But evidence that outcome is improved when sodium concentration is varied over the course of a treatment is scanty (Petitclerc *et al.*, 1996).

If the dialysate temperature is lowered then blood pressure is maintained, apparently due to vasoconstriction. Kaufman (1997) reduced the dialysate temperature so that the core arterial blood temperature decreased by 0.22°C, with patients appearing to maintain blood pressure despite a greater reduction in blood volume than in non-cooled patients.

A critical blood volume can be chosen as a point at which to slow down or temporarily stop ultrafiltration. While the feedback control of ultrafiltration based on changes in blood volume in this context is not FDA-approved in the USA, an alarm could indicate when the critical point has been reached.

What can reasonably be expected to improve the adequacy of dialysis?

The most likely substantial advance in adequacy is an increase in the number of dialyses per week. This will accomplish greater removal of uremic toxins and better control of phosphorus concentrations, permit smoother control of fluid balance, and more closely approximate the continuous characteristics of normal renal function. In order for this to occur at home, the current development of user-friendly machines needs to be perfected.

It seems unlikely that current systems of in-center dialysis could be expanded to daily dialysis. Possibly a fraction of patients could be treated in limited-care facilities with user-friendly machines and much lower patient to staff ratios. This could reduce the cost per treatment to a level closer to the current reimbursement structure. Earlier initiation of dialysis, before malnutrition and the adverse effects of uremia have affected the patient, could possibly improve long-term outcomes. The increasing use of hemodiafiltration will improve dialytic removal of small proteins, but it will require the development of resins or similar adsorptive substances with greater specificity to maximize this therapy.

The development of new vascular accesses should reduce the occurrence of underdialysis occuring with access failure and the use of temporary catheters. On-line clearance devices will optimize consistency of therapy. Ongoing studies will provide a greater understanding of the causes and consequences of cardiovascular disease in uremia, so that clinicians will be better able to correct lipid abnormalities and pro-oxidant stresses.

Finally, we suggest that compliance might increase and outcomes might be improved if renal replacement therapy is provided in the most patient-friendly environment possible. The conscientious dialysis team will provide the patient and family with as much information as possible on ESRD and on its proper treatment, and maximize opportunities for independence and rehabilitation.

NKF-DOQI guidelines

We include a short description of the National Kidney Foundation-Dialysis Outcomes Quality Initiative (NKF-DOQI), because it provides a great body of data on factors affecting dialysis adequacy. Readers seeking further information on this subject are directed to these guidelines, copies of which can be acquired from the National Kidney Foundation's headquarters in New York.

Over the years, four work groups have developed evidence-based clinical practice guidelines in the areas of hemodialysis adequacy, peritoneal dialysis adequacy, vascular access, and anemia. After selection of topic areas, the entire literature on each topic was examined, reviewing each paper for content and methods. Subsequently, a structured review was made of key or pertinent articles. The results of the literature review were compiled and quantitative data, when available, were aggregated. Guidelines were formulated with a rationale developed for each. The evidentiary basis for the rationales was clearly stated as being derived from empiric data or as the expert opinion of the individual work group. A three-stage, peer review process was instituted with Advisory Council Review, review by more than 50 ESRD-related organizations, and finally an open review by individuals ending in April 1997. Though the guidelines were published in 1997, their implementation is a continuing process. We include examples of several of the most relevant guidelines below.

The guidelines suggest that unless certain conditions are met, patients should be advised to initiate some form of dialysis when the weekly renal Kt/V_{urea} ($K_r t/ > V_{urea}$) falls below 2.0. The circumstance in which dialysis may not be necessary, even though the weekly $K_r t/V_{urea}$ is less than 2.0 is when all three of the following conditions apply to the patient:

(1) stable or increased edema-free body weight;
(2) nPNA (normalized appearance of protein nitrogen equivalent) $\geq$ 0.8 g/kg per day; and
(3) absence of any clinical signs or symptoms potentially attributable to uremia. A weekly $K_r t/V_{urea}$ of 2.0 approximates a renal urea clearance of 7 ml/min and a renal creatinine clearance that varies between 9 and 14 ml/min per 1.73 m^2. The glomerular filtration rate (GRF), will be approximately 10.5 ml/min per 1.73 m^2 when the $K_r t/V_{urea}$ is about 2.0.

The rationale suggests that it is illogical to prescribe a certain level of urea clearance for patients on dialysis and yet accept a lower level in the predialysis patient. This controversial recommendation suggests an earlier initiation of dialysis than that usually currently practised in North America.

Hemodialysis guidelines suggest the use of formal urea kinetic modeling using a single-pool, variable-volume model (rather than the urea reduction ratio or its derivatives, a minimum Kt/V delivered of at least 1.2 and monthly measurement of Kt/V).

Methods to draw pre- and post-BUN in an acceptable fashion are emphasized, including taking care not to dilute the specimens with saline and to draw the specimens at the exact initiation and the exact termination of the treatment. For the postdialysis specimens the dialysate flow is stopped, the UF rate is decreased to 50 ml/h, or switched off, and blood flow is reduced to 50–100 ml/min for 15 seconds before the specimen is taken. This methodology avoids the effect of access recirculation.

The guidelines also reinforce the AAMI Recommended Practice on dialyzer reuse, with an addition suggesting individual testing of the total cell volume before first use of all dialyzers.

Vascular access guidelines deal with the problem of a majority of USA dialysis facilities, i.e. choosing the creation of grafts rather than fistulas as initial procedures. The recommendation is that at least 50% of primary accesses should be AV fistulas, and an overall prevalence rate of at least 40%. Methods for detecting graft stenosis and potential fistula failure include the measurement of recirculation using a suitable slow-flow method, measurement of direct access flow (especially in grafts), and measurement of direct static and dynamic pressures.

Anemia guidelines emphasize appropriate iron stores and hematocrit levels when using erythropoietin.

Peritoneal dialysis (PD) guidelines emphasize a minimum weekly Kt/V of 2.0 (including residual renal function), with slightly higher figures for device-assisted nocturnal dialysis. Equivalent creatinine clearances are also provided. Both empiric and kinetic approaches to PD prescription are given in the guidelines.

Acknowledgment

We much appreciate the significant contribution to this chapter made by Jonathan Gross.

References

Bass, A. L., Strand, M. J., Uvelle, D. A., Multinovic, J., and Scribner, B. H. (1975). Quantitative description of dialysis treatment: a dialysis index. *Kidney International*, **7** (Suppl. 2), S23–S30.

Bloaembergen, W. E., Stannard, D. C., Port, F. K., *et al.* (1996). Relationship of dose of hemo-dialysis and cause-specific mortality. *Kidney International*, **20**, 557–65.

Chan, Y., and Green, G. (1994). Dietary compliance among young hemodialysis patients. *Dialysis and Transplantation*, **23**, 186–9.

Charra, B., Calemard, E., Ruffet, M., *et al.* (1992). Survival as an index of adequacy of dialysis. *Kidney International*, **41**, 1286–91.

Chertow, G., Burke, S., Lazarus, J., *et al.* (1997). Poly[allylamine hydrochloride] (Renagel): a noncalcemic phosphate binder for the treatment of hyperphosphatemia in chronic renal failure. *American Journal of Kidney Diseases*, **29**, 66–71.

Collins, A. J., and Kjellstrand, C. (1990). Shortening of the hemodialysis procedure and mortality in 'healthy' dialysis patients. *Transactions of the American Society of Artificial Internal Organs*, **36**, M145–M148.

Converse, R. L. J., Jacobsen, T. N., Jost, C. M. T., *et al.* (1992). Paradoxical withdrawal of reflex vasoconstriction and a cause of hemodialysis-induced hypotension. *Journal of Clinical Investigation*, **90**, 1657–65.

Daugirdas, J. (1992). Second generation logarithmic estimates of single-pool variable volume Kt/V: an analysis of error. *Journal of the American Society of Nephrology*, **4**, 1205–13.

Daugirdas, J., and Schneditz, D. (1995). Overestimation of hemodialysis dose (dKt/V) depends on dialysis efficiency (K/V) by regional blood flow and by concentional two-pool urea kinetic analyses. *American Society of Artificial Internal Organs Journal*, **41**, M719–M725.

Delmez, J. A., and Windus, D. W. (1992). Hemodialysis prescription and delivery in a metro-politan community. *Kidney International*, **41**, 1023–8.

Eknoyan, G., Levey, A., Beck, G., *et al.* (1996). The hemodialysis (HEMO) study: rationale for selection of interventions. *Seminars in Dialysis*, **9**, 24–6.

Fouque, D. (1997). Causes and interventions for malnutrition in patients undergoing main-tenance dialysis. *Blood Purification*, **15**, 112–20.

Gotch, F. (1996). Kinetic modeling in hemodialysis. In *Clinical dialysis* (3rd edn) (ed. A. R. Nis-senson, R. N. Fine, and D. E. Gentile), pp. 156–89. Appleton & Lange, Norwalk, Conn.

Gotch, F., and Sargent, J. A. (1985). A mechanistic analysis of the National Cooperative Dialysis Study (NCDS). *Kidney International*, **28**, 526–36.

Gotch, F., Sargent, J., Keen, M., Lam, M., Prowitt, M., and Grady, M. (1976). Clinical results of intermittent dialysis therapy (IDT) guided by ongoing kinetic analysis of urea metab-olism. *Transactions of the American Society of Artificial Internal Organs*, **22**, 175–89.

Gotch, F., Levin, N., Port, F., Wolfe, R., and Uehlinger, D. (1997). Clinical outcome relative to the dose of dialysis is not what you think: the fallacy of the mean. *American Journal of Kidney Diseases*, **30**, 1–15.

Haag-Weber, M., and Horl, W. H. (1994). Effect of biocompatible membranes on neutrophil function and metabolism. *Clinical Nephrology*, **42** (Suppl. 1), S31–S36.

Haag-Weber, M., Mai, B., Cahen, G., and Horl, W. H. (1994). A new view of uraemic toxicity. *Nephrology, Dialysis, Transplantation*, **9**, 346–7.

Hakim, R., Breyer, J., Ismail, N., and Schulman, G. (1994). Effects of dose of dialysis on morbidity and mortality. *American Journal of Kidney Diseases*, **23**, 661–9.

Hakim, R. M., Wingard, R. L., Husni, L., Parker, R. A., and Parker, T. F. 3rd. (1996*a*). The effect of membrane biocompatibility on plasma beta-2 microglobulin levels in chronic hemodialysis patients. *Journal of the American Society of Nephrology*, **7**, 472–8.

Hakim, R., Held, P., Stannard, D., Wolfe, R., *et al.* (1996*b*). Effect of dialysis membrane on mortality of chronic hemodialysis patients. *Kidney International*, **50**, 566–70.

Haklar, G., Yegenaga, I., and Yalcin, A. S. (1995). Evaluation of oxidant stress in chronic hemodialysis patients: use of different parameters. *Clinica Chimica Acta*, **234**, 109–14.

Harter, H. R. (1994). Excercise in the dialysis patient. *Seminars in Dialysis*, **7**, 192–8.

Held, P. H., Port, F. K., Wolfe, R. A., *et al.* (1996). The dose of hemodialysis and patient mortality. *Kidney International*, **50**, 550–6.

Hull, A., and Parker, T. (ed.) (1990). Proceedings from the morbidity, mortality and prescription of dialysis symposium. *American Journal of Kidney Diseases*, **15**, 375–515.

Jackson, P., Loughrey, C. M., Lightbody, J. H., McNamee, P. T., and Young, I. S. (1995). Effect of hemodialysis on total antioxidant capacity and serum antioxidants in patients with chronic renal failure. *Clinical Chemistry*, **41**, 1135–8.

Kaufman, A. M., Morris, A., Lavarias, V. *et al.* (1998). Effects of controlled blood cooling on hemodynamic stability and urea kinetics during high efficiency hemodialysis. *Journal of the American Society of Nephrology*, **9**, 877–83.

Kaysen, G. A., Rathore, V., Shearer, G. C., and Depner, T. A. (1995). Mechanisms of hypoalbuminemia in hemodialysis patients. *Kidney International*, **48**, 510–16.

Keshaviah, P., and Collins, A. (1989). High efficiency hemodialysis. *Contributions to Nephrology*, **69**, 109–19.

Kopple, J. D., and Massry, S. G. (ed.) (1997). *Nutritional management of renal disease*. Williams and Wilkins, Baltimore, MD.

Levin, N., Stannard, D., Gotch, F., and Port, F. (1995). Comparison of mortality risk by Kt/V single pool versus double pool analysis in diabetic and non-diabetic hemodialysis patients. *Journal of the American Society of Nephrology*, **6**, 606 (Abstract).

Leypoldt, J. K., Cheung, A. K., Steuer, R. R., Harris, D. H., and Conis, J. M. (1995). Determination of circulating blood volume by continuously monitoring hematocrit during hemodialysis. *Journal of the American Society of Nephrology*, **6**, 214–19.

Leypoldt, J. K., Cheung, A. K., Clark, W. R., *et al.* (1996). Characterization of low and high flux dialyzers with reuse in the Hemo Study. Interim report. *Journal of the American Society of Nephrology*, **7**, 1518 (Abstract).

Locatelli, F., Mastrangelo, F., Redaelli, B., *et al.* (1996). Effects of different membranes and dialysis technologies on patient treatment tolerance and nutritional parameters. *Kidney International*, **50**, 1293–302.

Loughrey, C. M., Young, I. S., Lightbody, J. H., McMaster, D., McNamee, P. T., and Trimble, E. R. (1994). Oxidative stress in hemodialysis. *Quarterly Journal of Medicine*, **87**, 679–83.

Lowrie, E., and Laird, N. (Guest ed.) (1983). Cooperative Dialysis Study. *Kidney International* (Suppl. 13), S1–S122.

Lowrie, E. G., and Lew, N. L. (1990). Death risk in hemodialysis patients: the predictive value of commonly measured variables and an evaluation of death rate differences between facilities. *American Journal of Kidney Diseases*, **14**, 458–83.

Maher, J. F., Schreiner, G. E., and Waters, T. J. (1961). Successful intermittent hemodialysis—

longer reported maintenance of life in true oliguria (181) days. *Transactions of the American Society of Artificial Internal Organs*, **6**, 123–6.

Miyata, T., and van Ypersele de Strihou, C. (1997). Beta2microglobulin, AGEs, and dialysis related amyloidosis—Where are we now? Implication of carbonyl stress in renal failure. *Nephrology*, **3** (Suppl. 1), S57 (Abstract).

Miyata, T., Hori, O., Zhang, J., *et al.* (1996). The receptor for advanced glycation end products (RAGE) is a central mediator of the interaction of AGE-beta2microglobulin with human mononuclear phagocytes via an oxidant-sensitive pathway. *Journal of Clinical Investigation*, **98**, 1088–94.

Murray, C. J. L. and Lopez, A. D. (1997). Mortality by cause for eight regions of the world: Global Burden of Disease Study. *Lancet*, **349**, 1269–76.

Oberley, E. (ed.) (1994). *Renal rehabilitation: bridging the barriers*. Medical Education Institute, Madison, Wis.

Owen, W., Lew, N., Liu, Y., Lowrie, E., and Lazarus, M. (1993). The urea reduction ratio and serum albumin concentration as predictors of mortality in patients undergoing hemodialysis. *New England Journal of Medicine*, **329**, 1001–6.

Parker, T., Laird, N., and Lowrie, E. (1983). Comparison of the study groups in National Co-operative Dialysis Study and a description of morbidity, mortality and patient withdrawal. *Kidney International*, **23** (Suppl. 13), S42–S49.

Parker, T., Husni, L., Huang, W., Lew, N., Lowrie, E., and Dallas Nephrology Associates (1994). Survival of hemodialysis patients in the United States is improved with a greater quantity of dialysis. *American Journal of Kidney Diseases*, **23**, 670–80.

Parker, T. F. 3rd, Wingard, R. L., Husni, L., Ikizler, T. A., Parker, R. A., and Hakim, R. M. (1996). Effect of the membrane biocompatibility on nutritional parameters in chronic hemodialysis patients. *Kidney International*, **49**, 551–6.

Petitclerc, T., Trombert, J. C., Coevoet, B., and Jacobs, C. (1996). Electrolyte modelling: sodium. Is dialysate sodium profiling actually useful? *Nephrology, Dialysis, Transplantation*, **11** (Suppl. 2), S35–S38.

Peuchant, E., Carbonneau, M. A., Dubourg, L., *et al.* (1994). Lipoperoxidation in plasma and red blood cells of patients undergoing hemodialysis: vitamins A, E, and iron status. *Free Radical Biology and Medicine*, **16**, 339–46.

Santoro, A., Mancini, E., Paolini, F., and Zucchelli, P. (1996). Blood volume monitoring and control. *Nephrology, Dialysis, Transplantation*, **11** (Suppl. 2), S42–47.

Sargent, J. A. (1990). Shortfalls in the delivery of dialysis. *American Journal of Kidney Diseases*, **15**, 500–10.

Sargent, J. A., and Gotch, F. (1975). The analysis of concentration dependence of uremic lesions in clinical studies. *Kidney International*, **7** (Suppl. 2), S35–S45.

Scribner, B. H. (1965). Discussion. *Transactions of the American Society of Artificial Internal Organs*, **11**, 29.

Scribner, B. (1996). *Replacement of renal function by dialysis* (4th edn) (ed. C. Jacobs, C. Kjellstrand, K. Koch, and J. Winchester), Forward. Kluwer Academic, Dordrecht.

Scribner, B. H., Buri, R., Caner, J. Z., Hegstrom, R., and Burnell, J. M. (1960). The treatment of chronic uremia by means of intermittent dialysis: a preliminary report. *Transactions of the American Society of Artificial Internal Organs*, **6**, 114–17.

Shapiro, F., and Umen, A. (1983). Risk factors in hemodialysis patient survival. *American Society of Artificial Internal Organs Journal*, **6**, 176–85.

Smye, S., Evans, J., Will, E., and Brocklebank, J. (1992). Pediatric haemodialysis: estimation of treatment efficiency in the presence of urea rebound. *Clin Phys Physiol Meas.*, **13**, 15–62.

Tattersal, J. E., DéTakats, D., Chamney, P., Greenwood, R. N., and Farrington, K. (1996). The post-hemodialysis rebound: predicting and quantifying its effect on Kt/V. *Kidney International*, **50**, 2094–102.

Teschan, P. E., Post, R. S., Smith, L. H., *et al.* (1955). Post traumatic renal insufficiency in military casualties. I. Clinical characteristics. *American Journal of Medicine*, **18**, 172–86.

Uehlinger, D. (1996). Another look at the relationship between protein intake and dialysis dose. *Journal of American Society of Nephrology*, **7**, 166–9.

Uehlinger, D., Keen, M., and Gotch, F. (1993). Patient survival with short-time high flux dialysis therapy (HFD). *Journal of the American Society of Nephrology*, **4**, 329.

USRDS (1994). *United States Renal Data System Annual Data Report*. The National Institutes of Health, National Institute of Diabetes and Digestive and Kidney Diseases, Bethesda, MD.

Vanholder, R., De Smet, R., Vogeleere, P., Hsu, C., and Ringoir, S. (1996). The uraemic syndrome. In *Replacement of renal function by dialysis* (4th revised edn) (ed. C. Jacobs, C. Kjellstrand, K. Koch, and J. Winchester), pp. 1–34. Kluwer Academic, Dordrecht.

Yawata, Y., and Jacob, H. S. (1975). Abnormal red cell metabolism in patients with chronic uremia: nature of the defect and its persistence despite adequate hemodialysis. *Blood*, **45**, 231–9.

Zocalli, C., Tripepi, G., Mallamaci, F., and Panuccio, V. (1997). The heart rate response pattern to dialysis hypotension in haemodialysis patients. *Nephrology, Dialysis, Transplantation*, **12**, 519–23.

11

Long hemodialysis: the key to survival?

Bernard Charra and Guy Laurent

Introduction

The obstinacy of the Seattle team (Scribner *et al.*, 1960) turned an experimental, acute-renal failure treatment (Kolff *et al.*, 1944) into a long-term maintenance therapy. The number of hours of each dialysis was then the only yardstick of the dialysis dose. When dialysis was increased from once to twice and ultimately thrice weekly, the session duration was decreased from 16 to 12 and then to 10 hours. This trial and error process led to a general agreement that the minimum requirement for an average-sized adult on a 60 g protein diet was 30 hours per week on the 1 square-meter Kiil dialyzer (Siddiqui and Kerr, 1971).

To cope with the growing number of patients and limited resources the session duration was reduced to 5 hours; this was shown to be clinically feasible in 1972 (Cambi *et al.*, 1972).

In the early 1980s the National Cooperative Dialysis Study (NCDS) showed that morbidity was mainly linked to the urea time-averaged concentration and dialysis time (Lowrie *et al.*, 1981). Some years later the NCDS Mechanistic Analysis by Gotch and Sargent (1985) (Gotch *et al.*, 1985) led to the measurement of the quantity of dialysis using the fractional clearance of urea (Kt/V). From a kinetic analysis device, the Kt/V became a prescription tool. The target Kt/V was initially set at 0.8–1.0; the authors suggesting that a higher Kt/V would convey no further benefit to the patient (Gotch, 1983). This 'all or nothing' adequate dose theory was not accepted by all (Henderson, 1988; Keshaviah and Collins, 1988), yet it was a justification for a further shortening of sessions to 3 hours or less using high-efficiency and high-flux dialysis (Collins and Keshaviah, 1988; von Albertini, 1988).

In 1990, the *Morbidity, Mortality and Prescription of Dialysis Symposium* in Dallas drew attention to the increasing mortality of dialysis patients in the USA (Hull and Parker, 1990). This alarming message was strengthened by the fact that Japan and Europe reported substantially better survival rates (Eggers, 1990). Since then, there has been a growing acceptance that dialysis prescription is often suboptimal, and that insufficient delivery of dialysis dose (Gotch *et al.*, 1990; Sargent, 1990) has often produced misery.

On the other hand, evidence is lacking about the respective effects of insufficient dose and session time on patient survival. Few centers around the world have maintained a long dialysis program for a very long time. In Tassin the same dialysis method has been maintained unchanged over the years. The following data illustrate our experience.

Dialysis in Tassin

Patients

Between May 1968 and January 1996 (5650 patient-years) 881 patients (296 females, 585 males) have been treated in Tassin. The mean age at start of dialysis was 51.1 (SD $\pm$ 16.0) years. The causes of end-stage renal disease (ESRD) are shown in Table 11.1. The population case-mix has strikingly changed over the years. The overall population was split into the five calendar cohorts shown in Table 11.2. The mean age at the start of dialysis was 40.8 years in the first cohort but 61.3 years in the last one. The proportion of 'high-risk causes' of ESRD (diabetes mellitus, nephrosclerosis, systemic diseases, and cancer) has increased dramatically from 11% to 55%. Over time, more patients started dialysis with antecedent cardiovascular events (i.e. angina, myocardial infarction, cerebrovascular accident or ischemia, peripheral vascular disease): 10.2% of the new patients in the first calendar cohort but 56.5% in the last one.

Table 11.1 Causes of renal failure in 881 patients on long dialysis

Cause of ESRD	Number	Per cent
Chronic glomerulonephritis	225	25.6
Interstitial nephritis	150	17.0
Nephrosclerosis/vascular	142	16.1
Diabetes mellitus	97	11.0
Polycystic kidney disease	88	10.0
Systemic diseases	36	4.1
Others	36	4.1
Malignant	15	1.7
Unknown	92	10.4

Table 11.2 Demographic features of 881 patients: Mean age at HD start, causes of chronic renal failure and prevalence (%) of cardiovascular antecedents†

Calendar years	< 1975	75–79	80–84	85–89	90–95
Patient no.	163	160	200	176	182
Mean age at start (years)	40.8	46.5	46.5	50.8	61.3
Diabetes (%)	2.4	4.5	4.8	12.1	22.2
Vascular disease* (%)	6.8	10.4	11.4	18.4	22.8
Others (%)	90.8	85.1	83.8	69.5	55.0
CV antecedents † (%)	10.2	22.6	26.4	39.5	56.5
≥ 2 antecedents (%)	2	8	10	18	29.0

*Vascular diseases: nephrosclerosis and other vascular diseases.

†Cardiovascular antecedents: myocardial infarction, angina, cerebrovascular accident, cerebral ischemia, peripheral ischemia.

The mean time spent on dialysis is 6.5 years over all the experience. At 1 January 1996, 221 patients had been treated for more than 10 years in the unit. Among them 42 have been treated for more than 20 years, and two for more than 30 years. The prevalent population under treatment in Tassin is stable (250 patients). Its mean age is presently 70.6 years.

Dialysis and treatment methods

The unit includes 65 stations in two different buildings: one of which is used to treat separately the (HBsAg) positive patients, and those with a high titer of HBs antibodies.

There are also two self-dialysis units. The home hemodialysis program, started in 1968, had treated up to 45% of patients in the mid-1980s, but, due to the increasing transplantation rate, multiplication of dialysis units all over the country, and casemix change, it has decreased steadily. Today, only 20% of patients are dialyzed at home or in the self-dialysis units. All patients dialyze for 8 hours, three times a week.

Cuprophan artificial kidneys have been used all along. The 1 m^2 Meltec® Micropoint Kiil dialyzers have been progressively replaced by Cuprophan disposable dialyzers (surface area $1.1–2.1 \text{ m}^2$), used presently for over 60% of patients. Dialysate flow is 500 ml/min; blood flow is 220 ml/min. Arteriovenous fistulas are used for 75% of the patients–their mean duration of patency is 7.5 years. Single-needle devices are never used. The buttonhole-sticking method with 14-gauge catheters has been used throughout the unit's experience (Laurent *et al.*, 1983) without the obvious drawbacks reported by others (Twardowski and Kubara, 1979). Vascular grafts and prostheses are seldom used.

Thomas femoral shunts (Thomas, 1969) are used for less than 10% of patients. Their life span is excellent; 142 femoral shunts have been used with a mean duration of patency of 7.7 years. Several of them have lasted over 20 years. They are particularly adapted to self-use at home. This good result is counterbalanced by the fact that they are more demanding in surgical skill, motivation, and availability, and require meticulous care by physician, nurse, and patient. Thomas femoral shunts must not used be as the 'last hope' access. They must also be avoided in patients at high risk of suicide.

Since 1988, internal jugular vein catheters have been used more extensively. Some have been functioning for over 6 years, but their life span is shorter than fistulas or Thomas shunts. Unless there is really no possibility for fistula creation, we consider them as temporary accesses.

The use of medications is restricted to a minimum. No antihypertensive medications are used after 3 months of dialysis (except in 2% of patients). Erythropoietin is used in about 15% of patients.

A high-protein, high-caloric, moderately low-salt diet is advocated. Determination and maintenance of dry weight is crucial. We have reported the method we use for the clinical assessment of dry weight elsewhere (Charra *et al.*, 1996a). At initiation of dialysis, 89% of the patients analyzed in this report were hypertensive in spite of antihypertensive medications. To normalize blood pressure and stop the antihypertensive medications the patients must get through a process of 'probing for dry weight'. A dry weight is permanently and systematically re-evaluated. A dialysis log chart summarizing line-by-line the last few weeks' sessions (weight, blood pressure, and intradialytic incidents) is an essential tool. Browsing through it gives, at a glance, a dynamic view of the extracellular volume (ECV) and blood pressure changes. In our practise, each preceding dialysis log must be validated by the physician in charge of the ward. If this is not done, a new dialysis sheet cannot be produced by the computer system.

Factors affecting long-term survival

The effective session time for individual patients was retrieved either from their chart or, over the last 8 years, from the computer program. The values of monthly Kt/V were computed from averaged pre-and postdialysis urea, mean weight loss, and dry weight according to Daugirdas (1989). The middle-molecule dialysis index (DI) (Babb *et al.*, 1975) was evaluated using *in-vivo* Vitamin B_{12} dialyzer clearance. The normalized protein catabolic rate (nPCR) was evaluated using the Gotch and Sargent formula. (Gotch and Sargent, 1985). The mean predialysis mean arterial pressure (MAP) was calculated for each patient from all the predialysis session blood pressure values (one-third of pulse pressure + diastolic blood pressure).

504 patients started dialysis before January 1st 1986, and they could therefore achieve 10 years of dialysis. Those who survived more than 10 years on dialysis (221 patients) were compared with those who did not (283 patients). The effects of changing the mode of treatment have been analyzed in two groups of patients. The effect of increasing the session time was analyzed in a group of 103 patients coming to Tassin from other units, usually to wait for a kidney transplantation in Lyon. They were unselected. All had been previously treated for 5 hours or less per session for 6 months or more. All were converted to our 3×8-hour schedule. When they came to us, 55 out of the 103 patients used antihypertensive medications.

Conversely, the effects of switching from 8 to 5 hours have been followed in 32 patients. To maintain a Kt/V value similar to that achieved during their long hemo-dialysis treatment, blood flow was increased to 300 ml/min and larger area dialyzers were used. These patients were selected: a reduction of the session time was used only in those patients who asked for it and who fulfiled two conditions: be normotensive on long hemodialysis without any antihypertensive treatment, and have a blood access providing a blood flow 300 ml/min or more.

Survival rates were determined using the Kaplan–Meier method (Kaplan and Meier, 1958). Comparisons of survival for the different groups was based on the log-rank test. The Cox proportional hazard model was used to evaluate the simultaneous effect of several covariates (Cox, 1972). The risk factors used in the Cox analysis were values observed at the start of treatment, except for blood pressure. For blood pressure, we used the value observed at the third month of dialysis, because, according to our experience, this is the delay needed by most patients to achieve dry weight. The standardized mortality ratio (SMR) (Wolfe *et al.*, 1992) has been calculated for eight successive calendar years, using the 1-year survival probability tables established by the United States Renal Data System (USRDS) for the American hemodialysis population adjusted for patient age, race, and cause of renal failure (USRDS, 1995).

An economic analysis was conducted for 1993. The 1989 Health Care Financing Administration (HCFA, 1990) report was used for comparison. A cost-comparison analysis of long vs. short hemodialysis over 20 years was conducted using a comparable French hemodialysis unit.

Numerical results are expressed as the means ± SD. For differences of means, the unpaired *t*-test was used, for comparing incidence rates, we used the Chi-square test. In all instances, a probability value of 0.05 or less was used to determine statistical significance.

Results

Delivered treatment

The mean effective dialysis time (± SD) was 23.8 (± 2.3) hours per week which is no different from the prescribed time. The compliance of patients was good, the number of missed or shortened sessions being negligible. The mean (± SD) dialysis dose values for the 881 patients were: *Kt/V*, 1.78 (± 0.42), and nPCR, 1.41 (± (0.32). The mean protein intake was 1.33 (± 0.42) g/kg body weight per day and the mean caloric intake 30.1 (± 5.2) kcal/kg per day, the mean NaCl intake was 4.5 g/day, and the mean interdialytic weight gain 1.6 kg.

Predialysis mean arterial pressure and postdialysis weight evolution over time are shown in Fig. 11.1. The mean initial predialysis MAP value was 123 (± 12.2) mmHg. After 3 months of dialysis it was down to 99 (± 10.9) mmHg, by which time antihypertensive treatment had been discontinued in 97% of patients. The lowest level of

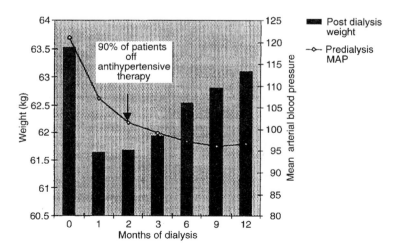

Fig. 11.1 Evolution of predialysis mean arterial pressure and postdialysis weight in 881 patients treated by long slow dialysis, Tassin 1968–1995.

dry weight was achieved after 1 month. Thereafter it increased regularly while the patient was rebuilding lean and fat body mass. The few weeks lag time between the change in weight and change in blood pressure fits well with the data of experimental (Guyton, 1991) and clinical studies (Comty *et al.*, 1964; Vertes *et al.*, 1969).

The overall population predialysis blood pressure was 128/79 mmHg, i.e. within the normal range (USRDS, 1993). Ambulatory blood pressure values of 91 randomly selected patients (Chazot *et al.*, 1995) were also within the normal range (Staessen *et al.*, 1991), but with a relative loss of circadian rhythm due to a reduced nocturnal dip in 22% of the patients.

Intradialytic incidents occur less often in long than in short dialysis. This is especially true for hypotension which was observed in 7.8% of long hemodialysis sessions vs. 20–40% reported on conventional hemodialysis (Daugirdas, 1991).

The mean hospitalization rate was 9.1 days per patient per year. The hospitalization rate was higher in diabetic patients (17.5 days per year vs. 6.8 for non-diabetics, $p < 0.001$) and in patients with cardiovascular antecedents (16.8 days per year vs. 6.4 for patients free of antecedent, $p < 0.001$).

The mean predialysis hematocrit of the total population was 29.6% ($\pm$ 6.9%). No systematic transfusion was used after 1968. The mean predialysis serum albumin was 41.6 ($\pm$ 4.8) g/l: the initial value was 36.6 g/l; increasing to 40.2 at the third dialysis month; reaching 41.9 at 18 months; remaining stable up to 30 years of dialysis.

A more precise analysis of the nutrition of 92 randomly selected patients (30 F/62 M) was performed in 1995 in our group of patients (Chazot, personal communication). Their mean age was 64.0 years and their mean dialysis duration was 118.5 months. The nPCR was 1.18, and the serum albumin concentration 40.4 g/l. The 3-day average energy and protein intake dietician evaluation were, respectively, 29.5 kcal and 1.2 g/kg. They were positively correlated with time on dialysis ($r = 0.36$ and 0.23; $p < 0.05$). The protein intake was less than 1 g/kg per day in 28% of patients and the caloric intake was less than 25 kcal/kg per day in 27% of patients. The vitamin B_6, C, and folic acid daily intakes were, respectively, 1.15 mg, 60.5 mg, and 236 μg per day.

Survival and mortality

The Kaplan–Meier survival data of all 881 patients are shown in Table 11.3. The population half-life was 14.6 years. The survival was shorter in older patients starting hemodialysis. Of the patients starting dialysis before 35 years of age 89% survived 5 years of dialysis versus only 29% of those starting at 75 years of age or later.

The etiology of renal failure has a significant impact on mortality. The patients with chronic glomerulonephritis, interstitial nephritis, or polycystic kidney disease had the best survival, diabetics had the worst. Type 1 diabetic patients had a better survival than type 2 (5-year survival 57% vs. 18%, $p < 0.01$).

Females had a slightly but statistically significant, longer survival than males. Survival was strongly affected by the cardiovascular comorbidity. There was a clear survival difference between 240 patients starting HD with prior cardiovascular event(s) and 641 patients free of such events. Their 10-year survival rates were, respectively, 33% and 73% ($p < 0.001$).

Table 11.3 Demographic and comorbid factors vs. survival at 5, 10, 15, and 20 years of dialysis

	Patient no.	% Patients surviving			
		5 years	10 years	15 years	20 years
Initial age (years):					
< 35	163	89	82	75	70
35–44	160	86	74	61	38
45–54	200	84	70	49	25
55–64	176	68	45	18	—
65–74	130	49	30	4	—
≥ 75	52	29	6	—	—
Etiology:					
Chronic GN	223	80	75	63	47
Interstitial nephritis	149	92	70	53	25
Polycystic kidneys	92	88	79	43	20
Nephrosclerosis	139	59	31	12	8
Diabetes	88	31	8	—	—
Systemic disease/diabetes	49	62	52	21	—
Other/unknown	141	74	62	15	—
Atheroma:					
antecedent	240	54	33	11	—
no antecedent	641	86	73	56	39
Total	881	83	69	49	34

Demographic and comorbid factors combine their effects to modify the outcome of treatment (Mailloux *et al.*, 1988; Collins *et al.*, 1990; Fernandez *et al.*, 1992). The crude mortality of our five calendar cohorts has been increasing (Table 11.4), although all patients have received exactly the same treatment. This demonstrates that it is misleading to infer the quality of a given dialysis treatment from a gross mortality analysis.

Table 11.4 The effect of increasing age on patient survival in successive cohorts

Calendar cohort	Patient no.	% Patients surviving			
		5 years	10 years	15 years	20 years
< 1975	163	89	76	59	38
1975–1979	160	81	70	50	—
1980–1984	200	82	61	—	—
1985–1989	176	67	45	—	—
≥ 1990	182	54	—	—	—

The SMR ratio has remained stable over the 8 years for which it has been calculated. It is 2–3-fold lower than the calculated SMR for similar risk patients (Wolfe *et al.*, 1992) having short dialysis times in the USA (Table 11.5).

Table 11.5   Standardized mortality ratio (SMR) in 8 calendar cohorts

Calendar year	O/E* deaths	SMR	P Value
1988	11/43.7	0.25	< 0.001
1989	23/43.7	0.53	< 0.005
1990	14/42.4	0.33	< 0.001
1991	18/44.7	0.40	< 0.001
1992	15/46.1	0.33	< 0.001
1993	23/47.7	0.48	< 0.001
1994	20/50.3	0.40	< 0.001
1995	23/57.0	0.40	< 0.001

*O = Observed, E = Expected for US patients (Wolfe *et al.*, 1992).

The most significant treatment-related factor influencing survival in our experience is mean arterial pressure. Splitting our population into two equal subgroups of
patients by the median value of predialysis MAP (97 mmHg) enables a comparison of
their survival to be made (Fig. 11.2). The lower MAP subgroup survived longer
($p = 0.003$). The difference in overall mortality was almost exclusively explained by
the difference in cardiovascular mortality (12.7 deaths vs. 28.1 per 1000 patient-years
at risk, $p < 0.001$).

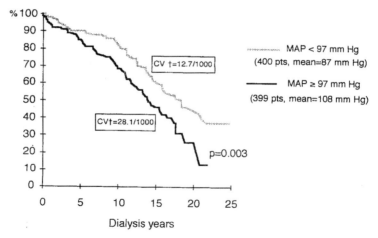

Fig. 11.2   Kaplan–Meier survival curve and cardiovascular mortality as a function of mean
arterial pressure (MAP). CVT, cardiovascular deaths.

The proportional hazard model analysis (Table 11.6) confirms the roles of age, etiology of renal failure, and cardiovascular comorbidity. It shows that blood pressure at 3
months'dialysis was a strong predictor of mortality: for each 1 mmHg increment of the
mean predialysis MAP the risk of death increased by 2.3%. The serum albumin concentration was also linked to mortality, but more weakly than to hypertension.

Table 11.6 Cox proportional hazards model of survival in 881 patients

Covariate	β coefficient	95% CI		Risk ratio	95% CI		P
Age at HD start	0.051	(0.029,	0.068)	1.052	(1.029, 1.070)		< 0.001
Cause of CRF							
(4 groups)	0.486	(0.172,	0.90)	1.626	(1.130, 2.23		< 0.01
CV antecedents*	0.928	(0.286,	1.561)	2.529	(1.343, 4.656)		< 0.01
MAP at 3 months							
of HD	0.023	(0.018,	0.048)	1.023	(1.018, 1.426)		< 0.001
Serum albumin	−0.086	(−0.159,	−0.014)	0.918	(0.853, 0.986)		< 0.02

*Angina, myocardial infarction, CVA, cerebral or peripheral ischemia.

Table 11.7 Causes of death expressed in % and for 1000 Patient-years of risk

	Number	% Deaths (of total)	Deaths/1000 patient-years
Cardiovascular causes	118	40.69	20.88
Cerebrovascular accident	22	7.59	3.89
Sudden death	44	15.17	7.79
Myocardial infarction	26	8.97	4.60
Cardiac failure	16	5.52	2.83
Peripheral vascular	6	2.07	1.06
Other cardiovascular	4	1.38	0.71
Infection	58	20.00	10.27
Cancer	29	10.00	5.13
Accident/suicide	21	7.24	3.72
Treatment stop	8	2.76	1.42
Various causes	35	12.07	6.19
Evolution coexistent disease	5	1.72	0.88
Dementia	4	1.38	1.24
Hemorrhage	5	1.72	0.88
Hyperkalemia	5	1.72	0.88
Postsurgical	10	3.45	1.77
Cachexia malnutrition	3	1.04	1.06
Iatrogenic	3	1.04	0.88
Unknown	21	7.24	3.72
Total/mean	290	100.00	51.33

Mortality data (Table 11.7) show that the major cause of death (20.9 deaths per 1000 patient-years) was cardiovascular (40.7%). Among cardiovascular causes of death, unexplained sudden death is the most frequent, followed by coronary and cerebrovascular deaths. Infection represents 20% of the deaths. The mortality rate due to infection in

Tassin (10.3 per 1000 patient-years) was lower than in France (15.5 per 1000 patient-years) (Degoulet *et al.*, 1982), and the USA (24.5 per 1000 patient-years) (USRDS, 1993).

There is only one detailed French study reporting mortality rates in dialysis patients available for comparison (Degoulet *et al.*, 1982). This multicenter study includes different dialysis modalities in a younger population than in Tassin (45.5 vs. 51.1, $p < 0.001$), and with less 'high-risk' etiologies of renal failure, i.e. diabetes and nephrosclerosis (18.1 vs. 27.3%). The overall mortality is higher in the multicenter study (97.4 vs. 51.3 deaths per 1000 patient-years), in spite of the favorable selection bias. The proportion of cardiovascular deaths is similar in both series, but the incidence of cardiovascular death is two-fold less in Tassin. The cerebrovascular and coronary death rates are particularly low in the Tassin series. On the other hand, the sudden unexplained deaths have been more frequent in Tassin than in the multicenter study.

Long-term survivors

As shown in Table 11.8, among the 504 patients starting dialysis before January 1st 1986 and therefore able to achieve 10 years or more of dialysis, 221 patients survived that term, 283 did not. Altogether 214 died, 203 were transplanted or lost to follow-up, and 87 are still on dialysis.

The survivors differed initially from the non-survivors. They were younger, had less high-risk causes of ESRD, less cardiovascular antecedents, and they were more often female. Their initial serum albumin and cholesterol levels were higher. They did not differ by size, the level of initial predialysis blood pressure, or the incidence of long-standing hypertension before dialysis. Their plasma urea and creatinine level were no different from the non-survivors.

The survivors had the same Kt/V and nPCR, but a higher middle-molecule index ($p < 0.001$). They also differed during treatment by a better nutritional index (plasma urea, creatinine, serum albumin, cholesterol, hematocrit) and by a better control of their blood pressure (mean predialysis MAP $p < 0.001$).

The causes of death in the two subsets of patients are reported in Table 11.9. The proportion of cardiovascular deaths was higher in long-term survivors, but their cardiovascular mortality was lower (21.7 vs. 29.2 cardiovascular deaths per 1000 patient-years). Compared to the group dialyzed for less than 10 years they suffered less deaths due to cerebrovascular accident and myocardial infarction, they showed the same incidence of unexplained sudden deaths, and more deaths due to cardiac failure and peripheral vascular disease. Infectious, malignant, accidental, and unknown or various causes of death were also less frequent in the long-term survivors.

Effect of increasing and decreasing the dialysis session time

In 103 unselected patients changed from ≤ 5 h to 8 h per session, the mean predialysis blood pressure fell from 162/98 to 126/74 mmHg after 9 months of long dialysis. The antihypertensive therapy was discontinued after 3 months in 54 out of 55 patients. The postdialysis weight dropped slightly in the first 3 months of long dialysis, but it increased by a mean of 2.5 kg after 9 months. This increased dry weight correlated with an increased appetite and an anabolic phase. The mean hematocrit rose from 24.4 to 29.4% after 9 months without erythropoietin, while the systematic transfusions had been stopped in the 26 patients who required them on short dialysis. The mean urea concentration increased from 29 to 31 mmol/l and the creatinine from 932 to 1024 μmol/l.

Table 11.8 Analysis of features of patients surviving less and more than 10 years

Patient group	< 10 years	> 10 years	*P* Value
Number of patients	283	221	—
Number deceased	120	94	—
Lost to follow-up or Tx	163	40	—
Mean HD follow-up time (years)	3.96 (2.98)	16.16 (4.6)	0.001
Group overall treatment time patient-years)	1110	3573	—
Situation at dialysis start			
Age (years)	46.5 (13.7)	42.6 (12.7)	0.001
Body mass index	22.4 (3.9)	22.2 (3.7)	N.S.
Sex male (%)	69	66	< 0.001
High-risk cause of CRF (%)[a]	27.3	10	< 0.001
Cardiovascular antecedents (%)[b]	32.4	12.5	< 0.001
Duration of HT before start > 5 years (%)	24.7	25.2	N.S.
Initial mean arterial pressure (mmHg)	126.4 (22.5)	123.7 (20.6)	N.S.
Initial urea (mmol/l)[c]	33.8 (7.8)	35.3 (7.1)	N.S.
Initial creatinine (μ mol/l)[c]	981 (182)	1002 (173)	N.S.
Initial serum albumin (g/l)[c]	38.7 (5.4)	40.8 (5.8)	0.03
Initial cholesterol (mmol/l)[c]	5.75 (1.60)	5.94 (1.83)	N.S.
During treatment (mean values)			
Mean Kt/V	1.71 (0.44)	1.72 (0.36)	N.S.
Mean Babb's dialysis index[d]	1.38 (0.31)	1.58 (0.44)	< 0.001
Mean hematocrit (%)	27.5 (6.0)	28.8 (5.8)	< 0.001
Mean arterial pressure (mmHg)	101.9 (15.2)	94.4 (15.1)	< 0.001
Mean nPCR[e]	1.50 (0.33)	1.44 (0.29)	N.S.
Mean predialysis plasma urea (mmol/l)	31.4 (6.8)	29.1 (4.9)	< 0.001
Mean predialysis plasma creatinine (μ mol/l)	838 (158)	892 (141)	< 0.01
Mean predialysis serum albumin (g/l)	40.7 (4.4)	41.9 (3.9)	<0.01
Mean predialysis serum cholesterol (mmol/l)	4.70 (1.56)	6.08 (1.36)	< 0.001

[a]High-risk causes of CRF: diabetes, nephrosclerosis, systemic and malignant disease.
[b]Cardiovascular antecedents: angina, myocardial infarction, cerebrovascular accident, cerebral ischemia, peripheral ischemia.
[c]Initial = mean of 3 first months of dialysis data.
[d]Mean Babb's dialysis index calculated using *in-vivo* Vit B_{12} clearance value corrected for ultra-filtration.
[e]nPCR calculated according to Gotch (Gotch *et al.*, 1985)
N.S., not significant.

Table 11.9 Causes of death (%) and mortality rate in cohorts surviving less and more than 10 years

Patient cohort	< 10 years (n = 283, 1110 patient-years)			> 10 years (n = 221, 3573 patient-years)		
	Number	% deaths	/1000 patient-years	number	% deaths	/1000 patient-years
Cardiovascular causes	35	29.17	26.72	33	36.67	21.67
Cerebrovascular accident	10	8.33	7.63	4	4.44	2.63
Sudden death	8	6.67	6.11	9	10.00	5.91
Myocardial infarction	11	9.17	8.40	6	6.67	3.94
Cardiac failure	3	2.5	2.29	9	10.00	5.91
Peripheral vascular	1	0.83	0.76	4	4.44	2.63
Other cardiovascular	2	1.67	1.53	1	1.11	0.66
Infection	26	21.67	19.85	18	20.00	11.82
Cancer	14	11.67	10.69	10	11.11	6.57
Accident/suicide	10	8.33	7.63	3	3.33	1.97
Treatment stop	7	5.83	5.34	6	6.67	3.94
Various causes	18	15.00	13.74	15	16.67	9.85
Evolution coexistent disease	5	4.17	3.82	0	0	0
Dementia	2	1.67	1.53	2	2.22	1.31
Hemorrhage	3	2.5	2.29	2	2.22	1.31
Hyperkalemia	3	2.5	2.29	0	0	0
Postsurgical	5	4.17	3.82	3	3.33	1.97
Cachexia malnutrition	0	0.00	0.00	4	4.45	2.63
Iatrogenic	0	0.00	0.00	4	4.45	2.63
Unknown	10	8.33	7.63	5	5.55	3.28
Total	120	100	91.61	90	100	59.1

Reducing the dialysis time in 32 patients led to changes in the opposite direction. Of the 32 patients, eight (25%) did not achieve 6 months of 5-h dialysis. This second 'selection' of the patients was due in three cases to difficulties in controlling dry weight and blood pressure; in the other five cases the patients themselves requested to go back to long dialysis, usually because they were feeling better, with less intra-dialytic incidents and with less dietary restriction.

Among the highly selected cohort of 24 patients who completed 9 months of 5-h dialysis, the mean predialysis blood pressure had slightly and not significantly increased (from 119/69 mmHg initially to 125/75 mmHg after 9 months). The mean post-dialytic weight, however, decreased from 58.7 to 56.5 kg. This was a real drop of body mass as evidenced by the evolution of their mean predialysis urea (23.8 to 20.9 mmol/l), creatinine (767 to 665 μmol/l), and hematocrit (32.2 to 29.4%).

Discussion

Is a longer dialysis session the key to survival?

Can we conclude that survival is better in Tassin long dialysis patients after taking into consideration the demographic and comorbid factors? If so, is the better survival linked to the reduction of some particular cause of death? If survival is longer, is this due to the length of the session *per se*, or to some specific 'center-effect' related to the other peculiarities of dialysis prescription or delivery in this unit? If long dialysis has better results because it is long, then what unique feature may explain it? This point is important because it can help to identify ways to improve the results of conventional dialysis.

Commentary on reported facts

We have described, in detail, the dialysis method used in Tassin for 28 years. The dose of dialysis, unusually large, the blood pressure control achieved for a great majority of patients, and significant laboratory data have been summarized.

The survival of this population as a whole is good. The mean half-life is almost 15 years. In part, this is due to the selection bias of the new patients at the early stage of the program. The increasing age at the start, the proportion of patients with comorbidity, and the proportion with causes of ESRD associated with an adverse outcome, all explain the worsening crude mortality in the successive calendar cohorts. But results over 8 years show that there has been no significant change in survival rate when the population at risk is standardized.

The Cox proportional hazard model confirms the independent and simultaneous effect of demographic and comorbid factors on survival. It illustrates the effect of the patients' initial nutritional state and, even more, of the mean predialysis arterial pressure achieved at 3 months. This effect of blood pressure control on survival is confirmed by the better survival of those patients whose mean arterial pressure is lower (Fig. 11.2). It is by far the most significant, dialysis treatment-related factor enhancing survival.

Comparing the causes of death with those of another French series (Degoulet *et al.*, 1982), the percentage who died from cardiovascular causes in both groups was high, but in long dialysis the cardiovascular mortality was halved, although patients were older with more risk factors. The difference is particularly obvious for cerebrovascular accidents which are associated with poor blood pressure control.

The comparison of the two cohorts surviving and not surviving for 10 years on the same treatment confirms the effects of age, risk factors, and antecedents. Interestingly it shows that mortality is in this case not linked to Kt/V, the surrogate marker of small molecule clearance, but strongly linked to the middle-molecule index (Table 11.8). Survival does not correlate with the initial blood pressure or the duration of hypertension before dialysis, but does so strongly with the mean of predialysis MAP values on dialysis. Some nutritional indices during treatment are linked significantly (serum albumin and cholesterol) to survival, but some are not (nPCR and plasma creatinine). The analysis of the causes of deaths before and after 10 years shows that the survivors subsequently died less from hypertension-related causes (cerebrovascular accident and myocardial infarction), but more often from cardiac failure and peripheral vascular disease. Infection, cancer, and various other causes were responsible for fewer deaths.

Our experience of increasing the dialysis session time in 103 patients, and decreasing it in 32 patients led to similar conclusions. When the same patient's dialysis session is longer, control of ECV (dry weight) can be achieved without antihypertensive medications. On the other hand, reducing the time, while maintaining the same dose delivery for small molecules made it difficult to maintain blood pressure control, and was associated with deterioration in nutrition, as suggested by the reduction in dry weight, plasma urea, creatinine, and hematocrit. One may speculate that this poor control of blood pressure and nutrition may, in the long-term, be responsible for an increased mortality rate.

Do patients really survive longer with long dialysis?

Survival data from Tassin have been widely published (Laurent *et al.*, 1983; Charra *et al.*, 1992*a*, 1996*b*). The facts reported here confirm this good survival.

They compare favorably with most reports issued by individual units or by registries. But comparing different units or registries is confusing. This is due to the different demographic and comorbid patterns of the compared populations (Collins *et al.*, 1990; Lowrie and Lew, 1990), to different transplant rates (Kjellstrand *et al.*, 1990), to different underlying mortality rates for the non-ESRD population, and to different methods in the use of the databases.

The standard mortality rates reveal a much lower mortality in Tassin than in the 'same risk' USRDS patients. SMR is not a perfect tool, the labeling of 'hypertension' as the cause of ESRD is imprecise (Mailloux, 1993), neither comorbidity nor the number of years spent on dialysis are included in the analysis factors, yet it is the simplest widely available tool for the indirect standardization of dialysis survival data to date.

What explains the longer survival of patients in Tassin?

The analysis of the causes of death provides a clear answer: cardiovascular mortality is the main difference compared to other series.

Furthermore, splitting the Tassin population into two cohorts as a function of pre-dialysis MAP shows that the lower the blood pressure the better the survival. This improved survival is explained almost exclusively by the difference in cardiovascular mortality.

Generally speaking, the cardiovascular causes of death are by far the greatest cause of mortality on dialysis (Anonymous, 1992). The incidence rate is higher than in the general population by a factor of 10 to 20 times, whatever the local baseline cardiovascular mortality (Raine *et al.*, 1992).

This may be explained by increased atherogenesis linked to risk factors present before and during ESRD therapy, such as hypertension, dyslipidemia, tobacco addiction, or lack of exercise (Lindner *et al.*, 1974; Haire *et al.*, 1978).

Reasons for the improved outcomes in long dialysis

If the better survival and lower cardiovascular mortality are not due to a favorable patient selection or to some center-effect, it must be due to the long, slow hemo-dialysis method *per se*.

Several questions must then be considered in turn, 'Is the long survival observed on long dialysis due to:

(1) the large dose of dialysis, for small and/or for middle molecules?
(2) or rather to good nutrition?
(3) or to satisfactory blood pressure level through control of ECV (dry weight) or some other mechanism(s)?
(4) or to a combination of those factors?
(5) or to some other reason(s)?

Dose of small-molecule dialysis (Kt/V)

In our Cox analysis, patient survival is not correlated to *Kt/V*. This seems surprising. But the variations of *Kt/V* from one patient to another in this population, where everybody received a very large dose of dialysis, may be not wide enough for a statistical significant difference to appear. No patient received a *Kt/V* of < 1.1.

Geographic comparisons of survival are misleading (Kjellstrand, 1994; Friedman, 1996), but they cannot be rejected as a whole. Wide mortality differences have been reported between the USA, where low doses of dialysis are used, and Europe (Held *et al.*, 1992) or Japan (Teraoka *et al.*, 1995), where higher doses of dialysis are delivered. Besides, in the USA (Collins *et al.*, 1994; Mailloux *et al.*, 1994a), Europe (Charra *et al.*, 1992a), South America (Fernandez *et al.*, 1992), and Asia (Iseki *et al.*, 1993), the longest survival rates have been reported for the largest doses of dialysis.

In the USA, between 1985 and 1990, reducing the dose of dialysis was associated with an increasing mortality (Eggers, 1990). In Europe, registry (Kramer *et al.*, 1982) and individual units (Wizemann and Kramer, 1987) data have shown increased mortality when session time and dialysis dose were reduced.

Conversely, increasing dialysis delivery by a combination of increased dialyzer surface, blood and dialysate flow, and dialysis time decreased the mortality, whether more 'biocompatible' membranes were used (Hakim *et al.*, 1994) or not (Collins *et al.*, 1994; Parker *et al.*, 1994).

Survival is linked to the dose of small molecule clearance. The question is what is the optimal dose of *Kt/V*? One of the main goals of the ongoing HEMO study (Eknoyan *et al.*, 1996) is to compare the outcomes of two quantities of dialysis: *Kt/V* of 1.0 vs. 1.4. These tested values are still much lower than the mean *Kt/V* of 1.78 delivered in Tassin. This factor alone could explain, in part, the good observed survival observed in Tassin.

Middle-molecule clearance rates

An adequate dose of dialysis should ensure the removal not only of small but also of higher molecular weight substances (Hakim, 1990; Vanholder *et al.*, 1995).

A deleterious effect of the NCDS mechanistic analysis (Gotch and Sargent, 1985) is that, by overemphasizing the role of urea alone, it has reintroduced the initial restrictive view of chronic renal failure as a purely small molecule-related disease, and neglected the possibility of a middle-molecule effect on morbidity and mortality (Cambi *et al.*, 1972).

The middle-molecule hypothesis has never suggested that small molecules were not toxic (Ahmad *et al.*, 1988), but it has added a new dimension to the toxicological concept of chronic renal failure.

Middle molecular weight substances are involved in changes in appetite (Bergström *et al.*, 1994), in immunodeficiency (Severini *et al.*, 1996), as well as in many other manifestations of chronic renal failure (Cheung, 1994). We observed a difference in the middle-molecules index between patients surviving 10 years of long dialysis or not.

Long hemodialysis is not, however, alone in delivering a large dose of middle-molecule clearance. This is achieved also by high-permeability membranes. A feature unique to long dialysis, though, is that it provides a longer time span thus allowing for a better transcellular shift of different solutes to maintain the concentration in blood entering the dialyzer.

Nutrition

Malnutrition is a leading cause of mortality on dialysis (Kopple *et al.*, 1981; Bergström, 1993). Adequate nutrition is unquestionably an important factor in survival on dialysis (Bergström, 1993; Owen *et al.*, 1993).

The required protein and energy intake targets (Kopple *et al.*, 1989) were met by 74 and 73% of long dialysis patients reported here. The mean intake values achieved were in the range of, or better than, many published data (Parfrey *et al.*, 1996). The large *Kt/V* (Lindsay and Spanner, 1989) and middle-molecule index (Heintz *et al.*, 1993) achieved may explain the satisfactory appetite and nutrition. Also, no restrictive diet is requested of the patient in long dialysis; indeed they are requested to eat a large amount of calories and proteins.

About one long dialysis patient out of four however, does not meet his theoretical necessary intake, and the usual recommended vitamin B_6, C, and folic acid allowances are often not met. Also, as Cuprophan membranes increase protein catabolism (Guiterez *et al.*, 1994) an even higher protein intake may be needed in our patients. Besides, caloric rather than protein deficiency predominates in stable hemodialysis patients (MacAllister and Vallance, 1996). We are far from the 35 kcal/kg per day theoretically recommended.

Serum albumin has a very strong positive correlation with survival (Owen *et al.*, 1993; Avram *et al.*, 1995). It is not only a strong predictor, but also a sensitive one: even a modest reduction in the serum albumin concentration correlates with an important increase in death risk (Schulman and Hakim, 1996). But a low serum albumin in hemodialysis patients is not synonymous with malnutrition, rather it may reflect an intercurrent disease or an acute-phase reaction (Kaysen, 1996) as suggested by the fact that C-reactive protein is the most powerful predictor of serum albumin in dialysis patients (Bergström *et al.*, 1995). On the other hand, a normal serum albumin level usually correlates with satisfactory nutrition. The fact that serum albumin remains over 40 g/l after 25 years of dialysis in the long dialysis patients does suggest overall good nutrition.

Good nutrition, however, is not specific to long dialysis. It is often also observed in shorter dialysis, and it does not seem that a difference in nutrition alone can explain the difference in survival.

Blood pressure

In long dialysis, cardiovascular mortality is lower than that usually reported. The pro-portion of cardiovascular deaths in Tassin is 40.7% of total deaths vs. 50–53% ob-served in Europe over the last 20 years (Raine *et al.*, 1992). Cardiovascular mortality, expressed in relation to risk exposure, appears to be even lower, 20.9 deaths per 1000 patient-years in Tassin long dialysis vs. 42.2 in conventional dialysis in France (Degoulet *et al.*, 1982).

The lower cardiovascular mortality in our series does not seem to be related to fac-tors such as a lower tobacco consumption or a lower rate of dyslipidemia. These atherogenic factors are no less prevalent in our population than in most other series (Charra *et al.*, 1992*b*). All pieces of evidence point to blood pressure control as being the most probable factor.

A steady reduction in cardiovascular mortality in the general population has been reported in the USA since 1968 (Sytkowski *et al.*, 1990). It is related to a reduction in the incidence of stroke and coronary events due to beneficial changes in life-style and to improved blood pressure control (Kaplan, 1994). In non-uremic individuals, hyper-tension is the major cause of cardiovascular morbidity and mortality (Kannel, 1975; Stamler *et al.*, 1993). This is probably the case in dialysis as well. As we have already demonstrated, in our long dialysis experience blood pressure is well controlled and cardiovascular mortality is low. Furthermore, the lowest cardiovascular mortality is observed in the cohort with the lowest blood pressure (Fig. 11.2).

Conversely, cardiovascular morbidity (Vincenti *et al.*, 1980; Neff *et al.*, 1983) and mortality (Lindner *et al.*, 1974; Lundin *et al.*, 1980; Parfrey *et al.*, 1996) are high in hyper-tensive dialysis patients. This is reinforced by observations such as the one made by

Tomita *et al.* (1995) who note, as in our Cox analysis, that the blood pressure during the maintenance period of dialysis is a better predictor of survival than blood pressure before or at the start of dialysis.

Blood pressure control by long hemodialysis is not a center-effect. It is observed in centers still using long dialysis (Covic *et al.*, 1996), and it was also observed worldwide when only long dialysis was used. In the early 1970s blood pressure was controlled in 90% of dialysis patients by ultrafiltration alone (Comty *et al.*, 1964; Blumberg *et al.*, 1967; Mailloux, 1992).

A smooth reduction in the extracellular fluid volume during long dialysis seems a critical ingredient to achieving a normal blood pressure. Adequate control of blood pressure without antihypertensive drugs is observed in daily hemodialysis (Buoncristiani *et al.*, 1985; Uldall *et al.*, 1994) as in continuous peritoneal dialysis (Mion *et al.*, 1986; Saldahana *et al.*, 1991). Conversely, hypertension is more difficult to control in twice-weekly dialysis (Degoulet *et al.*, 1982; Scribner, 1990). We conclude that hypertension is the single most important risk factor for cardiovascular morbidity and mortality in patients on dialysis (Degoulet *et al.*, 1982; Heyka and Paganini, 1989; Charra *et al.*, 1992*b*).

The relationship between blood pressure and cardiovascular mortality may not, however, be so clear-cut. Some groups report an inverse relationship between blood pressure and survival (Ritz and Koch, 1993; Lowrie *et al.*, 1994; Foley *et al.*, 1996). This paradoxical observation has several explanations:

1. At the initiation of dialysis, a variable proportion of patients with severe cardiac failure have a very low blood pressure (Foley *et al.*, 1996). Such patients with congestive heart failure have a very poor immediate prognosis (Santiago and Chazan, 1989). The weight of these subgroups of patients on the overall correlation analysis may be important.
2. The long-term evolution of blood pressure before and during dialysis is neither stable nor linear. Blood pressure tends to increase just before dialysis is started, and to decrease thereafter. The proportion of patients on different dialysis length within a population therefore impacts on the relationship.
3. The several years lag time between hypertension onset, target organ damage, and mortality explains that a large part of cardiovascular mortality observed on dialysis, especially in the first years, is dependent on patient selection rather than on the dialysis itself.
4. The proportion of patients receiving antihypertensive drugs is a very important factor in deciphering the mortality data; yet this information is not provided in many published cardiovascular mortality analyses.
5. Differences in study design bring about several confusing factors:
   (a) The initial 3 months of dialysis during which the blood pressure changes are the most prominent (Fig. 11.1) are excluded from the USRDS registry, but are included in the European and Japanese registries.
   (b) The blood pressure values used for a linear correlation or regression analysis may be systolic, diastolic, mean, or pulse blood pressures. They may be a mean of all, several, a few values, or a single value. The patient population may be split into 'normal' and 'hypertensive' subgroups according to different cut-off points.

Ambulatory blood-pressure monitoring studies show the relative value of casual predialysis blood pressure figures (Cheigh *et al.*, 1990; Simon *et al.*, 1992; Chazot *et al.*, 1995).

(c) Outcome variables are also different in different studies (crude mortality, cardiovascular mortality, coronary deaths, cardiac deaths including or not the sudden deaths, etc.).

6. In non-uremic patients the diluting effect of random fluctuations of blood pressure around the mean, the so-called regression dilution bias, cause a large underestimation of the true association between blood pressure and cardiovascular disease (MacMahon *et al.*, 1990). This also applies to uremic patients.

7. The ambiguous relationship between blood pressure and cardiovascular morbidity and mortality is illustrated in non-uremic patients by the J-curve relationship between blood pressure and coronary events (Cruickshank, 1988). This phenomenon can be explained by stiffer arteries and artifactually lowered diastolic blood pressure, or by a truly increased coronary death rate due to the poor coronary flow reserve combined to relative hypotension.

8. The difficulty in clearly demonstrating the relationship between blood pressure and cardiovascular mortality in chronic renal failure has been addressed by Ritz *et al.*, (1994) who suggest that the best explanation could be that the ideal target blood pressure is 'lower than realized in the past'.

The satisfactory blood pressure control on long hemodialysis contrasts with the poor control achieved using short dialysis. The incidence of hypertension increased as the dialysis duration was shortened (Wizemann and Kramer, 1987). Blood pressure is poorly controlled today in spite of the large use of antihypertensive medications (Cheigh *et al.*, 1992; Mailloux *et al.*, 1994*b*; Salem, 1995). Several explanations can be offered for this change:

1. Blood pressure control has been the 'neglected factor in hemodialysis treatment' (Scribner, 1994). There is indeed in the literature an amazing contrast between the number of papers concerning intradialytic hypotension and the relative scarcity of publications about hypertension on dialysis.

2. The pressure on the physician is unequal between, on the one hand, the acute hypotensive episodes, uncomfortable, noisy, and socially disturbing (but carrying no significant mortality risk) which are dramatically reported by the patient circle, and on the other hand, the chronic hypertension (the real killer) more often well tolerated, unnoticed by the patient, and which needs an uncomfortable treatment, i.e. returning to dry weight.

3. Another explanation lies in the dialysis time reduction itself. The high ultrafiltration rate required in short dialysis increases the intradialytic hypotension incidence and induces a vicious cycle perpetuating hypertension (Mailloux *et al.*, 1993; Charra *et al.*, 1996*b*). The prescribed dry weight cannot be achieved because hypotensive episodes lead the nurse to reduce the ultrafiltration rate, to give saline, or to disconnect the patient prematurely. Hypotensive episodes also induce the physician to erroneously re-evaluate the dry weight, and eventually to increase the dialysate sodium concentration. This, in turn, reduces the diffusive extraction

of sodium and makes the patient more thirsty, increasing the interdialytic weight gain. Altogether the patient becomes saline-overloaded and more hypertensive. To reduce this ECV-overload a higher ultrafiltration rate is needed, thus the intra-dialytic hypotension risk increases. When antihypertensive medications are pre-scribed they further increase the risk of intradialytic hypotension (Sulkora and Valek, 1988; Mailloux *et al.*, 1993; Salem, 1995). In addition, hypertension-induced left ventricular hypertrophy reduces the heart's adaptive capacity to sudden volemic changes (Ritz *et al.*, 1987).

4. Poor tolerance of ultrafiltration is becoming a prominent problem with the in-creasing proportion of patients exhibiting vascular disease in new patients cohorts.

Blood pressure regulation in maintenance hemodialysis is multifactorial (Zucchelli *et al.*, 1988; London *et al.*, 1996). Several factors could, apart from ECV control, explain the difficult control of blood pressure with short dialysis. The use of bicarbonate in-stead of vasodilating acetate, the higher sodium content of the dialysate, and the low clearance of the nitric oxide inhibitor dimethylarginine (Vallance *et al.*, 1992) are all relevant to the control of blood pressure. Middle molecular weight endothelin, arginine–vasopressin, sympathetic-activating uremic 'toxins' stimulating the renal afferent nerves (Converse *et al.*, 1992) could also be more adequately removed by a long hemodialysis. But so far the only strong body of evidence at hand points to ECV control as the most probable explanation of the better blood pressure control on long dialysis.

How does time work?

Increasing the dialysis time increases patients' survival. But there is no prospective randomized study analyzing the outcome for dialysis patients as a function of dialysis duration. The ongoing, National Institute of Health, HEMO study factorial design includes two factors, the *Kt/V* dose and the removal of middle molecules, but the time factor is kept between 2.5 and 4.5 hours (Eknoyan *et al.*, 1996). Another chance to disentangle the respective effects of time and dose is unfortunately going to be lost.

Separating, in our own 8 hours three times per week dialysis experience, the respective effect of time and dose is impossible. But our experience of increasing and decreasing the session duration in the same cohorts of patients indicates that many patients cannot get down to dry weight in 5 hours of dialysis, and that if they can do so, it is at the cost of their nutrition.

Increasing the dialysis session time has positive aspects other than simply improv-ing nutrition, extracellular volume, and blood pressure control. Long hemodialysis does not push every operational aspect of the treatment to its maximum, it leaves a great margin of safety for treatment delivery. Conversely, a high-quality, ultra-short dialysis is difficult to carry out properly. Recirculation is very common with the high flows used, and it has severe repercussions on dialysis delivery (Sherman, 1994).

Criticisms of long dialysis

These usually focus on its high cost and the time 'lost' by the patient.

We have reported that long dialysis is not significantly more expensive than a comparable shorter treatment. The long hemodialysis fee-for-service cost is high, but the per capita evaluation of the cost over 1 year is similar.

The time 'lost' on dialysis must be evaluated with care: most long dialysis patients get back to normal activities within 1 or 2 hours after the end of the session, while patients on very short schedules very often complain of a 'wash-out' period, when, exhausted, they are unable to get back to normal activity and must rest. The shorter the session the more the patient complains of the famous 'last hour' of dialysis . . . and the more he presses to reduce further the session duration. The length of the long hemodialysis session can be alleviated by using the night sleep hours whether at home or in the center.

Curiously, long hemodialysis is often accused of being responsible for the late amyloid 'complications'. That β_2-microglobulin amyloid complications increase with the time on dialysis has suggested that this pathology is linked to hemodialysis itself, and has justified the expression of 'dialysis-related amyloidosis'. Theoretical arguments about bioincompatible membranes have found some clinical support in the experience of some authors (Chanard *et al.*, 1989; Van Ypersele de Strihou *et al.*, 1991), but they are contested by others (Brunner *et al.*, 1990; Locatelli *et al.*, 1994 Kessler *et al.*, 1995). This syndrome is observed in patients treated by peritoneal dialysis (Gagnon *et al.*, 1988) or without dialysis at all (Zingraff *et al.*, 1990). There is strong evidence that the term dialysis-related amyloidosis should be replaced by uremic amyloidosis (Silberberg *et al.*, 1989).

Long dialysis is not perfect. One of the most worrying facts is that cardiovascular mortality remains higher than in the general population. This can be explained by left ventricular hypertrophy, an independent risk factor of death in renal failure (Silberberg *et al.*, 1989). In the Manchester series of long dialysis, normotensive patients (Covic *et al.*, 1996) as in Tassin (Leunissen, 1995), the proportion with left ventricular hypertrophy remains quite high. This could be due to persisting anemia and to several other factors, or some, as yet, unknown factors.

But long hemodialysis offers many benefits: long survival, low cardiovascular morbidity and mortality, low hospitalization rate, easy control of ECV, of blood pressure, and of anemia. Adequate nutrition, low use of medications, simplicity of material, good cost-effectiveness also make it worth spending some more hours on the machine. It has the outstanding quality for a treatment applied to a large population under very different conditions, of being very simple and easy to perform. Times are changing, the population on dialysis includes a decreasing number of transplantable patients. For the old and frail patients with increasing comorbidity a slow non-emotional dialysis is probably the best and easiest treatment type of dialysis.

In the 1990s the reduction of dialysis session time 'is no longer a primary objective' (Valderrabano, 1996). It is sad that, in the USA the dialysis time and dose are steadily increasing compared to 4 years ago (USRDS, 1995), but Europe shows the opposite trend, especially for elderly patients (Valderrabano, 1996; Jacobs and Selwood, 1995).

References

Ahmad, S., Blagg, C. R., and Scribner, B. H. (1988). Center and home chronic hemodialysis. In Schrier R. W., Gottshalk CW, eds. *Diseases of the kidney*, (IVth edn) Boston, (ed. R. W. Schrier and C. W. Gottshalk), pp. 3281–322.

Anonymous (1992). Report on management of renal failure in Europe. *Nephrology, Dialysis, Transplantation*, **7** (Suppl. 2), 5–48.

Anonymous. (1993). Fifth joint national committee on detection, evaluation, and treatment of high blood pressure. Fifth report. *Archives of Internal Medicine*, **153**, 154–93.

Anonymous. (1995). The cost effectiveness of alternative types of vascular access and the economic cost of ESRD. *American Journal of Kidney Diseases*, **26**, S140–S156.

Avram, M. M., Mittman, N., Bonomini, L., Chattopadhyay, J., and Fein, P. (1995). Markers for survival in dialysis: a seven-years prospective study. *American Journal of Kidney Diseases*, **26**, 209–19.

Babb, A. L., Popovich, R. P., Christopher, T. G., and Scribner, B. H. (1971). The genesis of the square meter–hour hypothesis. *Transactions of the American Society for Artificial Internal Organs*, **18**, 81.

Babb, A. G., Strand, M. J., Uvelli, D. A., Milutinovic, J., and Scribner, B. H. (1975). Quantitative description of dialysis treatment: a dialysis index. *Kidney International*, **7** (Suppl. 2), S23–S29.

Bergström, J. (1993). Nutrition and adequacy of dialysis in hemodialysis patients. *Kidney International*, **43** (Suppl. 41), S261–S267.

Bergström, J., Mamoun, H., and Anderstam, B. (1994). Middle molecules isolated from uremic ultrafiltrate and normal urine induce dose-dependent inhibition of appetite in rat. *Journal of the American Society of Nephrology*, **5**, 488.

Bergström, J., Heimbürger, O., Lindholm, B., and Qureshi, A. R. (1995). Elevated serum C-reactive protein is a strong predictor of increased mortality and low serum albumin in HD patients. *Journal of the American Society of Nephrology*, **6**, 573.

Blumberg, A., Nelp, W. D., Hegstrom, R. M., and Scribner, B. H. (1967). Extracelluar volume in patients with chronic renal disease treated for hypertension by sodium restriction. *Lancet*, **ii**, 69–73.

Brunner, F. P., Brynger, H., Ehrich, J. H. H., *et al.* (1990). Case control study on dialysis arthropathy: the influence of two different dialysis membranes: data from the EDTA Registry. *Nephrology, Dialysis, Transplantation*, **5**, 432–6.

Buoncristiani, U., Quintiliani, G., Cozzari, M., Giombini, L., and Ragaiolo, M. (1985). Daily dialysis: long term clinical metabolic results. *Kidney International*, **33** (Suppl. 24), S137–S140.

Cambi, V., Dall'Aglio, P., Savazzi, G., Arisi, L., Rossi, E., and Migone, L. (1972). Clinical assessment of haemodialysis patients with reduced small molecules removal. *Proceedings of European Dialysis and Transplantation Association*, **9**, 67–73.

Chanard, J., Bindi, P., Lavaud, S., Toupance, O., Maheut, H., and Lacour, F. (1989). Carpal tunnel syndrome and the type of dialysis membrane. *British Medical Journal*, 867–8.

Charra, B., Calemard, E., Ruffet, M., *et al.* (1992*a*). Survival as an index of adequacy of dialysis. *Kidney International*, **41**, 1286–91.

Charra, B., Laurent, G., Calemard, E., *et al.* (1992*b*). Risk factors involved in atherosclerotic events observed in HD patients. *Blood purification in perspective: new insights and future trends* II. Vol. 30 (ed. N. K. Man, J. Botella, and P. Zucchelli), pp. 83–8. ICAOT Press, Cleveland, Ohio.

Charra, B., Chazot, C., Laurent, G., *et al.* (1996*a*). Clinical assessment of dry weight. *Nephrology, Dialysis, Transplantation*, **11** (Suppl. 2), 16–19.

Charra, B., Calemard, E., and Laurent G. (1996*b*). Importance of treatment time and blood pressure control in achieving long-term survival on dialysis. *American Journal of Nephrology*, **16**, 35–44.

Chazot, C., Charra, B., Laurent, G., *et al.*, (1995). Interdialysis blood pressure control by long hemodialysis sessions. *Nephrology, Dialysis, Transplantation* **10**, 831–7.

Cheigh, J., Bui, D., Milite, C., *et al.* (1990). How well is hypertension controlled in hemodialysis patients. *Journal of the American Society of Nephrology*, **1**, 351 (Abstract).

Cheigh, J. S., Milite, C., Sullivan, J. F., Rubin, A. L., and Stenzel, K. H. (1992). Hypertension is not adequately controlled in hemodialysis patients. *American Journal of Kidney Diseases*, **19**, 453–9.

Cheung, A. K. (1994). Quantitation of dialysis: the importance of membrane and middle molecules. *Blood Purification*, **12**, 42–53.

Collins, A. J., and Keshaviah, P. R. (1988). Are there limitations to shortening dialysis treatment? *Transactions of the American Society for Artificial Internal Organs*, **34**, 1–5.

Collins, A. J., Hanson, G., Umen, A., Kjellstrand, C., and Keshaviah, P. (1990). Changing risk factor demographics in end-stage renal disease patients entering hemodialysis and the impact on long-term mortality: *American Journal of Kidney Diseases*, **15**, 422–32.

Collins, A. J., Ma, J., Umen, A., and Keshaviah, P. R. (1994). Urea index and other predictors of hemodialysis patient survival. *American Journal of Kidney Diseases*, **23**, 272–82.

Comty, C., Rottka, H., and Shaldon, S. (1964). Blood pressure control in patients with end-stage renal failure treated by intermittent dialysis. *Proceedings of the European Dialysis and Transplantation Association*, **1**, 209.

Converse, R. L., Jacobsen, T. N., Toto, R. D., *et al.* (1992). Sympathetic overactivity in patients with chronic renal failure. *New England Journal of Medicine*, **327**, 1912–18.

Covic, A., Goldsmith, D. J. A., Georgescu, G., Venning, M. C., and Ackrill, P. (1996). Echocardiographic findings in long-term, long-hour hemodialysis patients. *Clinical Nephrology*, **45**, 104–110.

Cox, D. R. (1972). Regression models and life tables (with discussion). *Journal of the Royal Statistical Society*, **34**, 187–220.

Cruickshank, J. M. (1988). Coronary flow reserve and the J curve relation between diastolic blood pressure and myocardial infarction. *British Medical Journal*, **297**, 1227–30.

Daugirdas, J. T. (1989). Bedside formulas for urea kinetic modeling. *Contemporary Dialysis and Nephrology*, **10**, 23–5.

Daugirdas, J. T. (1991). Dialysis hypotension: a hemodynamic analysis. *Kidney International*, **39**, 233–46.

Degoulet, P., Legrain, M., Reach, I., *et al.* (1982). Mortality risk factors in patients treated by chronic hemodialysis. *Nephron*, **31**, 103–10.

Eggers, P. W. (1990). Mortality rates among dialysis patients in Medicare's end-stage renal disease program. *American Journal of Kidney Diseases*, **25**, 414–21.

Eknoyan, G., Levey, A. S., Beck, G. J., *et al.* (1996). The hemodialysis (HEMO) study: rationale for selection of interventions. *Seminars in Dialysis*, **9**, 24–33.

Fernandez, J. M., Carbonell, M. E., Mazzuchi, N., and Petrucelli, D. (1992). Simultaneous analysis of morbidity and mortality factors in chronic hemodialysis patients. *Kidney International*, **41**, 1029–34.

Foley, R. N., Parfrey, P. S., Harnett, J. D., Kent, G. M., Murray, D. C., and Barre, P. E. (1996). Impact of hypertension on cardiomyopathy, morbidity and mortality in end-stage renal disease. *Kidney International*, **49**, 1379–85.

Friedman, E. A. (1996). End-stage renal disease therapy: an American success story. *Journal of the American Medical Association*, **275**, 1118–22.

Gagnon, R. F., Lough, J. O., and Bourgouin, P. (1988). Carpal tunnel syndrome with $\beta2$-microglobulin containing amyloid during continuous ambulatory peritoneal dialysis. *Canadian Medical Association Journal*, **139**, 753–5.

Gotch, F. A. (1983). Dialysis of the future. *Kidney International*, **33** (Suppl. 24), S100–S104.

Gotch, F. A. and Sargent, J. A. (1985). A mechanistic analysis of the National Cooperative Study (NCDS). *Kidney International*, **28**, 526–34.

Gotch, F. A., Yarian, S., and Keen, M. (1990). A kinetic survey of U. S. hemodialysis prescriptions. *American Journal of Kidney Diseases*, **XV**, 511–15.

Gutierez, A., Alvestrand, A., Bergström, J., Beving, H., Lantz, B., and Henderson, L. W. (1994). Biocompatibility of hemodialysis membranes: a study in healthy subjects. *Blood Purification*, **12**, 95–105.

Guyton, A. C. (ed.) (1991). *Textbook of medical physiology*, (8th ed) Saunders, Philadelphia.

Haire, H. M., Sherrard, D. J., Scardapane, D., Curtis, F. K., and Brunzell, J. D. (1978). Smoking, hypertension and mortality in a maintenance dialysis population. *Cardiovascular Medicine*, **3**, 1163–8.

Hakim, R. A. (1990). Assessing the adequacy of dialysis. *Kidney International*, **37**, 822–32.

Hakim, R. M., Breyer, J., Ismail, N., and Schulman, G. (1994). Effects of dose of dialysis on morbidity and mortality. *American Journal of Kidney Diseases*, **23**, 661–9.

HCFA (1991). Health Care Financing Administration, research report, end-stage renal disease. *Health Care Financing Administration*, 59–71.

Heintz, B., Königs, F., Dakshinamurty, K. V., *et al.* (1993). Response of vasoactive substances to intermittent ultrafiltration in normotensive hemodialysis patients. *Nephron*, **65**, 266–72.

Held, P. J., Blagg, C. R., Liska, D. W., Port, F. K., Hakim, R., and Levin, N. (1992). The dose of hemodialysis according to dialysis prescription in Europe and the United States. *Kidney International*, **42** (Suppl. 38), S16–S21.

Henderson, L. W. (1988). Of Time TAC urea and treatment schedules. *Kidney International*, **33** (Suppl. 24), 105–6.

Heyka, R. L., and Paganini, E. P. (1989). Blood pressure control in chronic dialysis patients. In *Replacement of renal function by dialysis*, (3rd ed) (ed. J. F. Maher), pp. 772–87. Kluwer Academic Publishers, Dordrecht.

Hull, A. R., and Parker, T. F. (1990). Proceedings from the morbidity, mortality and prescription of dialysis symposium, Dallas, Texas, September 1989: introduction and summary. *American Journal of Kidney Diseases*, **15**, 375–83.

Iseki, I., Kawazoe, N., Ozawa, A., and Fukiyama, K. (1993). Survival analysis of dialysis patients in Okinawa, Japan (1971–1990). *Kidney International*, **43**, 404–9.

Jacobs, C., and Selwood, N. H. (1995). Renal replacement therapy for ESRF in France: current status and evolutive trends over last decade. *American Journal of Kidney Diseases*, **25**, 188–95.

Kannel, W. B. (1975). Role of blood pressure in cardiovascular disease: the Framingham study. *Angiology*, **26**, 1–14.

Kaplan, N. M. (1994). *Clinical hypertension* (6th eds.) Williams & Wilkins, Baltimore, MD.

Kaplan, E. L., Meier, P. (1958). Non parametric estimation from incomplete observations. *Journal of the American Statistical Association*, **53**, 457–81.

Kaysen, G. A. (1996). Hypoalbuminemia in dialysis patients. *Seminars in Dialysis* **9**, 249–56.

Keshaviah, P., and Collins, A. (1988). A re-appraisal of the National Cooperative study (NCDS). *Kidney International*, **33**, 227.

Kessler, M., Hestin, D., Aymard, B., *et al.* (1995). Carpal tunnel syndrome with β-2 amyloid deposits and erosive arthropathy of the wrist and spine in a uremic patient before chronic hemodialysis. *Nephrology, Dialysis, Transplantation*, **10**, 29.

Kjellstrand, K. M. (1994). International comparisons of dialysis survival are meaningless to evaluate differences in dialysis procedure. In *Death on hemodialysis: preventable or inevitable?* (ed. E. A. Friedman), pp. 55–68. Kluwer Academic, Dordrecht.

Kjellstrand, C. N., Hylander, B., and Collins, A. C. (1990). Mortality on dialysis—on the influence of early start, patient characteristics, and transplantation and acceptance rates. *American Journal of Kidney Diseases*, **15**, 483–90.

Kolff, W. J., Berk, H. T. J., ter Welle, M., van der Ley, A. J. W., van Dijk, E. C., and van Noordwijk, J. (1944). The artificial kidney, a dialyzer with a great area. *Acta Medica Scandinavica*, **117**, 121–8.

Kopple, J. D., Henry, D. A., Roberts, C. E., Goodman, W. G., and Blumenkrantz, M. J. (1981). Relationship between nutritional status of patients undergoing maintenance hemodialysis and duration of dialysis therapy. In *Uremia. pathobiology of patients treated for 10 years or more* (ed. C. Giordano E. A., Friedman), pp. 25–31. Wichtig, Milan.

Kopple, J. D., Shinaberger, J., Coburn, J., and Sorensen, M. (1989). Optimal dietary protein treatment during chronic hemodialysis. *Transactions of the American Society for Artificial Internal Organs*, **15**, 302–8.

Kramer, P., Broyer, M., Brunner, F. P., Brynger, H. (1982). Combined report on regular dialysis and transplantation in Europe. *Proceedings of the European Dialysis and Transplantation Association*, **19**, 4–59.

Laurent, G., Calemard, G., and Charra, B. (1983). Long dialysis: a review of fifteen years experience in one center: 1968–1983. *Proceedings of the European Dialysis and Transplantation Association*, **20**, 122–9.

Leunissen, K. M. L. (1995). Fluid status in hemodialysed patients. *Nephrology, Dialysis, Transplantation*, **10**, 153–5.

Lindner, A., Charra, B., Sherrard, D., Blagg, C., and Scribner, B. H. (1974). Accelerated atherosclerosis in prolonged maintenance hemodialysis. *New England Journal of Medicine*, **290**, 697–701.

Lindsay, R. M., and Spanner, E. (1989). A hypothesis: the protein rate is dependent upon the type and amount of treatment in dialysed uremic patients. *American Journal of Kidney Diseases*, **13**, 382–9.

Locatelli, F., Mastrangelo, F., Redaelli, B., Ronco, C., Marcelli, D., and Orlandini, G. (1994). The effects of different membranes and dialysis technologies on the treatment tolerance and nutritional parameters of hemodialysis patients. Design of a prospective randomised multicentre trial. *Journal of Nephrology*, **7**, 123–9.

London, G., Marchais, S., and Guerin, A. P. (1996). Blood pressure control in chronic hemodialysis patient. In *Replacement of renal function by dialysis* (ed. C. Jacobs, C. M. Kjellstrand, K. M. Koch, and J. F. Winchester), pp. 969–89. Kluwer Academic, Dordrecht.

Lowrie, E. G., and Lew, N. L. (1990). Death risk in hemodialysis patients: the predictive value of commonly measured variables and an evaluation of death rate differences between facilities. *American Journal of Kidney Diseases*, **15**, 458–82.

Lowrie, E. G., Laird, N. M., Parker, T. F., and Sargent, J. A. (1981). Effect of the hemodialysis prescription on patient morbidity. Report from the National Cooperative Study. *New England Journal of Medicine*, **305**, 1176–81.

Lowrie, E. G., Huang, W. H., Lew, M., and Liu, Y. (1994). The relative contribution of measured variables to death risk among hemodialysis patients. In *Death on hemodialysis: preventable or inevitable?* (ed. E. A. Friedman), pp. 121–41. Kluwer Academic, Dordrecht.

Lundin, A. P., Adler, A. J., Feinroth, M. V., Berlyne, G. M., and Friedman, E. A. (1980). Maintenance hemodialysis. Survival beyond the first decade. *Journal of the American Medical Association*, **244**, 34–40.

MacAllister, R. J., and Vallance, P. (1996). Systemic vascular adaptation to increases in blood volume: the role of the blood-vessel wall. *Nephrology, Dialysis, Transplantation*, 11, 231–40.

MacMahon, S., Peto, R., Cutler, C., *et al.* (1990). Blood pressure, stroke, and coronary heart disease. Part 1: Prolonged difference in blood pressure: prospective observational studies corrected for the regression dilution bias. *Lancet*, 335, 765–74.

Mailloux, L. U. (1992). More dialysis leads to better survival: a point of view. *Seminars in Dialysis*, 5, 224–6.

Mailloux, L. U. (1993). What is hypertensive ESRD? The need for stricter clinical definitions. *Seminars in Dialysis*, 6, 141–2.

Mailloux, L. U., Bellucci, A. G., and Mossey, R. T. (1988). Predictors of survival in patients undergoing dialysis. *American Journal of Medicine*, 84, 855–62.

Mailloux, L. U., Herbert, L., and Mossey, R. T. (1993). Interdialytic hypertension. *Seminars in Dialysis*, 6, 409–10.

Mailloux, L. U., Bellucci, A., Napolitano, B., Mossey, R. T., Wilkes, B. M., and Bluestone, P. A. (1994a). Survival estimates for 683 patients from 1970 through 1989: identification of risk factors for survival. *Clinical Nephrology*, 42, 127–35.

Mailloux, L. U., Bellucci, A. G., Napolitano, B., and Mossey, R. T. (1994b). The contribution of hypertension–to dialysis patients outcomes, a point of view. *American Society for Artificial Internal Organs Journal*, 40, 130–7.

Mion, C., Slingeneyer, A., and Canaud, B. (1986). Pathophysiology and management of hypertension in continuous ambulatory peritoneal dialysis patients. *Contributions to Nephrology*, Ed. Maschio, G., Campese, V. M., Valvo, E., Oldrizzi, L. Vol. 54, pp. 202–9. Karger, Basel.

Neff, M. S., Eiser, A. R., Slifkin, R. F., *et al.* (1983). Patients surviving 10 years of hemodialysis. *American Journal of Medicine*, 74, 996–1004.

Owen, W. F., Lew, N. L., Yan Lu, S. M., Lowrie, E. G., and Lazarus, J. M. (1993). The urea reduction ratio and serum albumin concentration as predictors of mortality in patients undergoing hemodialysis. *New England Journal of Medicine*, 329, 1001–6.

Parfrey, P. S., Foley, R. N., Harnett, J. D., Kent, G. M., Murray, D., and Barre, P. E. (1996). Outcome and risk factors of ischemic heart disease in chronic uremia. *Kidney International*, 49, 1428–34.

Parker, T. F., Husni, L., Huang, W., Lew, M., Lowrie, E. G., and the Dallas Nephrology Associates (1994). Survival of hemodialysis patients in United States is improved with a greater quantity of dialysis. *American Journal of Kidney Diseases*, 23, 670–80.

Raine, A. E. G., Margreiter, R., Brunner, F. P., *et al.*, (1992). Report on management of renal failure in Europe XXII. *Nephrology, Dialysis, Transplantation*, (Suppl. 2), 7–35.

Ritz, E., and Koch, M. (1993). Morbidity and mortality due to hypertension in patients with renal failure. *American Journal of Kidney Diseases*, 21, (Suppl. 2), 113–18.

Ritz, E., Ruffman, K., Rambausek, M., Mall, G., and Schmidli, M. (1987). Dialysis hypotension: is it related to diastolic left ventricular malfunction? *Nephrology, Dialysis, Transplantation*, 2, 293–7.

Ritz, E., Wiecek, A., and Rambausek, M. (1994). Cardiovascular death in patients with end-stage renal failure. Strategies for prevention. *International yearbook of Nephrology, Dialysis and Transplantation*, (ed. V. E. Andreucci and L. G. Fine), pp. 120–8.

Saldahana, L. F., Weiler, E. W. K., and Gonnick, H. C. (1991). Effect of continuous ambulatory peritoneal dialysis on blood pressure control. *American Journal of Kidney Diseases*, 21, 184–8.

Salem, M. M. (1995). Hypertension in the hemodialysis population: a survey of 649 patients. *American Journal of Kidney Diseases*, 26, 461–8.

Santiago, A., and Chazan, J. A. (1989). The cause of death and co-morbid factors in 405 chronic hemodialysis patients. *Dialysis and Transplantation*, 18, 484–8.

Sargent, J. A. (1990). Shortfalls in the delivery of dialysis. *American Journal of Kidney Diseases*, 15, 500–10.

Schulman, G., and Hakim, R. M. (1996). Improving outcomes in chronic hemodialysis patients: should dialysis be initiated earlier. *Seminars in Dialysis*, 9, 225–8.

Scribner, B. H. (1990). A personalized history of chronic hemodialysis. *American Journal of Kidney Diseases*, 6, 511–19.

Scribner, B. H. (1994). Blood pressure control: the neglected factor that affects survival of dialysis patients. In *Death on hemodialysis: preventable or inevitable?* (ed. E. A. Friedman), pp. 195–7. Kluwer Academic, Dordrecht.

Scribner, B. H., Buri, R., Caner, J. E. Z., Hegstrom, R. M., and Burnell, J. M. (1960). The treatment of chronic uremia by the means of intermittent dialysis: a preliminary report. *Transactions of the American Society for Artificial Internal Organs*, 6, 114–19.

Severini, G., Diana, L., Giovanndrea, R., and Sagliaschi, G. (1996). Influence of uremic middle molecules on *in vitro* stimulated lymphocytes and interleukin-2 production. *American Society for Artificial Internal Organs Journal*, 42, 64–7.

Sherman, R. A. (1994). Recirculation in the hemodialysis access. In *Principle and practice of dialysis*, (ed. W. L. Heinrich), pp. 38–46.

Siddiqui, J., and Kerr, D. N. S. (1971). Complications of renal failure and their response to dialysis. *British Medical Bulletin*, 27, 153–9.

Silberberg, J. S., Barre, P. E., Pritchard, S. S. and Sniderman, A. D. (1989). Impact of left ventricular hypertrophy on survival in end-stage renal disease. *Kidney International*, 36, 286–90.

Simon, P., Benziane, A., Cam, G., Ghali, N., Ang, K., and Charasse, C. (1992). Intérêt de la mesure ambulatoire de la pression artérielle (MAPA) chez l'urémique hypertendu et traité par dialyse péritonéale continue ambulatoire. *Le Bulletin de Dialyse Péritonéale* 2, 128–36.

Staessen, J. A., Fagard, R. H., Lijnen, P. J., Thijs, L., Van Hoof, R., and Amery, A. K. (1991). Mean and range of the ambulatory blood pressure in normotensive subjects from a meta-analysis of 23 studies. *American Journal of Cardiology*, 67, 723–7.

Stamler, J., Stamler, R., and Neaton, J. D. (1993). Blood pressure, systolic and diastolic, and cardiovascular risks: US population data. *Archives of Internal Medicine*, 153, 598–615.

Sulkova, S., and Valek, A. (1988). Role of antihypertensive drugs in the therapy of patients on regular dialysis treatment. *Kidney International*, 34, (Suppl. 25), S198–S200.

Sytkowski, P. A., Kannel, W. B., and D'Agostino, R. B. (1990). Changes in risk factors and the decline in mortality from cardiovascular disease. The Framingham Heart Study. *New England Journal of Medicine*, 322, 1635–41.

Teraoka, S., Torna, H., Nihei, H., Ota, K., *et al.*, (1995). Current status of renal replacement therapy in Japan. *American Journal of Kidney Diseases*, 25, 151–64.

Thomas, G. I. (1969). A large vessel applique ateriovenous shunt for hemodialysis. *Transactions of the American Society for Artificial Internal Organs*, 15, 288–92.

Tomita, J., Kimura, G., Inoue, T., *et al.* (1995). Role of systolic blood pressure in determining prognosis of hemodialysis patients. *American Journal of Kidney Diseases*, 25, 405–12.

Twardowski, Z. J., and Kubara, H. (1979). Different sites versus constant sites in needle insertion into arteriovenous fistulas for treatment by repeated dialysis. *Dialysis and Transplantation*, 8, 978–80.

Uldall, R., Francoeur, R., Ouwendyk, M., *et al.* (1994). Simplified nocturnal home hemodialysis a new approach to renal replacement therapy. *Journal of the American Society of Nephrology*, 5, 428.

USRDS (1993). *U.S. Renal Data System, 1993 Annual data report*. The National Institutes of Health, National Institute of Diabetes and Digestive and Kidney Diseases, Bethesda, MD.

USRDS (1995). *U.S. Renal Data System, 1995 annual data report*. The National Institutes of Health, National Institute of Diabetes and Digestive and Kidney Diseases, Bethesda, MD.

Valderrabano, F. (1996). Weekly duration of dialysis treatment—does it matter for survival? *Nephrology, Dialysis, Transplantation*, **11**, 569–72.

Vallance, P., Leone, A., Calver, A., Collier, J., and Moncada, S. (1992). Accumulation of an endogenous inhibitor of nitric oxide synthesis in chronic renal failure. *Lancet*, **339**, 572–5.

van Ypersele de Strihou, C., Jadoul, M., Malghem, J., Maldague, B., and Jamart, J. (1991). Effect of dialysis membrane and patient's age on signs of dialysis related amyloidosis. *Kidney International*, **39**, 1012–19.

Vanholder, R., de Smet, R., Vogeleere, P., and Ringoir, S. (1995). Middle molecules: toxicity and removal by hemodialysis and related strategies. *Artificial organs*, **19**, 1120–5.

Vertes, V., Cangiano, J. L., Berman, L. B., and Gould, A. (1969). Hypertension in end-stage renal disease. *New England Journal of Medicine*, **280**, 978–81.

Vincenti, F., Amend, W. J., Abele, J., Feduska, N. J., and Salvatierra, O. (1980). The role of hypertension in hemodialysis-associated atherosclerosis. *American Journal of Medicine*, **63**, 363–9.

Von Albertini, B. (1988). High efficiency hemodialysis: an overview. *Contributions to Nephrology*, **61**, 37–45.

Wizemann, V., and Kramer, W. (1987). Short-term dialysis, long-term complications. *Blood Purification*, **5**, 193–201.

Wolfe, R. A., Gaylin, D. S., Port, F. K., Held, P. J., and Wood, C. L. (1992). Using USRDS generated mortality tables to compare local ESRD mortality rates to national rates. *Kidney International*, **42**, 991–6.

Zingraff, J. J., Noël, L. H., Bardin, T., *et al.* (1990). β-2Microglobulin amyloidosis in chronic renal failure. *New England Journal of Medicine*, **323**, 1070–1.

Zucchelli, P., Santoro, A., and Zuccala, A. (1988). Genesis and control of hypertension in hemodialysis patients. *Seminars in Nephrology*, **8**, 163.

12

Long-term vascular access

Peter J. Conlon and Steve J. Schwab

Introduction

Despite the enormous technological advances in dialysis since its inception 35 years ago, there continues to be a very high annual mortality for patients with end-stage renal disease (ESRD). It is an extremely small minority of patients who develop ESRD who remain on life-sustaining hemodialysis for longer than 10 years. In the United States of America the annual mortality from ESRD approaches 20%. After 10 years of ESRD the majority of patients will have either have succumbed to a complication of the disease process which caused their kidneys to fail, will have died from a complication of uremia, or will have undergone renal transplantation. Table 12.1 summarizes the US Renal Data System results for 10-year survival on dialysis with censoring at the time of renal transplantation. It can be seen that only a little over 4% of patients who start dialysis between the ages of 65 to 74 years will be alive 10 years later. Overall 2.5% of patients will still be on dialysis 10 years after starting hemodialysis, with black patients probably faring significantly better than white patients and females faring slightly better than males. Patients with diabetes as the primary cause of renal disease have the poorest prognosis, with less than 1 in 50 patients surviving on dialysis to 10 years. Patients with primary kidney diseases have the best prognosis, with close to 1 in 20 patients remaining on dialysis for their 10th anniversary of initiating renal replacement therapy.

Despite these poor statistics there are a group of patients who, through personal choice or for immunological reasons, will not have undergone successful renal transplantation and who remain continuously on dialysis for longer than 10 years. One can anticipate that this group will become bigger if the current trend of the increasing waiting time for cadaveric organs continues, and as the treatment of ESRD improves with reductions in annual mortality.

In 1983, Dr Gutman, from this institution, carried out a survey of seven renal replacement centers in the USA and Sweden to identify those patients who had been maintained on hemodialysis for longer than 14 years (Gutman, 1983). In this survey Dr Gutman identified 25 patients. None of the patients were able to remember the number of vascular access procedures they had undergone because they had been so numerous. All but one of the patients had used an external shunt at some stage in their past, and six were using an external shunt at the time of the survey. Vascular access difficulty was described as 'overwhelming' in two cases. In the ensuing 13 years the technology of vascular access has advanced considerably, but the maintenance of vascular access for prolonged periods remains a considerable technical challenge to this day.

Table 12.1 Ten-year survival probability: from day 1 to 10 years for patients 65 and over at the start of ESRD therapy by age race, sex, and primary cause of ESRD (± standard error); censored at time of transplantation

Age	
65–74	4.02 ± 0.18
75 plus	1.01 ± 0.17
Race	
Black	3.67 ± 0.28
White	2.15 ± 0.12
Other	4.91 ± 1.16
Sex	
Male	2.5 ± 0.17
Female	2.85 ± 0.18
Primary diagnosis	
Diabetes	1.47 ± 0.21
Hypertension	2.79 ± 0.22
Glomerulonephritis	4.6 ± 0.47
Other cause	3.70 ± 0.23
Total adjusted probability	2.63 ± 0.12

The nephrologist caring for patients with chronic renal failure and ESRD has to deal with many important issues, but none are as important as the careful planning and pre-emptive management of vascular access, for without adequate access to the circulation, dialysis will be impossible and the patient will die.

Types of permanent vascular access

Primary fistula

In 1962 Cimino and Brescia described the technique of anastomosing the radial artery to the adjacent veins (Brescia *et al.* 1996, Cimino and Brescia, 1994). This technique allowed the repeated puncturing of veins for dialysis access. In this series of 14 attempted fistula creations, 2 failed immediately postoperatively, and the remaining 12 appeared to work for their required duration of 110 patient-dialysis months. To this day, the Cimino–Brescia arteriovenous (AV) fistula remains unrivaled when compared to any other form of long-term vascular access for either complication-free function or patency. Estimates of long-term graft survival rates vary enormously (Mennes *et al.*, 1978; Munda *et al.*, 1983; Palder *et al.*, 1985*a*; Kherlakian *et al.*, 1986; Fan and Schwab,

1992; Windus, 1994). Cumulative primary fistula patency rates vary considerably between dialysis centers. The differences probably reflect multiple factors such as the demographics of the local dialysis population, the expertise of the dialysis staff, and the skill and preference of the vascular surgeons. The most frequent problem with AV fistulas is failure to mature, as manifested by early thrombosis or inadequate flow rates. The reported incidence of a primary AV fistula failure to mature to a functional hemodialysis vascular access is between 9% (Winsett and Wolma, 1979) and 30% (Kinnaert *et al.*, 1977). The upper arm brachial–cephalic fistula can mature in most patients, even in those who have failed radial–cephalic placement. Thus aggressive attempts at an upper arm AV fistula creation are frequently rewarding in the avoidance of the long-term complications of prosthetic grafts. Once the AV fistula has matured and begun to be used successfully, many authors have documented their excellent long-term use. Winsett and Wolma (1979) reported that after 2 years' dialysis 90% of primary fistulas were functioning, with 80% still functioning at 3 years. At our center the 3-year cumulative patency for native AV fistulas is 80%. There is no data on the 10-year cumulative patency rates.

PTFE grafts

Polytetrafluoroethylene (PTFE) was introduced as a material for vascular bypass grafts in 1976 (Rapaport *et al.*, 1981). Since that time, this material has become the mainstay for dialysis vascular access when an autologous AV fistula is either believed to be technically impossible or has failed to mature. Using PTFE as a conduit, a fistula is created between an upper limb artery and vein. Such a graft accounts for more than 80% of the vascular procedures performed in the USA (Windus, 1993). In other parts of the world the reverse is the case, with more than 80% of patients receiving a primary AV fistula. The major reason for the discrepancies in the use of primary AV fistulas between the USA and other parts of the world probably relates to the older age of the USA population and the increased proportion of patients in the USA with diabetes and poor quality veins for vascular access surgery. In addition, more than 40% of patients who present with ESRD in the USA have not had a vascular access created prior to the need for hemodialysis. Studies looking at the survival of PTFE grafts have noted cumulative patency rates (Table 12.2) for PTFE grafts of between 63% and 90% at 1 year and between 50% and 77% at 2 years; fewer than 50% of synthetic fistulas survive beyond 3 years (Rapaport *et al.*, 1981; Munda *et al.*, 1983; Palder *et al.*, 1985*a*, *b*). Most of these studies defined patency as persistent graft function, regardless of whether or not the graft had undergone revision or thrombectomy. Unassisted graft patency (that is graft patency without graft revision, thrombectomy, or angioplasty) has been reported by a number of authors (Winsett and Wolma, 1979; Palder *et al.*, 1985*b*). Sabanayagam *et al.* (1980) reported the unassisted PTFE graft patency of 77% at 1 year, while Palder *et al.* (1985*b*) reported an unassisted graft patency of 51% at 1 year. There are no systematic studies of the survival of PTFE grafts beyond 3–4 years. At our center we have a 78%, 3-year cumulative patency rate for PTFE grafts. This is made possible by the development of a rigorous, prospective intervention plan. This prospective treatment plan is discussed in detail later in the chapter. Nonetheless, compared with native AV fistulas the intervention rate to maintain this patency rate is 5-fold greater than for native AV fistulas.

Table 12.2   Comparison of survival rates between native AV fistulas (AVF) and PTFE grafts at years 1, 2, and 3

Study	1 Year		2 Years		3 Years	
	AVF	PTFE	AVF	PTFE	AVF	PTFE
Kinnaert *et al.*, 1977	88	—	88	—	82	—
Kherlakian *et al.*, 1986	71	75	66	61	64	50
Palder *et al.*, 1985*a*	60	80	53	68	45	68
Jenkins *et al.*, 1980	—	68	—	65	—	64
Munda *et al.*, 1983	—	67	—	50	—	—
Mean	73	72	69	61	64	61

Dual-lumen cuffed catheters

Although a far inferior choice for vascular access than either a primary AV fistula or PTFE graft, dual-lumen cuffed catheters have assumed an important role in the provision of vascular access for ESRD patients in the USA (Schwab *et al.*, 1988*a*; Shusterman *et al.*, 1989; Moss *et al.*, 1990; Gibson and Mosquera, 1991). These catheters may be employed in a number of circumstances, as an initial vascular access while waiting for an access to mature, or as a bridge between one access that has failed acutely and the establishment of an alternative. In addition, there is a group of patients in whom all alternative sites have been exhausted. These catheters are most commonly placed in the jugular veins, but they may also be placed for varying times in the femoral veins, into the superior vena cava, or by a translumbar route into the inferior vena cava. In addition, dual-lumen cuffed catheters may be used in patients with severe coronary artery disease or congestive heart failure who cannot tolerate the approximately 10% increase in cardiac output which an AV fistula will induce.

The two major reasons for failure of dual-lumen cuffed catheters is either thrombosis (Caruana *et al.*, 1987) or infection. There are a number of relatively simple strategies that will successfully prolong the life of the catheter when it presents with poor flow. The first approach should be to instill 5000 U of urokinase made up to the same volume as the catheter's internal lumen and allowed to stand for up to 30 minutes. This technique should be successful in restoring flow to the catheter in approximately 75% of cases. If this technique is unsuccessful, flow can almost always be restored with the assistance of interventional radiology. A gooseneck snare can be introduced through the femoral vein and fibrin sheaths stripped off the tip of the catheter, this restores flow in 95% of cases (Crain *et al.*, 1994; Suchocki *et al.*, 1996).

The major reason for permanent catheter failure is their high rate of infection. We have noted approximately four catheter-related bacteremias per 1000 patient-days. In general, when patients become bacteremic as a result of a catheter-related infection, the catheter should be removed at the earliest opportunity. Patients should receive between 2 and 4 weeks of appropriate antibiotics following removal of the catheter. In a prospective trial at our institution, attempts to 'salvage' the catheter by treating with antibiotics for prolonged periods resulted in only 22% of catheters being salvaged. These catheters, although excellent for intermediate access, have a very limited role as permanent access. At our center the use-life of catheters intended for permanent use is 12.7 months (Suchocki *et al.*, 1996). Most catheters are removed secondary to tunnel-tract infection or catheter-mediated bacteremia.

We believe that, whenever possible, some form of vascular access other than a cuffed catheter should be sought for any patient who has a prognosis of more than 6 months. In our opinion, the role of the cuffed catheter is to act as a 'bridge' between other permanent AV access and to allow those patients who present with ESRD to have adequate time for an AV fistula to mature.

Reasons for access failure

AV access thrombosis

Thrombosis is the leading cause of AV access loss. A thrombosis that occurs within 1 month of vascular access placement is due either to technical errors in the fistula construction or to the premature use of the access. After the first month, the thrombosis rate is approximately 0.5–0.8 episodes per patient per year. Access type greatly affects access thrombosis rates: synthetic grafts clot much more frequently than do native fistulas. The major predisposing factor to graft thrombosis is anatomical venous stenosis, being responsible for 75–80% of thromboses (Table 12.3) (Beathard, 1992; Fan

Table 12.3 Causes of prosthetic PTFE graft loss

Thrombosis
  Anatomical etiology
  Anastomotic stenosis
  Central venous stenosis
  Intra graft thrombosis
Non-anatomical etiology
  'Low-flow' state
  Disturbed procoagulant/anticoagulant equilibrium
  Undetected anatomical lesions
Infection
Pseudoaneurysm
Perigraft hematoma or seroma
Graft attrition

and Schwab, 1992; Kanterman *et al.*, 1995). The majority of venous stenoses develop at or within 2–3 cm of the vein graft anastomoses, and are due to progressive fibromuscular intimal hyperplasia and perivenous fibrosis (Swedberg *et al.*, 1989). The remainder are located in more proximal veins, including central veins. Subclavian vein stenosis may account for up to 20% of venous stenoses (Barrett *et al.*, 1988; Kanterman *et al.*, 1995). Previous subclavian vein cannulation, particular if the catheter became infected, is the major risk factor associated with subclavian vein stenosis (Barrett *et al.*, 1988; Schwab *et al.*, 1988*b*). Arterial stenosis accounts for less than 2% of graft failures.

About 15–20% of late-access thromboses occur in the absence of an identifiable anatomical lesion (Galbraith *et al.*, 1992). Hypotension, intravascular volume depletion, and prolonged compression of the fistula during sleep or by inexperienced nursing staff, may lead to a markedly decreased fistula flow and subsequent thrombosis. Indeed, one of the chief causes of fistula thrombosis, in the absence of identifiable anatomical stenosis, is from the patient or dialysis staff using excessive compression on the vascular access in an attempt to achieve rapid hemostasis following hemodialysis.

The question as to whether the increased hematocrit brought about by the use of erythropoietin is associated with increased rates of graft thrombosis has been controversial. The Canadian erythropoietin study demonstrated a higher rate of graft thrombosis among patients with higher hematocrits compared with control patients (Canadian Erythropoietin Study Group, 1990), although other authors have failed to confirm this observation (Tang *et al.*, 1992).

A number of recent studies have addressed the question of whether specific subgroups of patients are at increased risk for vascular access thrombosis (Table 12.4) (Windus, 1994). Most of these studies have focused specifically on patients with PTFE grafts. There is now substantial evidence that patients with diabetes mellitus are at greater risk than non-diabetics for prosthetic fistula thrombosis for up to 2 years after graft placement (Windus *et al.*, 1992). This observation has been confirmed in a recent analysis of the USRDS data (Lerner and Weinstein, 1996). Subjects of black race and female sex have also been observed to have an increased incidence of graft thrombosis (Lerner and Weinstein, 1996). The Canadian Hemodialysis Morbidity Study also identified a serum albumin level of below 3 g/dl as a risk factor for graft thrombosis (Feldman *et al.*, 1993). The mechanism of this is unclear, but it may be related to decreased intravascular oncotic pressure.

Table 12.4   Comorbid conditions reported to be associated with increased fistula thrombosis

---

Type of vascular access:
   Prosthetic graft fistula
   History of prior subclavian catheter

Diabetes mellitus

Black race

Hypoalbuminemia

Increased liopoprotein (a)

Antiphospholipid antibodies

A number of articles have reported increased graft thrombosis rates in subjects with hypercoagulable states, such as antiphospholipid antibody syndrome and protein-S or protein-C deficiency states (Garcia–Martin *et al.*, 1991; Macdougal *et al.*, 1991). In general, these are uncommon causes of graft thrombosis and should probably only be looked for in patients who develop recurrent graft thrombosis in the absence of an identifiable anatomical lesion on fistulography.

Vascular access infection

Access infection is the most common reason for access failure when cuffed silastic catheters are used for long-term access, and is the second most common cause of graft failure when PTFE grafts are used. Failure of a primary AV fistula due to infection is extremely unusual. Synthetic fistula and catheter infections account for 20% of all vascular access complications, and for the majority of episodes of bacteremia in hemodialysis patients (Bhat *et al.*, 1980).

Antibiotic prophylaxis for vascular access infection has been attempted in the past, aimed primarily at staphylococcal infections, with a variety of oral, topical, and intravenous agents (Boelaert *et al.*, 1989, 1994). Unfortunately, most have had minimal or only transient effects on staphylococcal skin or nasal carriage. Even an effective anti-staphylococcal agent such as rifampicin, has only limited clinical utility because of the emergence of resistant strains. Indeed, in view of the recent pandemic of vancomycin-resistant enterococci, nephrologists must be extremely cautious with the overliberal use of this agent. It is unlikely that newer antibiotics will function as effective prophylaxis agents for bacterial infection in prosthetic graft infections.

Pseudoaneurysm formation

AV access that functions for prolonged periods will frequently fail due to aneurysm and pseudoaneurysm formation. The reported incidence of aneurysm formation has been reported as 0.16 per 100 graft-months (Sabanayagam, 1995). The average hemodialysis patient will have two dialysis needles inserted per treatment, with three treatments per week. For each year on dialysis, the graft or fistula will undergo 312 needle cannulations. By 5 years this number will have reached 1570 needle insertions, which is more than most PTFE grafts can stand before they 'wear out'.

Strategies to prolong the life of PTFE and primary AV fistulas

As we have previously pointed out, stenosis at the graft–vein anastomosis accounts for in excess of 80% of PTFE graft failures. It therefore makes sense to develop strategies to predict prospectively the occurrence of graft thrombosis, so that prophylactic interventions can be undertaken using either surgical or endoluminal techniques such as angioplasty. There are currently four techniques that have proved useful for detecting high-grade venous stenosis: venous dialysis pressure measurement (Schwab *et al.*, 1989; Beathard, 1992), urea recirculation (Sherman and Levy, 1991; Levy *et al.*, 1992; Sherman, 1993), colour Doppler evaluation (Middleton *et al.*, 1989; Tordoir *et al.*, 1990; Nonnast *et al.*, 1992), and, recently, access flow measurement (Depner and Krivitski, 1995, 1996). Clinical features such as arm edema, pain over the access, and prolonged bleeding after hemodialysis are relatively non-specific, but may also also herald impending graft thrombosis.

Early correction of venous stenosis with angioplasty or fistula revision reduces thromboses rates and prolongs access viability (Schwab *et al.*, 1989; Windus *et al.*, 1990; Levy *et al.*, 1992; Kanterman *et al.*, 1995; Ziegler *et al.*, 1995). In a prospective study at our institution, the rate of fistula thrombosis among patients who underwent pro-spective monitoring for venous stenosis, and treatment of venous stenosis when detected, was reduced from 1.4 episodes of fistula thrombosis among those patients who refused such intervention to 0.15 episodes per year (Schwab *et al.*, 1989).

It is important to measure dynamic venous dialysis pressure (VDP) according to established protocols, as many factors such as the rate of extracorporeal blood flow and the compliance characteristics of the tubing and needle size can affect this value. We therefore adopted a protocol in which VDP is measured in every patient at the initiation of dialysis for 2 min using 15-or 16-gauge needles prior to increasing to maximum blood flow. Such a protocol costs nothing and may be performed at every dialysis treatment. Trends in venous dialysis pressure are more predictive than absolute pressure values. Static VDPs measured at zero blood flow are even more predictive, but require specialized machinery and are cumbersome to perform (Besarab *et al.*, 1995). Venous pressure measurements are indirect measures of access flow. When direct measures of access flow become reliable and clinically useful they should be even more predictive.

Urea recirculation

Hemodialysis access recirculation occurs when dialyzed blood returning through the venous needle re-enters the extracorporeal circuit through the arterial needle. Recir-culation is usually caused by a venous stenosis proximal to the venous needle which produces retrograde blood flow into the arterial needle. Recirculation can be quanti-fied using the formula (systemic BUN − dialyzer arterial BUN)/(systemic BUN − dialyzer venous BUN). Prospective screening for an abnormally elevated urea recir-culation will also allow the detection of venous stenosis. As with dialysis pressure, many factors influence recirculation. Urea recirculation is dependent on factors such as needle position, extracorporeal blood flow, cardiac output, intravascular volume, and venous and arterial stenosis. When performed in a standardized fashion, urea recirculation prospectively detects venous stenosis.

In recent years the measurement of access recirculation has been revolutionized by the development of sophisticated devices for measuring access recirculation without the need to draw blood. Such devices will undoubtedly prove more reprodu-cible, and predictive of venous stenosis than the currently employed BUN method of detecting dialysis recirculation (Canaud *et al.*, 1994; Lindsay *et al.*, 1996). However, it is likely that any recirculation technique will detect impending access failure later rather than earlier because of the critical decrease in flow that must occur to develop recirculation.

Color–Doppler evaluation

Doppler ultrasound may also be useful for detecting stenosis in vascular access grafts (Middleton *et al.*, 1989; Tordoir *et al.*, 1990; Nonnast *et al.*, 1992). The major drawbacks of this technique are the degree of variability obtained between operators and the expense of the procedure. Thus far no study has prospectively assessed its utility in preventing fistula thrombosis. A potential application that avoids many of the pitfalls, involves the sequential measurement of fistula blood flow velocity. When fistula blood flow velocity decreases significantly below a previously established baseline then a venous stenosis may be present. Shackleton and colleagues (1987) demonstrated that a Doppler flow of less than 450 ml/min had a sensitivity of 83% and a specificity of 75% for the development of PTFE–graft thrombosis within 2–6 weeks. The effects of prophylactic correction of these lesions on thrombosis rates has not been tested.

Access flow

Several new techniques have been developed to measure access flow. These include ultrasound and hemoglobin dilution techniques using a modified 'Fick' principle. Preliminary observations show these techniques for access flow to be more reproducible than Doppler flow. Depner and Krivikski (1995, 1996) have reported that access flows of <600 ml/min were associated with access thrombosis, while access flows greater than 600 ml/min were unlikely to lead to thrombosis.

A fistulogram is the 'gold standard' for the assessment of vascular access patency as it provides detailed visualization of the fistula lumen, venous anastomosis, and proximal venous system (Table 12.5). A fistulogram is of limited utility as a screening test because of its expense and because the overall prevalence of venous stenosis is relatively low. Screening techniques such as VDP and access recirculation are used to select cases for fistulography.

Table 12.5   Indications for fistulogram

Graft thrombosis
Prolonged bleeding
Fistula arm edema
Pain in arm with dialysis
Elevated venous pressures
Elevated fistula recirculation
Unexplained decrease in delivered dialysis dose
Decreased access flow

Treatment of venous stenosis

Treatment of venous stenosis with at least short-term maintenance of the vascular access is important clinically because it preserves other potential sites for future use. Percutaneous transluminal angioplasty, which is an outpatient procedure, corrects over 80% of stenoses in both native and synthetic fistulas, and in both venous and arterial outflow tracts (Schwab *et al.*, 1987; Davidson *et al.*, 1991). Prospective angioplasty of all venous stenoses that narrow the lumen by more than 50% improves fistula function and prolongs access survival (Schwab *et al.*, 1989). Angioplasty can be performed on both anastomotic and more proximal lesions, including central stenosis.

The use of angioplasty requires continued monitoring because of the high stenosis recurrence rates (55–70% at 12 months). Recurrent lesions can be corrected by repeat angioplasty. The complication rate of each angioplasty procedure has averaged less than 5%. Lesions unsuitable for percutaneous transluminal angioplasty can be surgically revised. Surgical fistula revision of stenotic venous and arterial lesions remains the gold standard. It has the lowest recurrence rate, but has generally been replaced (in the first instance) by angioplasty because of the disadvantages of requiring hospitalization and of extending the fistula site further up the involved extremity.

Insertion of an endovascular stent has been advocated as a method of preventing recurrent stenosis after angioplasty (Gunther *et al.*, 1989; Beathard, 1993). However, recent controlled trials have been unable to demonstrate a benefit in most patients (Beathard, 1993). In contrast, use of a Gianturco stent at the vein–fistula anastomosis was associated with a faster recurrence rate than with angioplasty alone (Beathard, 1993). Similar findings have been noted with central vein stenoses, with improved patency seen only in elastic stenoses (which comprised 23% of lesions) (Kovalik *et al.*, 1994). Thus, stents usually accelerate endothelial hyperplasia when placed into an abnormal endothelial bed.

Pharmacological and other strategies to prolong access survival

A number of early trials demonstrated that antiplatelet agents can prevent graft thrombosis in external shunts (Kaegi *et al.*, 1974, 1975; Harter *et al.*, 1979; Fiskerstrand *et al.*, 1985; Grontoft *et al.*, 1985). More recently, Hakim and colleagues studied the effect of aspirin and dipyrimadole in prolonging the time to the first thrombosis in PTFE grafts. These authors demonstrated a highly significant reduction in the number of graft thromboses in patients treated with aspirin and dipyrimadole compared to those treated with placebo (Sreedhara *et al.*, 1994). *In-vitro* data also suggest that the angiotensin-converting enzyme inhibitors may have a significant effect in reducing intimal hyperplasia (Powell *et al.*, 1989). To date there are no clinical trials addressing this issue.

Recently, endovascular irradiation has been studied as a technique to reduce intimal hyperplasia which develops at the site of coronary angioplasty. There is now extensive animal and some preliminary human data suggesting that intravascular radiation applied to the site of angioplasty effectively reduces the degree of coronary restenosis after coronary angioplasty. The mechanism of coronary artery restenosis after coronary angioplasty and intimal hyperplasia at the graft–vein anastomosis appears to be similar and there remains the possibility, as yet untested, that the application of low doses of radiation to graft–vein anastomosis will reduce the development of intimal hyperplasia and subsequent graft thrombosis. There is also recent interest in the development of novel pharmacological agents and even the possibility of gene transfer techniques to retard the progression of intimal hyperplasia (Sukhatme, 1996).

Treatment of thrombosed vascular access

Once thromboses have developed, the therapeutic options include surgical thrombectomy, thrombolytic agents, and mechanical dissolution. If these modalities are successful, a fistulogram can then be performed and detected stenoses treated with angioplasty or surgical revision (Hurt *et al.*, 1983; Munda *et al.*, 1983; Palder *et al.*, 1985*b*; Fan and Schwab, 1992; Windus, 1993).

Surgical thrombectomy, using a Fogarty embolectomy catheter, requires a small incision to be made in the hemodialysis fistula. Any clot is then removed by expansion of the catheter. This outpatient procedure is quick and has a very low complication rate.

Attempts to treat fistula thrombosis with thrombolytic agents, such as urokinase and streptokinase, originally yielded disappointing results (Young *et al.*, 1985). Access patency could be re-established in fewer than 60% of patients, nearly all of whom required hospitalization. The initial trials were also marked by significant bleeding complications. However, recent dosing adjustments and technical advances have improved the success rate and reduced the incidence of bleeding in patients in whom there is no contraindication to thrombolytic therapy (such as a bleeding disorder, a recent bleeding episode, or severe hypertension) (Valji *et al.*, 1991; Ahmed *et al.*, 1993). As an example, use of the pulse spray technique, which combines thrombolytic therapy with mechanical clot disruption, rapidly established access patency in over 90% of cases with minimal complications (Valji *et al.*, 1991). At 1 year, 50% of these fistulas remained patent. Commonly present venous stenoses should be corrected.

More recently Beathard and others have reported on the mechanical disruption of a clot in the graft without the use of any lytic agent (Beathard, 1994; Trerotola *et al.*, 1994). These investigators found a similar rate of success in opening the thrombosed grafts between mechanical thrombolysis and surgical thrombectomy. However, the grafts which had undergone mechanical thrombectomy achieved considerably higher long-term patency (Beathard, 1994). In our view, however, the safety of allowing the thrombus from the interior of the graft to float to the lungs has not yet been settled, and we do not, at present, practise these techniques. Similar results have been reported with the use of a high-speed rotating device, which pulverizes the clot into tiny particles, compared with surgical thrombectomy (Taber *et al.*, 1994).

Thrombolytic therapy is also useful in central venous thrombosis, where it is the only available choice. Advancing an infusion catheter into the clot with progressive dissolution is the preferred technique in this setting (Newman *et al.*, 1991).

Non-traditional vascular access

In general, the principle when planning vascular access should be 'as distal as possible for as long as possible'. Once both upper arms have been exhausted, for both upper and lower arm PTFE grafts, there are a variety of more difficult options. These options include: axillary–axillary or axillary–jugular grafts, femoral grafts, or less commonly axillary–femoral grafts. If all these procedures are exhausted the option of conversion to peritoneal dialysis should be seriously considered.

Our preference for the management of patients who have truly run out of all sites on their upper limbs for vascular access is to create a graft from the axillary artery to the axillary vein on the opposite side. In 1978, Garcia-Rinaldi and Von Koch described the technique of axillary artery to axillary vein graft using a bovine hetero-graft. PTFE is presently the preferred conduit. This procedure has the following advantages: (a) technical ease of construction (for surgeon and patient); (b) the graft lies in a gentle curve and not in a loop; (c) the size of the vessels permits a larger graft (8 mm) than can be used in the forearm, (d) the graft is in a position that makes cannulation easy for the dialysis technician. Problems associated with this approach are the difficulty in securing needles on the chest wall, problems with hemostasis after removal of the dialysis needles, and the fact that the graft may frequently produce an unwanted cosmetic result. Results reported by Garcia-Rinaldi and Von Koch (1978) showed that 10 out of 10 grafts were patent up to 18 months with excellent flow for hemodialysis. The axillary–axillary AV graft may also be positioned on one side of the chest, as described by Haimov (1982).

The groin is clearly not a preferred site for angio-access grafts due to increased infection as well as patient discomfort and inconvenience. In extreme cases of upper extremity vascular or infectious complications, a loop thigh PTFE or saphenous vein AV graft may be constructed. The use of the saphenous vein from the upper leg, as a dialysis conduit in the thigh, was popularized in the early 1970s either as a loop saphenofemoral shunt (Firlit and Canning, 1972) or as a straight popliteal–saphenous graft (Blakeley, 1974). Both techniques involve transposing the arterialized saphenous vein to a more superficial location to facilitate the use of the graft by the dialysis staff. While sporadic good results with autologus saphenous vein grafts for hemodialysis have been noted, the modern consensus is that due to stricture, pseudoaneurysm formation, infection, and thrombosis, as well as the preferential preservation of the saphenous vein for peripheral and coronary revascularization, this autologous conduit is not recommended for hemodialysis access (Anderson *et al.*, 1995). When other options will not suffice, it is acceptable to use lower extremity AV grafts

We prefer the use of the axillary graft to any form of femoral graft, since we have noted fewer infectious complications with this approach.

Long-term complications of vascular access

Overt, vascular access related, cardiac decompensation occurs rarely, even in patients with underlying cardiac dysfunction. However, cardiac hypertrophy is a very frequent complication of long-term dialysis even with the optimal correction of anemia using recombinant erythropoietin (Low *et al.*, 1989; Goldberg *et al.*, 1992). It is probable that part of the cardiac hypertrophy associated with ESRD is related to the increased cardiac output which is related to the vascular access AV fistulas. In patients on dialysis for long periods a primary AV fistula may become enormously dilated and aneurysmal, with large fractions of the cardiac output passing through the fistula (Brescia *et al.*, 1966; Anderson *et al.*, 1976; Mennes *et al.*, 1978). Patients with cardiomyopathy can develop high-output heart failure with lesser blood flows through the fistula. Limiting fistula flow by banding, or tying off some of the draining veins, may be attempted, but they frequently result in access thrombosis. Some of these patients may tolerate the creation of a new smaller fistula on the contralateral arm. However, patients unable to tolerate a hemodialysis fistula should be converted to peritoneal dialysis or hemodialyzed through a permanent indwelling cuffed catheter.

Experience at Duke University in maintaining vascular access in long-term survivors of hemodialysis

Fig. 12.1 shows the length of time patients have survived on dialysis at the Duke University Medical Center and its affiliated dialysis units. Table 12.6 summarizes the vascular access procedures performed on those patients who have been maintained on hemodialysis for more than 10 years. In these units we practice a policy of aggressive, prospective monitoring of grafts for impending graft failure, by measuring venous dialysis pressure at the beginning of each dialysis treatment, measuring

Table 12.6 Vascular access history of 17 patients who have currently been on hemodialysis for longer than 10 years

Patient	Duration of HD (years)	Previous access	Current access
1	10	Forearm PTFE	Upper arm PTFE graft
2	11	Forearm PTFE	Upper arm PTFE graft
3	11	None	Primary AV fistula
4	11	Multiple failed upper limb PTFE grafts	Axillary–axillary PTFE graft
5	15	None	Primary AV fistula
6	12	Two upper arm PTFE grafts	Lower arm PTFE graft
7	13	None	Primary fistula
8	16	Lower arm PTFE graft	Upper arm PTFE graft
9	12	Lower arm PTFE	Upper arm PTFE graft
10	20	Bilateral failed primary fistulas and PTFE grafts	Ipsilateral axillary–jugular graft
11	14	Primary AV fistula	Primary AV fistula
12	13	Lower arm PTFE	Upper arm PTFE graft
13	12	Bilateral upper and lower arm PTFE grafts	Axillary–axillary PTFE graft
14	14	Bilateral upper and lower arm PTFE grafts	
		Bilateral subclavian vein thrombosis	Femoral permcath
15	10	None	Primary AV fistula
16	11	Upper arm PTFE	Lower arm PTFE graft
17	19	Lower arm PTFE graft	Upper arm PTFE graft

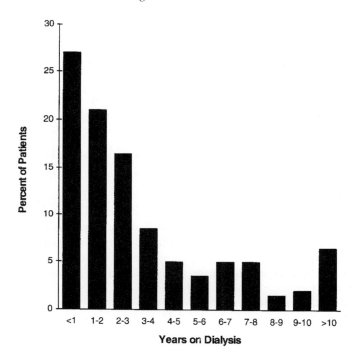

Fig. 12.1 Frequency distribution of the length of time patients at Duke University Medical Center have been on dialysis.

access recirculation four times a year, and sending patients for early angioplasty or graft revision. It can be seen that 5 of the 17 patients have had the good fortune to have a successful primary AV fistula for longer than 10 years, thereby allowing them trouble-free repetitive dialysis. In addition, four patients have exhausted traditional vascular access sites, two are now being effectively dialyzed via an axillary–axillary graft, and one is currently dialyzed via a femoral dialysis catheter.

Conclusions

The maintenance of vascular access in patients who require very prolonged periods of dialysis is a major challenge to the renal caregiver and requires a coordinated plan of action between the nephrologist, vascular surgeon, dialysis nurse, and interventional radiologist in order to achieve the maximum life out of each individual vascular access device. The formation of a primary AV fistula is the cornerstone of access management. The placement of brachial–cephalic fistulas in patients in whom radiocephalic fistulas have failed is an essential step towards long-term access management. However, even if it is not possible to fashion a primary arteriovenous fistula and a PTFE graft is placed, through aggressive prospective monitoring and intervention for vascular access incipient failure, much can be done to maintain adequate vascular access for a decade or more.

References

Ahmed, A., Shapiro, W. B., and Porush, J. G. (1993). The use of tissue plasminogen activator to declot arteriovenous accesses in hemodialysis patients. *American Journal of Kidney Diseases*, **21**, 38.

Anderson, R. C., and DeBord, J. R. (1995). Exotic vascular access. In *Vascular access for hemodialysis*, (ed. M. L. Henry and R. M. Ferguson), pp. 118–30. W. L. Gore & Associates, Inc., Precept Press, Columbus, Ohio.

Anderson, C. B., Codd, J. R., Graff, R. A., Groce, M. A., Harter, H. R., and Newton, W. T. (1976). Cardiac failure and upper extremity arteriovenous dialysis fistulas. Case reports and a review of the literature. *Archives of Internal Medicine*, **136**, 292–7.

Baethard, G. A. (1992). Percutaneous transvenous angioplasty in the treatment of vascular access stenosis. *Kidney International*, **42**, 1390.

Baethard, G. (1993). Gianturco self-expanding stents in the treatment of stenoses in dialysis access grafts. *Kidney International*, **43**, 872.

Baethard, G. A. (1994). Comparison of mechanical thrombolysis and surgical thrombectomy for the treatment of thrombosed dialysis access grafts. *Journal of the American Society of Nephrology*, **5**, 407 (Abstract).

Barrett, N., Spencer, S., McIvor, J., and Brown, E. A. (1988). Subclavian stenosis: a major complication of subclavian dialysis catheters. *Nephrology, Dialysis, Transplantation*, **3**, 423–5.

Besarab, A., Sullivan, K. L., Ross, R. P., and Moritz, M. J. (1995). Utility of intra-access pressure monitoring in detecting and correcting venous outlet stenosis prior to thrombosis. *Kidney International*, **47**, 1364–73.

Brescia, M. J., Cimino, J. E., Appel, K., Harwich, C. J. (1966). Hemodialysis using venipuncture and a surgically created arteriovenous fistula. *New England Journal of Medicine*, **275**, 1089–92.

Bhat, D. J., Tellis, V. A., Kohlberg, W. I., *et al.* (1980). Management of sepsis involving expanded PTFE grafts for hemodialysis. *Surgery*, **87**, 445.

Blakeley, W. (1974). Current surgical management of fistulae for dialysis: methods and improvisations. *American Surgery*, **40**, 168–71.

Boelaert, J. R., DeSmedt, R. A., De Baere, Y. A., *et al.* (1989). The influence of calcium mupirocin nasal ointment on the incidence of *Staphyloccus aureus* infections in hemodialysis patients. *Nephrology, Dialysis, Transplantation*, **4**, 278–81.

Boelaert, J. R., Van Landuyt, H. W., De Baere, Y. A., *et al.* (1994). Epidemiologie et prevention des infections a *Staphylococcus aureus* en hemodialyse. *Nephrologie*, **15**, 157–61.

Brescia, M. J., Cimino, J. E., Appel, K., and Hurwich, B. J. (1966). Chronic hemodialysis using venipuncture and a surgically created arteriovenous fistula. *New England Journal of Medicine*, **275**, 1089–92.

Canadian Erythropoietin Study Group. (1990). Association between recombinant human erythropoietin and quality of life and exercise capacity of patients receiving hemodialysis. *British Medical Journal*, **300**, 573–8.

Canaud, B., Tetta, C., Bosc, J. Y., Berti, M., Mazzocchi, B., and Mion, C. (1994). Routine on-line evaluation of access recirculation without blood sampling. *Journal of the American Society of Nephrology*, **5**, 411.

Caruana, R. J., Raja, R. M., Zeit, R. M., Goldstein, S. J., and Kramer, M. S. (1987). Thrombotic complications of indwelling central catheters used for prolonged use. *American Journal of Kidney Diseases*, **9**, 497–501.

Cimino, J. E., and Brescia, M. J. (1994). The early development of the arteriovenous fistula needle technique for hemodialysis. *American Society for Artificial Internal Organs Journal*, **40**, 923–7.

Crain, M. R., Mewissen, M. W., and Fueredi, G. A. (1994). Fibrin sleeve stripping for maintenance of failing hemodialysis catheters. *Journal of the American Society of Nephrology*, 5, 412.

Davidson, C. J., Newman, G. E., Sheikh, K., *et al.* (1991). Mechanisms of angioplasty in hemodialysis fistula stenosis evaluated by intravascular ultrasound. *Kidney International*, 40, 91.

Depner, T. A., and Krivitski, N. M. (1995). Access flow measured from recirculation of urea during hemodialysis with reversed blood lines. *Journal of the American Society of Nephrology*, 6, 486.

Depner, T. A., and Krivitski, N. M. (1996). Clinical measurement of blood flow in hemodialysis access fistulae and grafts by ultrasound dilution. *American Society for Artificial Internal Organs Journal*, 41, M745–749.

Fan, P. Y., and Schwab, S. J. (1992). Vascular access: concepts for the 1990s. *Journal of the American Society of Nephrology*, 3, 1–11.

Feldman, H. L., Held, P. J., and Hutchinson, J. T. (1993). Hemodialysis vascular access morbidity in the United States. *Kidney International*, 43, 1091–6.

Firlit, C., and Canning, J. (1972). Saphenofemoral shunt its application in long term hemodialysis. *Archives of Surgery*, 104, 854–5.

Fiskerstrand, C. E., Thompson, I. W., Burnet, M. E., Williams, P., and Anderton, J. L. (1985). Double-blind randomized trial of the effect of ticlopidine in arteriovenous fistulas for hemodialysis. *Artificial Organs*, 9, 61–63.

Galbraith, S., Fan, P., Collins, D., *et al.* (1992). Hemodialysis fistula thrombosis: a prospective evaluation of anatomic versus nonanatomic causes. *Journal of the American Society of Nephrology*, 3, 365 (Abstract).

Garcia-Martin, F., De Arriba, G., and Carrascosa, T. (1991). Anticardiolipin antibodies and lupus anticoagulant in end-stage renal disease. *Nephrology, Dialysis, Transplantation*, 6, 543–7.

Garcia-Rinaldi, R., and Von Koch, L. (1978). The axillary artery to axillary vein bovine graft for circulatory access. *American Journal of Surgery*, 135, 265–8.

Gibson, S. P., and Mosquera, D. (1991). Five years experience with the quinton permcath for vascular access. *Nephrology, Dialysis, Transplantation*, 6, 269–74.

Goldberg, N., Lundin, A. P., Delano, B., Friedman, E. A., and Stein, R. A. (1992). Changes in left ventricular size, wall thickness, and function in anemic patients treated with recombinant human erythropoietin. *American Heart Journal*, 124, 424–7.

Grontoft, K. C., Mulec, H., Gutierrez, A., and Olander, R. (1985). Thromboprophylactic effect of ticlopidine in arteriovenous fistulas for haemodialysis. *Scandinavian Journal of Urology and Nephrology*, 19, 55–7.

Gunther, R. W., Vorwerk, D., Bohndorf, K., *et al.* (1989). Venous stenosis in dialysis shunts: treatment with self-expanding metallic stents. *Radiology*, 170, 401.

Gutman, R. A. (1983). Characteristics of long-term (14 years) survivors of maintenance dialysis. *Nephron*, 35, 111–15.

Haimov, M. (1982). Vascular access for hemodialysis—New modifications for the difficult patient. *Surgery*, 92, 109–10.

Harter, H. R., Burch, J. W., Majerus, P. W., *et al.* (1979). Prevention of thrombosis in patients on hemodialysis by low-dose aspirin. *New England Journal of Medicine*, 301, 577–9.

Hurt, A. V., Batello-Cruz, M., Skipper, B. J., *et al.* (1983). Bovine carotid artery heterografts versus polytetrafluorethylene grafts. *American Journal of Surgery*, 146, 844.

Jenkins, A. M., Buist, T. A. S., and Glover, S. D. (1980). Medium-term follow-up of forty autogenous vein and forty polytetrafluoroethylene (Gore-tex) grafts for vascular access. *Surgery*, 88, 667–72.

Kaegi, A., Pineo, G. F., Shimizu, A., Trivedi, H., Hirsh, J., and Gent, M. (1974). Arteriovenous-shunt thrombosis. Prevention by sulfinpyrazone. *New England Journal of Medicine*, 290, 304–6.

Kaegi, A., Pineo, G. F., Shimizu, A., Trivedi, H., Hirsh, J., and Gent, M. (1975). The role of sulfinpyrazone in the prevention of arterio-venous shunt thrombosis. *Circulation*, **52**, 497–9.

Kanterman, R. Y., Vesely, T. M., Pilgram, T. K., Guy, B. W., Windus, D. W., and Picus, D. (1995). Dialysis access grafts: anatomic location of venous stenosis and results of angioplasty. *Radiology*, **195**, 135–9.

Kherlakian, G. M., Roedersheimer, L. R., Arbaugh, J. J., Newmark, K. J., and King, L. R. (1986). Comparison of autogenous fistula versus expanded polytetrafluoroethylene graft fistula for angioaccess in hemodialysis. *American Journal of Surgery*, **152**, 238–43.

Kinnaert, D. N., Vereerstraeten, P., Toussaint, C., and Van Geertruyden, J. (1977). Nine years' experience with internal arterio-venous fistulas for hemodialysis: a study of some factors influencing the results. *British Journal of Surgery*, **64**, 242–6.

Kinnaert, P., Vereerstraeten, P., Toussaint, C., and Van Geertruyden, J. (1977). Nine years experience with internal arteriovenous fistulas for hemodialysis: a study of some factors influencing the results. *British Journal of Surgery*, **64**, 242–6.

Kovalik, E., Newman, G., Suchocki, P., *et al.* (1994). Correction of central venous stenosis: use of angioplasty and vascular wall stents. *Kidney International*, **45**, 1177.

Lerner, P. I., and Weinstein, L. (1966). Infective endocarditis in the antibiotic era. *New England Journal of Medicine*, **274**, 199–206.

Levy, S. S., Sherman, R. A., and Nosher, J. L. (1992) Value of clinical screening for detection of asymptomatic hemodialysis vascular access stenoses. *Angiology*, **43**, 421–4.

Lindsay, R. M., Burbank, J., Brugger, J., Bradfield, E., Malek, P., and Blake, P. G. (1996). A device and a method for rapid and accurate measurement of access recirculation during hemodialysis. *Kidney International*, **49**, 1152–60.

Low, I., Grutzmacher, P., Bergmann, M., and Schoeppe, W. (1989). Echocardiographic findings in patients on maintenance hemodialysis substituted with recombinant human erythropoietin. *Clinical Nephrology*, **31**, 26–30.

Macdougal, I. C., Davies, M. E., Hallet, I., *et al.* (1991). Coagulation studies and fistula blood flow during erythropoietin therapy in hemodialysis patients. *Nephrology, Dialysis, Transplantation*, **6**, 862–7.

Mennes, P. A., Gilula, L. A., Anderson, C. B., Etheredge, E. E., Weerts, C., and Harter, H. R. (1978). Complications associated with arteriovenous fistulas in patients undergoing chronic hemodialysis. *Archives of Internal Medicine*, **138**, 1117–21.

Middleton, W., Picus, D., Marx, M., and Melson, G. (1989). Color doppler sonography of hemodialysis vascular access: comparison with angiography. *American Journal of Radiology*, **152**, 633.

Moss, A. H., Vasilakis, C., Holley, J. L., *et al.* (1990). Use of silicone, dual lumen catheter with a dacron cuff as a long-term vascular access for hemodialysis patients. *American Journal of Kidney Diseases*, **16**, 211–15.

Munda, R., First, M. R., Alexander, J. W., *et al.* (1983). PTFE graft survival in hemodialysis. *Journal of the American Medical Association*, **249**, 219.

Newman, G. E., Saeed, M., Himmelstein, S., *et al.* (1991). Total central vein obstruction: resolution with angioplasty and fibrinolysis. *Kidney International*, **39**, 761.

Nonnast, B., Martin, R., Lindert, O., *et al.* (1992). Color doppler ultrasound assessment of hemodialysis fistulas. *Lancet*, **339**, 143.

Palder, S. B., Kirkman, R. L., Whittemore, A. D., *et al.* (1985a) Vascular access for hemodialysis. Patency rates and results of revision. *Annals of Surgery*, **202**, 235–9.

Palder, S. B., Kirkman, R. L., Whittemore, A. D., *et al.* (1985b) Vascular access for hemodialysis. *Annals of Surgery*, **202**, 235.

Powell, J., Clozel, J., Muller, R., *et al.* (1989). Inhibitors of angiotensin converting enzyme prevent mild intimal proliferation after vascular injury. *Science*, **245**, 186.

Rapaport, A., Noon, G. P., and McCollum, C. H. (1981). Polytetrafluorethylene (PTFE) grafts for hemodialysis in chronic renal failure: assesment of durability and function at three years. *Australian and New Zealand Journal of Surgery*, **51**, 562–7.

Sabanayagam, P. (1995). 15-year experience with tapered (4–7 mm) and straight (6 mm) PTFE angio-access in the ESRD patient. In *Vascular access for hemodialysis*, (ed. M. L. Henry and R. M. Ferguson), pp. 159–68. W. L. Gore & Associates, Inc., Precept Press, Columbus, Ohio.

Sabanayagam, P., Schwartz, A. B., Soricelli, R. R., Chintz, J. L., and Lyons, P. (1980). Experience with one hundred reinforced expanded PTFE grafts for angioaccess in hemodialysis. *Transactions of the American Society for Artificial Internal Organs*, **26**, 582–3.

Schwab, S. J., Saeed, M., Sussman, S. K., McCann, R. L., and Stickel, D. L. (1987). Transluminal angioplasty of venous stenoses in polytetrafluoroethylene vascular access grafts. *Kidney International*, **32**, 395–8.

Schwab, S. J., Buller, G. L., McCann, R. L., Bollinger, R. R., and Stickel, D. L. (1988 *a*). Prospective evaluation of a dacron cuffed hemodialysis catheter for prolonged use. *American Journal of Kidney Diseases*, **11**, 166–9.

Schwab, S. J., Quarles, L. D., Middleton, J. P., Cohan, R. H., Saeed, M., and Dennis, V. W. (1988*b*) Hemodialysis-associated subclavian vein stenosis. *Kidney International*, **33**, 1156–9.

Schwab, S. J., Raymond, J. R., Saeed, M., Newman, G. E., Dennis, P. A., and Bollinger, R. R. (1989). Prevention of hemodialysis fistula thrombosis. Early detection of venous stenoses. *Kidney International*, **36**, 707–11.

Shackelton, C. R., Taylor, D. C., Buckley, A. R., Rowley, V. A., Cooperberg, P. L., and Fry, P. D. (1987). Predicting failure in polytetrafluoroethylene vascular access grafts for hemodialysis: a pilot study. *Canadian Journal of Surgery*, **30**, 442–4.

Sherman, R. A. (1993). The measurement of dialysis access recirculation. *American Journal of Kidney Diseases*, **22**, 616–21.

Sherman, R. A., and Levy, S. S. (1991). Rate-related recirculation: the effect of altering blood flow on dialyzer recirculation. *American Journal of Kidney Diseases*, **17**, 170–3.

Shusterman, N. H., Kloss, K., and Mullen, J. L. (1989). Successful use of double-lumen, silicone rubber catheters for permanent hemodialysis access. *Kidney International*, **35**, 886–90.

Sreedhara, R., Himmelfarb, J., Lazarus, M., and Hakim, R. (1994). Anti-platelet therapy in graft thrombosis; Results of a prospective, randomized, double-blind study. *Kidney International*, **45**, 1477.

Suchocki, P., Conlon, P. J., Schwab, S. J., and Knelson, M. H. (1996). Management of hemodialysis catheter dysfunction. *American Journal of Kidney Diseases*, **627**, 379–86.

Sukhatme, V. P. (1996). Vascular access stenosis: prospects for prevention and therapy. *Kidney International*, **49**, 1161–74.

Swedberg, S. H., Brown, B. G., Rigley, R., *et al.* (1989). Intimal fibromuscular hyperplasia at the venous anastomosis of PTFE grafts in hemodialysis patients. Clinical, immunocytochemical, light and electron microscopic assesement. *Circulation*, **80**, 1726.

Taber, T. E., Gaylord, G. M., Ehrman, K. O., Porter, D. J., and Brown, P. B. (1994). Thrombus removal in PTFE dialysis access grafts with the TRAC catheter system. *Journal of the American Society of Nephrology*, **5**, 427.(Abstract).

Tang, I. Y., Vrahnos, D., Valaitis, D., and Lau, A. H. (1992). Vascular access thrombosis during recombinant human erythropoietin therapy. *American Society of Artificial Internal Organs Journal* M528–M531.

Tordoir, J. H., Hoeneveld, H., Eikelboon, B. C., and Kitslaar, P. J. (1990). The correlation between clinical and duplex ultrasound parameters and the development of complications in arterio-venous fistulae for hemodialysis. *European Journal of Vascular Surgery*, **4**, 179.

Trerotola, S. O., Lund, G. B., Scheel, P. J., Savader, S. J., Venbrux, A. C., and Osterman, F. A. (1995). Thrombosed dialysis access grafts: percutaneous mechanical declotting without uroki-nase *Radiology*, **191**, 721–6.

Valji, K., Bookstein, J., Roberts, A., *et al.* (1991). Pharmacomechanical thrombolysis and angio-plasty in the management of clotted hemodialysis grafts: early and late results. *Radiology*, **178**, 243.

Windus, D. (1993). Permanent vascular access: a nephrologist's view. *American Journal of Kidney Diseases*, **21**, 457.

Windus, D. W. (1994). The effect of comorbid conditions on hemodialysis access patency. *Advances in Renal Replacement Therapy*, **1**, 148–54.

Windus, D. W., Audrain, J., Vanderson., R., *et al.* (1990). Optimization of high-efficiency hemo-dialysis by detection and correction of fistula dysfunction. *Kidney International*, **21**, 337.

Windus, D. W., Jendrisak, M. D., and Delmez, J. A. (1992). Prosthetic fistula survival and compli-cations in hemodialysis patients: effects of diabetes and age. *American Journal of Kidney Dis-eases*, **19**, 448–52.

Winsett, O. E., and Wolma, F. J. (1979). Complications of vascular access for hemodialysis. *South-ern Medical Journal*, **66**, 23–8.

Young, A. T., Hunter, D. W., Zuniga, W. P., *et al.* (1985). Thrombosed synthetic hemodialysis access fistulas: failure of thrombolytic therapy. *Radiology*, **154**, 639.

Ziegler, T. W., Safa, A., Amarillis, K., *et al.* (1995). Prolonging the life of difficult hemodialysis access using thrombolysis, angiography, and angioplasty. *Advances in Renal Replacement Ther-apy*, **2**, 52–9.

13

Long-term peritoneal dialysis: does a spell of peritoneal dialysis prolong survival on hemodialysis?

Norbert Lameire and Wim Van Biesen

Introduction

Since the inception of peritoneal dialysis (PD) as a form of long-term renal replacement therapy, the number of PD patients has continued to grow and PD therapy is steadily increasing throughout Europe and the USA at an annual rate of 15%. (Worldwide Registry Update, 1994; Blagg and Mailloux, 1996). This increase in the total dialysis population has been partly related to the inclusion of much higher risk populations (the elderly, those with diabetes mellitus, and those with cardiovascular and multisystem diseases).

A recent review of frequently quoted studies published between 1988 and 1992, concludes that mortality and morbidity 'do not seem to differ greatly in dialysis patients' (Maiorca and Cancarini, 1994). Furthermore, the latest Canadian Organ Replacement Register report (1995) shows significantly lower risks of death with continuous ambulatory peritoneal dialysis (CAPD) compared to hemodialysis (HD) for diabetics and non-diabetics, in a variety of age groups.

The selection of patients on any mode of dialysis treatment should, by and large, be based on medical, social, and patient preference criteria. Provided the survival and morbity results are the same for both dialysis modes, then the percentage of patients on the various modalities would be similar around the world. However, the facts are different: the utilization of PD in various countries ranges from 5% to 90%. Such a vast discrepancy in usage cannot be entirely related to medical, social, and patient-related factors. Financial and reimbursement policies and poor patient, as well as physician, education turn out to be the most important of five non-medical factors that have an impact on end-stage renal disease (ESRD) modality selection (Nissenson *et al.*, 1993). For example, there is a higher incidence of PD in those countries where there is state funded National Health Service. In countries where financial aspects are less prominent, other factors such as physician bias and social mores take on greater importance. Poor education of patients and physicians about available dialysis options also has an important impact on modality selection. Well-informed patients with ESRD prefer PD to HD, providing they are referred to the dialysis unit in time (Ahlmen *et al.*, 1993; Prichard, 1996). On average, only 75% of ESRD patients were referred early enough to six Western European dialysis centers to be informed about the therapeutic dialytic possibilities. Whereas PD was selected in the majority of early referred patients, the majority of the late referrals were treated in an emergency by HD and they remained on this modality without a further option for choice (Lameire 1997). It should further be stressed that patient information and education can only be adequate when both nurses and doctors are similarly convinced that all dialysis therapies should be considered at the same level, as patient decision is strongly influenced by the opinion of the treating staff. The best outcome of any dialysis treatment is achieved in patients referred to a specialist center before dialysis is required (Innes *et al.*, 1992).

Besides these financial and educational issues there is an important bias, based on a number of concerns still present among nephrologists. These concerns include the long-term survival of PD patients compared with HD patients, the high transfer of patients from PD to HD, and the morbidity in PD patients compared with HD patients. There is also a great need for future technical developments in PD, including more physiological solutions, small cyclers that produce solutions from concentrates, trouble-free peritoneal access, and completely fail-safe connections. Finally, there is a great need for future developments in the clinical applications of PD, such as a better definition of adequacy, precise nutritional targets, optimization of the dose of dialysis at a cost within reimbursement levels, and the standardization of exit-site care.

The growing number of PD patients should thus not create a false impression that long-term PD is a well-established and accepted dialysis therapy without major problems.

Problems with peritoneal dialysis

In this chapter, a number of issues related to the long-term patient and technique survival of PD will be discussed. Where possible, solutions to eventual problems will be suggested and arguments for a better integration of PD in the overall therapeutic approach to the patient with ESRD will be put forward.

Long-term patient and technique survival

The observations showing a similar overall prognosis between PD and HD patients (Maiorca and Cancarini, 1994) have been challenged in a analysis from the United States Renal Data System of dialysis patients over three successive years (Bloembergen *et al.*, 1995). In this report, CAPD patients had a 19% higher mortality rate than those receiving any form of HD. European data confirmed that PD patients, when compared with HD patients, have a higher risk of death even after correction for sex, age, underlying disease, comorbidity, and malignancy (Locatelli *et al.*, 1995). A recent analysis of the Canadian registry (Ferton *et al.*, 1997) and a re-analysis of the USRDS data (Vonesh *et al.*, 1998), using incident instead of prevalent patients, show no difference in survival between PD and HD patients. Indeed in the first two to three years after starting dialysis, survival on PD is better than on HD.

Cardiovascular diseases are, as in hemodialysis patients, by far the most common cause of death in PD patients (Lameire *et al.*, 1994, 1996a in press), and the burden of disease resulting from the clinical consequences of cardiomyopathy and ischemic heart disease in chronic uremia is high (Parfrey *et al.*, 1995; Amman and Ritz, 1996).

It is remarkable that the high rate of cardiovascular morbidity and mortality in ESRD patients is occurring at a time when the prevalence of coronary disease is declining, at least in the general Western European population.

Still today, many dialysis programs preferentially reserve PD for the cardio-vascularly handicapped patient, on the premise that this continuous dialysis technique offers some advantages over intermittent HD. Because heart disease, or at least several of its risk factors, often antedates dialysis or even precedes renal failure, the high mortality due to cardiovascular causes in the PD population could be explained by the acceptance of these high-risk patients who are given a dialysis opportunity despite adverse odds. In a previous analysis (Lameire, 1993), an overall correlation between patient survival and the number of cardiovascular risk factors at the onset of PD was found, but it was further observed that the prevalence of the cardiovascular risk factors changes with time in the PD population, suggesting that there is an additional and continuous impact of PD *per se* on the cardiovascular status of the patient. The influence of continuous PD on cardiovascular hemodynamics, the survival of patients with heart failure, and the known alterations of lipoprotein metabolism have been recently reviewed (Lameire *et al.*, 1994; Alpert *et al.*, 1995; Culleton and Parfrey, 1996) and will therefore not be discussed further.

The conflicting results obtained in the several comparisons of survival achievable with HD and PD, instead of shedding light on the subject rather create confusion. According to Churchill (1996*a*) all studies suffered from either a modality selection bias, a censoring bias, or a missing data bias. Many of these data were obtained at a time when for CAPD therapy, the delivery of dialysis was inadequate, the importance of residual renal function (RRF) was poorly understood, and the contribution of the severity of eventual comorbid conditions was not taken into account. In no study was RRF or adequacy of dialysis considered as an independent variable in the multivariate analysis. The importance of dialysis dose in patient survival in both HD and PD has been well established (Gotch and Sargent, 1985; Churchill *et al.*, 1996*b*).

Using data from the CANUSA study (Churchill *et al.* 1996) and their own data from the RKDP Minneapolas database, Keshaviah *et al.* (1995) have recently compared 2-year survival data for those patients on HD with those on continuous PD, the dose of dialysis being matched according to the peak urea concentration hypothesis. Survivals were adjusted for age, diabetic status, weekly clearance of urea normalized to total body water (Kt/V urea), and serum albumin. HD and PD survivals were similar at equivalent Kt/V urea doses and declined in both HD and PD at lower levels of Kt/V urea. These results not only support the peak urea hypothesis but provide evidence that small clearance doses influence survival. When well-dialyzed PD patients are compared with well-dialyzed HD patients, survival results are similar.

Comparisons of technique survival on PD and HD usually favor HD. However, many reports addressing technique failure contain patients who commenced dialysis prior to the introduction of the disconnect technology. In the past, peritonitis and catheter problems, such as exit-site and tunnel infections, have been the major areas of focus, these being the predominant reasons for converting patients from PD to HD. Peritonitis can cause permanent damage to the peritoneal membrane, and the attendant physical and psychological suffering often discourages the patient and his/

her family from continuing PD. With the advent of disconnect systems, a significant reduction in the incidence of peritonitis has been observed, with a consequent favorable impact on therapy survival (Bernardini *et al.*, 1991). Peritonitis is nowadays responsible for only 15% of the technique failures in the United States of America (Nolph, 1994), and a similar trend has been reported in the 1993 Canadian Register (Canadian Organ Replacement register, 1995). Catheter-related problems, including both mechanical problems as well as catheter-related infections, are today the most common cause of CAPD dropout (Jindal, 1995). Several successful exit-site care techniques, better training methods, new designs of catheters, and new catheter implantation techniques will, in the future, succeed in improving the technique survival of PD such that it approaches that of HD (Dasgupta, 1995; Jindal, 1995). The infectious problems may have masked the problems of inadequate dialysis and of decreasing peritoneal ultrafiltration capacity in the past, but this may no longer be the case in the future.

Today, one of the most important issues in the long-term survival of PD is the, as yet, unanswered question of whether this technique will be able to maintain adequate dialysis for a considerable length of time.

The problem of long-term adequacy

Whilst adequacy can be defined and assessed in a number of ways, the capacity to maintain fluid balance, a normal blood pressure, to remove adequate amounts of solutes, and to restore normal electrolyte and acid–base balance form the basis of adequacy evaluation. The classical dose of dialysis in CAPD is four exchanges of 2 l per day, although the mathematical model for CAPD, originally proposed by Popovich *et al.* (1976) required a sufficient RRF before allowing this dose. It took some years before it was realized that declining RRF has a major impact on the ability to deliver adequate dialysis.

A comparison of the weekly clearances that are achieved by standard HD, hemofiltration, CAPD, and the natural kidneys for a wide range of solute sizes reveals that the solute clearances with CAPD are lower than those of hemofiltration or high-flux HD, but are equal or exceed those of standard HD for all but the small molecular weight solutes, such as urea and creatinine (Keshaviah, 1992). These findings explain why concern about the adequacy of CAPD should focus on small solute clearances rather than on middle molecular size solutes.

Although it is widely recognized that urea is not a direct uremic toxin, it is a good marker for the assessment of small solute clearance because the link between Kt/V and uremic symptoms and morbidity in HD patients is well established. When CAPD patients manifest uremic symptoms, increasing the number or the volume of the exchanges causes a significant increase in small solute clearances and is an effective approach to alleviating the symptoms, as long as the patients complies with the increased number of the exchanges.

Clinical criteria alone of inadequate dialysis are subjective and appear too late. More objective criteria, largely inspired by what has been realized in HD, have now been introduced for PD. The targets for both adequate PD and adequate nutrition include the determination and follow-up of creatinine clearances, Kt/V urea index, urea appearance rate, dialysis index or dialysis efficacy number, and the calculation of parameters such as the protein catabolic rate (PCR)—or better named the protein equivalence of nitrogen appearance (PNA)—and monitoring of the serum albumin, transferrin, and prealbumin levels. The most frequently used parameters are the weekly creatinine clearance and the Kt/V urea index.

Weekly creatinine clearances have to be calculated on 24-hour collections of urine and dialysate and should, according to recent data, have a minimal value of 60–70 l/ week, normalized to 1.73 m^2 body surface (Nolph *et al.*, 1992). Each 1 ml/min due to 'glomerular filtration', adds 10 l/week of creatinine clearance. Taking into account that a patient in terminal renal failure at the start of CAPD usually has a residual endogenous creatinine clearance of 5 ml/min, corresponding roughly to 50 l/week, it is relatively easy to meet the target with a standard CAPD treatment, as long as the patient's RRF is maintained between 1 and 3 ml/min creatinine clearance.

Follow-up of the weekly creatinine clearances over 7 years of uninterrupted PD in 23 CAPD patients showed that the total creatinine clearance, i.e. the sum of urine and peritoneal clearances, decreased over time, only because of the progressive fall in RRF. At the end of follow-up, a value of 55–60 l/week was still achieved in these patients. It is of interest to note that in these patients the peritoneal creatinine clearance did not decrease with time. The D/P (dialysate/plasma) creatinine ratio after of a mean of 6 hours of dwell-time remained constant at a value ranging between 0.8 and 0.85. The progressive fall in residual renal creatinine clearance was translated into a progressive rise in the serum creatinine level (Faller and Lameire, 1994).

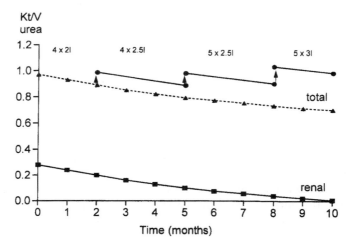

Fig. 13.1 Evolution over 5 years of total and renal Kt/V urea in 16 CAPD patients dialyzed with a constant dialysis dose of 4×2 l per day. Calculation of the dose adaptation to maintain the initial Kt/V urea.

The Kt/V urea index is the ratio between the total clearance of urea over a given treatment time, and the distribution volume of urea. Figure 13.1 illustrates the evolution of the Kt/V urea index in 16 CAPD patients, dialyzed with a constant dialysis dose over 5 years. The index was corrected to be comparable to a thrice-weekly HD treatment. The Kt/V urea index falls with time and this is due to two factors: the first is the decline in RRF with a progressive decrease in the renal contribution to the total index. This contribution decreased from 22% to virtually zero after 5 years. For each 1 ml/min of residual urea clearance, it can be calculated that 0.25 is added to the total weekly Kt/V urea for a 70 kg male. The second reason for the decrease in Kt/V urea was the evolution of the calculated urea distribution volume in these patients. The urea distribution volume in CAPD is calculated as either a fixed percentage of the dry body weight or by anthropomorphic data, obtained by Watson *et al.* (1980). In the Watson formulas, the impact of the evolution of body weight is less important, since age, sex, and height of the patients is also taken into account. Since the dry body weight in the patients on CAPD increases substantially with time due to the continuous transperitoneal absorption of glucose (Lameire *et al.*, 1992), the increase in the distribution volume is less when it is calculated by the Watson formulae than by the fixed percentage of body weight. Comparing the weekly Kt/V urea indices of a HD and CAPD patient reveals an important paradox (Keshaviah *et al.*, 1989; Ronco *et al.*, 1994). In an example of a 70-kg patient with a volume of distribution of 40 l, a weekly urea Kt/V is calculated as 1.5. This value translates into a HD weekly equivalent of roughly 0.5, a value that in a HD patient should be associated with a very high treatment failure and significant morbidity. The absence of such morbidity in the majority of the CAPD patients despite such a low Kt/V urea index poses a paradox and calls into question the validity of the Kt/V index as an assessment of CAPD adequacy.

One solution to this paradox is given by the peak urea concentration hypothesis (Keshaviah *et al.*, 1989). According to this hypothesis, the major difference is that CAPD is a continuous treatment whereas HD is intermittent. The body levels of the various uremic toxins are relatively constant in CAPD but follow a sawtooth profile with peaks and valleys in HD. At the same weekly clearance or Kt/V, a patient on HD will have the same time-averaged concentrations (TAC) as the steady-state urea and, presumably, other uremic toxins in CAPD. However, the HD patient will have toxin concentrations higher than the TAC values for approximately half of the week and lower body toxin concentrations for the other half of the week. If uremic symptoms and lesions are dependent upon peak urea concentrations (or whatever solute for which urea is a surrogate), then the ability of CAPD to deliver adequate therapy at lower Kt/V urea values is a function of the lower steady-state solute concentrations in CAPD at any comparable value of Kt/V urea in HD. We were able to show that the Kt/V urea index did correlate with some parameters of outcome in these patients (Lameire *et al.*, 1992; Faller and Lameire, 1994). There was a negative correlation between the number of hospitalization days and the overall Kt/V urea index; i.e. the higher the index, thus the more efficient the dialysis, the lower the morbidity. Perhaps more important, but, in view of the limited number of patients, more difficult to interpret is the observation that the Kt/V urea index over the first year of treatment predicted the evolution of the motor nerve conductivity during the other 4 years of follow-up in these patients (Lameire *et al.*, 1992).

The recently published CANUSA study has confirmed the correlation between several of the adequacy parameters and 2-year patient survival, and it is now recommended to aim for a weekly Kt/V urea of 2.1 (Churchill *et al.*, 1996).

The correct dialysis dose

In the absence of catabolic factors such as acidosis and infection, the main determinants of dialysis dose include the volume of drained dialysate, the D/P creatinine ratio at the end of a dwell period, body size, and the residual renal solute clearance.

It can easily be calculated that with an average peritoneal permeability for creatinine, corresponding to an average 24-hour D/P creatinine ratio of 0.80, the total 24-hour dialysate flow should be at least 9 l for an idealized body surface of 1.73 m^2. As pointed out above, this 'ideal' body surface is almost never present in the average PD population after 5 years of treatment. It is easy to understand that in an anuric patient it becomes problematic to achieve the minimum creatinine clearance target of 60 l/1.73 m^2 body surface at the standard dialysis dose of 4×2 l per day. Starting patients on CAPD with a residual creatinine clearance of 5 ml/min means that a value of 50 l/week in the first 6–12 months will be achieved by the renal function alone. However, after the complete disappearance of residual renal function, usually after 3–5 years of treatment, the creatinine clearance is totally dependent on peritoneal creatinine clearance. At that moment it becomes more problematic to achieve the minimum creatinine value of 50 l week and virtually impossible to obtain the actually accepted target value of 60–70 l creatinine clearance per week.

Peritoneal transport characteristics are also important in determining the actual creatinine clearance achieved. In anuric CAPD patients with slow diffusive creatinine transport (low D/P creatinine), a target of 60–70 l/week creatinine clearance per 1.73 m^2 will be very difficult to achieve, even if the body weight is below average.

The time has come for individualizing the dose of dialysis prescribed for CAPD according to the needs of the patient. As shown in Table 13.1, taken from Keshaviah (1996), for an anephric patient with a body weight of 70 kg, body water volume of 40 l, body surface area of 1.8 m^2, and average peritoneal transport characteristics, the weekly Kt/V urea and creatinine clearance per 1.73 m^2 are 1.66 and 53.4 l, respectively. According to the CANUSA data (Churchill *et al.*, 1996), this may represent under- dialysis. However, if this same patient is treated with 4×2.5 l exchanges per day, the increased volume of dialysate and the concomitant increase in membrane surface area, available for transport, results in a marked improvement in both Kt/V and weekly creatinine clearance (Keshaviah *et al.*, 1994). According to the CANUSA data, this improvement in Kt/V would translate into an improvement in 2-year survival from 71% to 81%. It is virtually impossible to obtain a reasonably adequate Kt/V urea index of 1.9 weekly, with a dialysis dose of less than 12 l per day in an anuric patient of more than 80 kg body weight.

Table 13.1   Influence of exchange volume on dialysis dose in CAPD

	2 l × 4 exch.	2.5 l × 4 exch.
Kt/V	1.66	2.08
Weekly creatinine clearance/1.73 m^2	53.4 l	67.3 l

It is worthwhile recalling that in the prospective cohort of the CANUSA study, no attempt was made to compensate the dialysis dose for the declining renal function, and over 90% of the patients remained on 4×2 l exchanges daily throughout the study period. According to Blake (1996), what CANUSA has shown is not that increased dialysis dose is associated with a lower mortality rate but, rather, that patients with more residual renal function live longer! In most long-term, non-interventional studies on CAPD, no changes in peritoneal clearances have been realized and almost all the variations in Kt/V urea or creatinine clearance represented variations in RRF.

As shown in Fig. 13.1, it has been calculated that in order to maintain the initial Kt/V urea index in our previously published series of patients, the dialysis dose should, after 5 years, have been changed to 5×3 l per day, a dose hardly achievable with manual exchanges in a standard CAPD program. A recent study by Tattersall *et al.* (1994) also emphasized the difficulty of providing adequate dialysis to all CAPD patients over a period of time. By progressively increasing the exchange volumes in an effort to keep pace with the reduction in renal function, CAPD was unable to provide Kt/V urea values of 1.75/week in more than 40% of the patients, despite individualization of the dialysis prescription. Johnston *et al.* (1995) found that, despite increasing the prescribed volume by 22% using 2.5-litre exchanges, the decline in RRF resulted in an overall increase in Kt/V urea by only 6%, and 1% for creatinine clearance after a 6-month period.

Cycler-assisted automated peritoneal dialysis should, at least theoretically, be able to increase the clearances and improve the adequacy of dialysis by increasing the number of exchanges and/or increasing the intraperitoneal volumes, but some of the results achieved have been disappointing. According to Diaz-Buxo and Suki (1994) almost no single cycler technique succeeds in achieving the same weekly clearances as CAPD. De Fijter *et al.* (1994) found, after a follow-up period of 2 years, that the indices of adequacy (total creatinine clearances and Kt/V urea) were no better in continuous cyclic peritoneal dialysis (CCPD) than in CAPD patients. Brunkhorst and his associates (1994) have extensively studied 104 patients treated with automated peritoneal dialysis (APD). Patients were successively treated with nightly intermittent peritoneal dialysis (NIPD) alone, in the presence of a substantial residual renal clearance; however, the more the residual renal clearance decreased the more frequent the association of NIPD with additional manual CAPD exchanges became necessary. In complete anuria, CCPD had to be combined with one or two additional CAPD exchanges per day in order to achieve a weekly creatinine clearance of 50–55 l. Twardowski and Nolph (1996) have suggested that in the presence of anuria, dialysis efficiency could be increased by using nightly tidal PD, combined with high-volume exchanges during the day. However, it is doubtful if many patients will prefer this demanding regimen above a transfer to hemodialysis.

An important parameter in the prescription of APD is the characteristics of the peritoneal transport. A high transporter (D/P creatinine > 0.81, at 4 hours of dwell-time) can be treated by nightly intermittent peritoneal dialysis (NIPD) or nocturnal tidal peritoneal dialysis (NTPD); the high average transporter (D/P creatinine 0.65–0.81) by continuous cycling peritoneal dialysis (CCPD), NIPD, or TPD; the low average transporter (D/P creatinine 0.5–0.65) by CCPD; whereas the low transporters (D/P creatinine < 0.5) are not good candidates for any of the APD techniques.

Hybrid systems, based on both automated and manual PD techniques are often necessary to provide the long-term solute removal, once the patient becomes anuric. This need is accentuated when the patient is large and muscular. With the typical D/P urea ratio in the range of 0.6 to 0.7 in APD, it would require a daily drain volume of 19–23 l to achieve the optimal Kt/V urea of 2.3/week (0.328 daily) in an anuric, 70-kg patient. Although current technology can achieve this goal, the nearly threefold increase in dialysate cost is clearly prohibitive and probably unacceptable to most patient's lifestyles in terms of immobility. If PD is to survive as a credible long-term therapy for ESRD patients, it must have the capacity to deliver optimal renal replacement therapy at a cost within the reimbursement levels.

Adequacy and cardiovascular mortality

In view of the findings that deaths from cardiovascular disease are the most common cause of patient mortality, it is logical to assume that failure to achieve targets of adequacy in PD patients is in some way associated with an increased risk of adverse cardiovascular events. Some hemodynamic studies show that CAPD patients, compared with HD patients, are constantly overhydrated. This overhydration is demonstrated by a higher mean pulmonary arterial pressure measured before kidney transplantation and by a remarkable reduction in 'dry' body weight and a significant decrease in diastolic blood pressure after transferring CAPD patients to HD (Rottembourg, 1993; Lameire *et al.*, 1996*b*).

Recent studies indicate that the blood pressure can be readily controlled in CAPD patients during the first 2–3 years, but once the RRF is very low or absent the control becomes more difficult and the patients need a higher number of antihypertensive drugs (Saldanha *et al.*, 1993; Faller and Lameire, 1994). At least in HD patients, rigorous control of the blood pressure and normalization of the extracellular volume status with long, slow HD were the two most important factors influencing patient outcome in Tassin (Charra *et al.*, 1992, 1996). There is no reason to believe that this would be different in PD patients.

Symptomatic fluid gain occurs in 25% of CAPD patients; peripheral edema (100%), pulmonary congestion (80%), pleural effusions (76%), and systolic and diastolic hypertension were the most common manifestations (Tzamaloukas *et al.*, 1995). A hyperpermeable membrane with high, peritoneal solute transport is a risk factor for this complication as high, peritoneal solute transfer is associated with poor ultrafiltration which would be expected to exacerbate poor cardiac function. Latent overhydration is particularly frequent in patients with diabetic nephropathy (Mulec *et al.*, 1995). One may speculate that the superior survival among CAPD patients with a higher RRF is indeed related to the better control of the fluid balance. This is supported by the recent findings of Davies *et al.* (1996) who found that the dialysis dose was associated with outcome in patients with ischemic heart disease, but not in those with left ventricular dysfunction, which is an independent predictor of mortality in CAPD patients. These patients fared significantly worse if they had a high solute transfer and a low plasma albumin.

Thus, besides the decline in RRF, loss of the peritoneal ultrafiltration, which is not infrequent in PD, becomes an important prognostic factor. Heimburger *et al.* (1990) reported that by 6 years' CAPD, 31% of their patients had problems with fluid removal. Whether this was due to low pH, high lactate or dextrose dialysate, recurrent peritonitis, or was completely unrelated to dialysate composition, is unknown. Similarly, Faller and Lameire (1994) found that peritoneal ultrafiltration declined as a result of the previous use of a dialysate containing acetate rather than lactate. However, a gradual increase in the daily use of more hypertonic bags was also noted in patients who were never exposed to acetate. Selgas *et al.* (1994) have followed the long-term peritoneal function of 56 patients who had been on CAPD for at least 3 years. It was concluded that after 5–11 years, the human peritoneum showed functional stability in patients with a low peritoneal inflammation rate. However, patients with frequent and/or prolonged peritonitis showed a significant decrease in ultrafiltration capacity and an increase in peritoneal creatinine diffusion capacity. Similar results were obtained in a more recent analysis, including 38 patients with at least 5 years' CAPD (Selgas *et al.*, 1995). Importantly, the loss of ultrafiltration in association with peritoneal hyperpermeability (ultrafiltration loss type I), may recover by introducing 4-week peritoneal 'rest periods'.

The most severe form of peritoneal inflammation resulting in an adverse outcome of PD is sclerosing encapsulating peritonitis. This complication has appeared several to many months after transfer to HD or renal transplantation. Although the cause of this dramatic disease is unknown, postulated causes include acetate-containing dialysates, recurrent or severe peritonitis, formaldehyde, chlorhexidine, plastic particles, interleukin-1 production, frequent use of hypertonic dialysates, and beta-blockers. The best prevention of this dreadful disease is early removal of the catheter in severe and/or prolonged peritonitis, reduction in the use of hypertonic dialysates to avoid exposure of the naked stroma of the membrane to the effects of glucose, and resting the peritoneum, if feasible, to allow remesothelialization. (Moncrief *et al.*, 1994).

A discussion of the problem of the bioincompatibility of the dialysis fluids and their *in-vitro* effects on peritoneal structure and function, and the attempts that are being made to modify the fluid to make it more biocompatible, is beyond the scope of this chapter. This topic has recently been extensively summarized by Jörres *et al.* (1994) and Coles (1995). It is sufficient to say that the currently available fluids are bioincompatible *in vitro*, mainly due to their acidity and/or hyperosmolality, but the potential clinical relevance of these findings, especially regarding the long-term outcome of PD, is unclear. Besides the *in-vitro* adverse effects of the solution, glucose as the osmotic agent may contribute to the formation of advanced glycosylation end products (AGEs) in the peritoneal cavity (Yamada *et al.*, 1994). *In vitro*, AGEs inhibit mesothelial cell growth (Kumano *et al.*, 1994), and one may speculate that exposure of the submesothelial layer to glucose during the denudation caused by peritonitis may impair the structural and functional recovery of the membrane (Dobbie, 1992).

The problem of malnutrition

Another concern in the long-term survival of PD patients is the occurrence of malnutrition. Protein malnutrition especially is a common and serious problem in

CAPD patients. In a large multicenter study in the USA, it was calculated that mild malnutrition occurred in 32% and severe malnutrition in 8% of all CAPD patients (Young *et al.*, 1991). The most simple and predictive method for the continuous monitoring of the nutritional state is the follow-up of the serum albumin values. Although it is debatable if albumin is a marker of nutrition (Heimburger *et al.*, 1994), the strong correlation between the level of albumin and patient survival has recently been confirmed in the CANUSA study (Churchill *et al.*, 1996). It is important to realize that the absolute value of the serum albumin is dependent on the method of determination (Koomen *et al.*, 1992; Blagg *et al.*, 1993).

In view of the strong relationship between malnutrition and patient survival and morbidity, it is not surprising that multiple interventions have been tried either to prevent or to treat this complication. These interventions include: optimization of the dialysis dose, use of biocompatible dialysate solutions, intensive nutritional counseling, intradialytic parenteral and enteral nutritional supplements, and growth factors such as recombinant human growth hormone (rHGH) and recombinant insulin-like growth factor-1 (rHIGF-1). Recent findings with growth hormones suggest a favorable effect on protein turnover, lean body mass, and total body muscle measurements (Ikizler *et al.*, 1994; Kang *et al.*, 1994). Many studies, summarized by Jones (1995), have also been performed with amino-acid dialysates in order to prevent or treat protein malnutrition in PD patients. The use of intraperitoneal amino acids has been shown to improve nutritional status over the short term in malnourished patients. Its long-term benefits are however unknown.

The main questions arising around the use of amino acids are related to their nutritional effect. Although extra elements are made available for protein synthesis, excess availability will result in their breakdown through gluconeogenesis, and in the retention of extra nitrogen metabolites in the blood. This process is inevitable when amino acids are not combined with extra caloric intake (Lameire and Faict, 1994). It should also be taken into consideration that their use is counterbalanced by a loss of appetite, especially if many non-essential amino acids are used, accumulation of excess nitrogen metabolites, and acidosis. A final pitfall is the cost of these solutions. These are additional reasons to use amino acids only intermittently, and not during the whole day (Vanholder and Lameire 1996).

Role of CAPD in the management of ESRD

It can be concluded from all the studies so far discussed that patients treated with any form of PD can be maintained in reasonably good health as long as there remains at least a minimum of RRF and body weight is not excessively high. In patients who do not experience recurrent episodes of severe infections, either peritonitis or serious catheter infections, the peritoneal diffusive transport and ultrafiltration capacities can be maintained for at least 7 to 8 years. In the remaining sections of this chapter, the problems of maintaining RRF for as long as possible, the decision on the time of commencenment of dialysis, and the integration of PD in an overall program of ESRD treatment will be discussed.

The maintenance of the residual renal function

Following the initial observation of Rottembourg and his associates (1983), several other groups have observed that RRF is better maintained in CAPD patients compared to patients on intermittent HD (Nolph, 1990; Lysaght *et al.*, 1991; Rottembourg, 1993). Table 13.2 summarizes some of the reasons why RRF is better preserved in CAPD than in HD. Some studies have observed that in HD patients suffering from glomerular diseases, the fall in RRF in the first 3 months after starting dialysis was more rapid than in patients suffering from non-glomerular diseases (Iest *et al.*, 1989). This could not be confirmed in our CAPD population. On the other hand, CAPD could exert positive effects on renal function, such as a greater hemodynamic stability with less abrupt fluctuations in volume and osmotic load and less drastic modification in the hemodynamic status of the patients (Lysaght *et al.*, 1991). These can probably maintain a stable glomerular capillary pressure, leading to a more constant glomerular filtration rate. In this regard, the recent demonstration that RRF declined more rapidly on intermittent APD compared with CAPD is very relevant (Hiroshige *et al.*, 1996).

Table 13.2 Reasons for better preservation of RRF during CAPD compared to HD (adapted from Rottembourg, 1993)

- Constant overhydration of the CAPD patient
- Less exposure to inflammatory mediators
- Less hemodynamic instability
- More routine prescription of diuretics to CAPD patients

It has also been suggested that inflammatory mediators, such as interleukin-1, generated by the extracorporeal circulation of hemodialysis, may be nephrotoxic in their repeated exposure to native kidneys (Lysaght *et al.*, 1991). However, patients dialyzed with biocompatible membranes such as polysulfone or polyacrylonitrite were observed to lose residual creatinine clearance at a rate similar to patients dialyzed with bioincompatible Cuprophan membranes (Caramelo *et al.*, 1994). However, as pointed out before, we believe that a more important factor is the continuously volume-expanded state that is often associated with the CAPD treatment.

What is the clinical importance of a better preservation of the RRF in CAPD patients? It can be presumed that in the presence of a preserved excretory renal function the non-excretory, endocrine function will also be better preserved, resulting in the maintenance of erythropoietin synthesis (Caro *et al.*, 1979; Zappacosta *et al.*, 1982; Chandra *et al.*, 1988), conversion of vitamin D into its active form (Jongen *et al.*, 1984), and in a better elimination of β_2-microglobulin (Blumberg and Burgi, 1987; Rottembourg *et al.*, 1987; Thielemans *et al.*, 1988; Acchiacardo *et al.*, 1989; Scalamogna *et al.*, 1989). Serum β_2-microglobulin levels are reportedly lower in PD patients with RRF, and inverse correlations between serum β_2-microglobulin levels and serially measured creatinine clearances or residual diuresis have been demonstrated (Montenegro *et al.*, 1992; Amici *et al.*, 1993; Catizone *et al.*, 1993).

In view of the importance of the preservation of RRF in PD, the question can be asked whether measures can be taken that contribute to its maintenance. Some of these measures are summarized in Table 13.3. The routine use of high doses of loop diuretics can, without doubt, contribute to the maintenance of the residual diuresis. In the collaborative Colmar and Gent study, the evolution of residual diuresis was different between the two patient groups (Faller and Lameire, 1994). Because of a more rapid loss of peritoneal ultrafiltration, the French patients maintained a better diuresis thanks to the routine prescription of his high doses of frusemide. However, controversial results with the prescription of loop diuretics have been described in CAPD patients (Scarpioni *et al.*, 1982), and, based on studies with high doses of loop diuretics in preterminal renal failure patients, the increase in diuresis and natriuresis is not accompanied by an increase in creatinine clearance (Lameire and Rosenkranz, unpublished results). Furthermore, because diuretic-induced volume depletion occurs during therapy, the drug's effectiveness diminishes over time (Grantham and Chonko, 1978). One may wonder whether continuous stimulation of the diuresis is not detrimental for the RRF. On the other hand, careful use of loop diuretics could be beneficial to PD patients in order to maintain a more normal extracellular volume resulting in a reduced need for the use of hypertonic glucose solutions.

Table 13.3   Recommendations to preserve RRF in CAPD

- Avoid NSAID, ACE inhibitors
- Avoid repetitive administration of aminoglycosides, vancomycin
- Avoid excessive ultrafiltration
- Start with CAPD and introduce APD as late as possible
- Routine prescription of loop diuretics (?)

The time of commencement of peritoneal dialysis

Traditionally, the presence of clinical symptoms of uremia and of fluid overload and/or the biochemical indices of advanced renal failure, such as the blood levels of urea, creatinine, anemia, hyperkalemia, hyperphosphatemia, acidosis, etc., have assumed great importance in the decision to start dialysis at the appropriate time. As recently pointed out by Shulman and Hakim (1996), dialysis should, at least theoretically, be started very early, probably before any clear-cut benefits could be ascribed to it. Bonomini has suggested beneficial effects of an early start of dialysis (residual creatinine clearance as high as 15–20 ml/min) on outcome and rehabilitation of HD patients (Bonomini *et al.*, 1984; Bonomini, 1987). However, any form of dialysis is expensive, disrupts a patient's life, and entails a number of risks. Thus the issue of the appropriate time to initiate dialysis therapy is an important one.

Whereas there is no discussion over the absolute and relative indications for starting dialysis (Schulman and Hakim, 1996), the criteria are more subtle and subjective in relatively asymptomatic patients with slowly progressive chronic renal failure. Besides medical reasons, the decision as to the correct time to commence renal replacement therapy also depends on the availability of facilities, including a sufficient number of trained nephrologists. In this regard, it is worrying that in some European countries the numbers of nephrologists and trained nurses are low and, if this trend continues, may become in itself a limiting factor in the availability of renal replacement therapy.

Recently, Tattersall *et al.* (1995) have used urea kinetic modeling to predict the optimum timing of commencement of dialysis. At the initiation(i) of dialysis, the residual daily Kt/V urea (Kt/V_i urea) calculated according to the Watson formulas, was significantly lower than the total daily Kt/V urea recorded in the same patients when they had been receiving CAPD or hemodialysis for 6 months. Daily Kt/V_i urea was only 0.15, a figure which, if recorded in a CAPD patient, would be taken to indicate severe underdialysis. After 6 months of CAPD and hemodialysis, the total daily Kt/V urea had increased to 0.35 ± 0.12 and 0.49 ± 0.08, respectively. Even more important was that Kt/V_i was inversely correlated with the hospital admission rate and with the number of inpatient days. Kt/V_i was significantly lower and age and comorbidity indices significantly higher in the group of patients who subsequently died than in survivors.

A similar calculation in our series of 16 patients (Lameire *et al.*, 1992) revealed a Kt/V_i urea of 0.124 and an increase to a total Kt/V urea after 6 months of CAPD to 0.40. This corresponds with a weekly Kt/V_i urea of 0.87 and a total weekly Kt/V urea of 2.8 after 6 months of CAPD. According to the latest insights into dialysis adequacy, a weekly Kt/V urea in CAPD of 2.0 to 2.1 is accepted as adequate, thus a starting daily Kt/V_i of around 0.3 should be considered. Depending on the distribution volume of urea, and thus on the patient's body size, this should roughly correspond with a creatinine clearance between 10 and 15 ml/min. The findings of Tattersall *et al.* (1995) and the present calculations suggest that patients may well benefit from the earlier commencement of dialysis, perhaps at a time when Kt/V_i has declined to the point at which CAPD would be considered inadequate. The same reasoning also applies to the time of starting HD. Commencing dialytic therapy earlier would also decrease the danger of malnutrition that develops during the predialysis periods in many patients with ESRD. Based on anthropometric measurements, a sometimes precarious nutritional status was apparent in patients newly initiated on dialysis (Blumenkrantz *et al.*, 1980). One of the reasons for this malnutrition is the either spontaneous or therapeutic decrease in dietary protein intake during the predialysis period in order to slow the progression of renal failure.

Taking into account that RRF and its contribution to the total Kt/V urea and creatinine clearance decreases more slowly in PD than in HD, a period of 3–5 years on PD should not compromise the general health status of the patient too much, before he/she needs to be transferred to HD. It is clear that in patients who present a number of absolute and relative medical or social contraindications to any of the dialysis techniques (PD or HD) the choice, although limited, is easier to make. The relatively few absolute contraindications to PD are well known and have been described in recent textbooks (Burkart and Nolph, 1996; Churchill, 1996*b*). The relative contraindications range from very strong to minor, and the selection of PD must be determined by weighing the advantages and disadvantages for a given clinical situation and by

Long-term peritoneal dialysis

patient preference. The choice between PD, HD, or pre-emptive transplantation is not always easy, and a number of psychological, social, and financial factors determine the choice in the patient without major medical contraindications for any of the dialysis techniques.

Integration of PD in an overall ESRD program

Renal replacement therapy should be seen as a continuum of treatments in which, at a given time in the patient's life, one or other mode of therapy will be more appropriate. Free and easy transfer of the patient from one renal replacement program to another without restriction will probably be the best option that the nephrologist can offer in the near future. All three options must therefore be integrated in one program of ESRD treatment. Surprisingly few studies are available on the outcome of patients who converted from PD to HD, and vice versa. We recently performed such an analysis summarized in Table 13.4. (Van Biesen *et al.*, 1998)

Table 13.4 Transfer of patients from one dialysis modality to another (Gent 1979–1994)

	CAPD population	HD population	Transfer CAPD→HD	Transfer HD→CAPD
n	200	276	35	45
Age + range (years)	56 (8–81)	53 (14–84)	54 (15–79)	56 (15–79)
M/F	96/104	153/123	11/24	19/26
Dialysis time before transfer (patient months)	—	—	21.4	37.5

From a group of 200 previously non-dialysed CAPD patients who were maintained for at least 3 months on this modality between 1979 and 1994, 35 patients (17.5%) were subsequently transferred to HD after a mean follow-up of 21.4 patient-months on CAPD. In the same period, 276 patients started thrice-weekly HD. From this group, 45 patients (16.3%) were transferred to CAPD after a mean follow-up of 37.5 patient-months on HD. The reasons for the transfer from CAPD to HD were recurrent peritonitis in 13 patients, loss of ultrafiltration and solute clearance in 11 patients, psychosocial problems in 9 patients, abdominal access problems after surgery in 1 patient, and hydrothorax in 1 patient, The reasons for the transfer from HD to CAPD, were personal choice in 6 patients, cardiovascular problems in 12 patients, vascular access failure in 18 patients, intractable arterial hypertension in 3 patients, cerebro-vascular accident in 2 patients, and diabetes in 4 patients. Kaplan–Meier survival curves of the transferred patients are compared in Fig. 13.2 with the survival curves of the patients who remained on the original modality. Transplantation was regarded as being lost to follow-up.

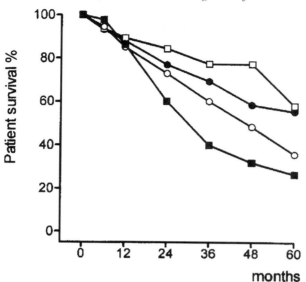

Fig. 13.2 Cumulative 5-year patient survival in four groups of patients (Gent 1979–1994).
-●-: HD patients remaining on HD(n = 276);
-○-: CAPD patients remaining on CAPD (n = 200);
-■-: HD patients converted to CAPD (n = 45);
-□-: CAPD patients converted to HD (n = 56).

After 5 years' treatment, the survival rate for those patients remaining on CAPD was 36%, which was significantly lower than the survival of 55% in the group maintained on HD. The same figure depicts some interesting differences in patient survival of the transferred populations. The patient survival 5 years after transfer in the group that converted from CAPD to HD was 58%; in contrast, only 27% of the patients who changed from HD to CAPD survived for 5 years after transfer. It should be stressed that the majority of the patients who converted from HD to PD had completely lost their RRF. The results obtained in the CAPD group that transferred to HD are no different than in the HD population that remained on this modality. On the other hand, the survival of the patients who converted from HD to CAPD was worse compared to the group that was initially treated with this modality. Although these results do not allow us to make any conclusion whether an initial spell on CAPD improves the survival rate on HD, they do suggest that converting CAPD patients to HD does not compromise their survival after the transfer.

Taking into account this effective integration of all treatment forms, for some patients (e.g. elderly, newborns, and small children) PD may first of all offer a unique opportunity for treatment, since these patient categories may encounter potential hazards and logistical problems with other dialysis modalities or renal transplantation. In addition, children may benefit from PD at home as this allows them to continue their school education.

The expected duration of dialysis is also an important factor to consider. Short-term candidates for renal transplantation, with a cadaver or living related donor, may be easily treated with PD without the need for creating a vascular access. It is now well established that both patient as well as graft survival are the same in both PD as in HD patients (Winchester *et al.*, 1993; Maiorca *et al.*, 1994). Although transplantation is often considered as the optimum therapeutic option, it has advantages and disadvantages. The long-term results of renal transplantation in patients aged 15–29 years at the start of renal replacement therapy show an overall graft loss of approximately 50%, 10 years after transplantation (data presented by van Renthengbus at the XXXIIIrd Congress of the ERA–EDTA in June 1996, Amsterdam). Furthermore Carpenter (1995) pointed out the marked divergence between the early and long-term graft survival curves between the years 1975 and 1991, these indicated a progressive improvement in the 1-year graft survival, but no evolution in the 7–8-year half-life of graft loss.

A majority of these successfully transplanted patients will thus return to dialysis before they can obtain a second (or third) graft. In a number of these patients further transplantation may be difficult due to the formation of cytotoxic antibodies and the greater difficulty in achieving a satisfactory match in a second graft as opposed to a first one. For patients who are unlikely to receive a transplant and who are suitable for either hemodialysis or PD, the choice by the well-informed patient becomes the major determinant.

Are there medical arguments to suggest that some patients could be advised to start with peritoneal dialysis at the beginning of their career with ESRD? In view of the evidence described earlier in this chapter that small solute clearance influences morbidity and mortality of the dialysis patient, there are several arguments that suggest that PD could be recommended as the initial dialysis modality. The longer maintenance of RRF may have implications in the control of β_2-microglobulin with its associated amyloidosis. Symptomatic amyloidosis is uncommon before 10 years on HD treatment, and, although few PD patients have been maintained on treatment for this length of time, the better total elimination of β_2-microglobulin over a longer period compared to HD may be a potential benefit. A recent multicenter study in Japan found an incidence of carpal tunnel syndrome in only 5 out of 5050 patients, treated exclusively by CAPD (Nomoto *et al.*, 1995).

Assuming that PD can provide adequate dialysis for 3–5 years (the time that RRF completely disappears), creation of a vascular access is not necessary during that period and peripheral veins can be preserved for the future creation of an arterio-venous fistula in case HD ultimately becomes necessary. In patients who present late in renal failure and who need immediate dialysis treatment, PD can be commenced in an emergency without the need for a temporary central venous dialysis catheter.

During the first 2–3 years of PD, hypertension and cardiac complications are effectively controlled and antihypertensive drug intake can be reduced. Thus, a previous spell on PD is not harmful for cardiac function and will not compromise the evolution of the cardiovascular status when the patient continues on HD. However, a word of caution is warranted here. PD, and notably CAPD, may have an adverse effect on peripheral vascular disease because of its propensity for accelerating atherosclerosis due to the continuous absorption of glucose from the dialysis fluid and its effect on carbohydrate and lipid metabolism (Lameire *et al.*, 1988). The introduction of alternative osmotic agents in the near future, possibly leading to a reduction of the glucose burden for the patient, will certainly play a major role.

Most forms of PD, with the exception of the now rarely used intermittent PD, are ideally suitable for home treatment. In the well-selected patient, PD offers specific advantages in providing good chances for effective rehabilitation. The patient's social and working life may be less hindered compared with in-center hemodialysis and PD, as self-care treatment offers more possibilities for planning holidays and travelling. This can contribute to better patient compliance and makes the acceptance of dialysis treatment in the early years psychologically easier.

To achieve a complete integration of PD in the treatment of ESRD a detailed analysis of the costs should be undertaken. It was considered that PD with its lack of a need for sophisticated expensive equipment would be much cheaper than HD. This is now recognized to be only partly true. In some countries of Central and Eastern Europe, the introduction of PD is rather slow because of the high costs of the dialysis fluids that have to be imported and often have to be paid for in foreign currency. However, the effective integration of PD may provide the means to correctly allocate the available resources. PD represents an important buffer which avoids further expansion of the dialysis center. Despite the continuous growth of the number of dialysis patients, by using PD the number of HD stations can be kept constant, and medical and nursing staff can remain adequate.

Another considerations is travel. For some patients living a long way from a hospital, home PD may represent a unique solution in certain clinical and logistical conditions (Ronco *et al.*, 1996). The time needed to travel to and from the dialysis centers is avoided, which can amount to a considerable saving particularly for patients in rural areas.

Conclusions

We believe that PD is a very useful mode of dialysis that can compete in many aspects with HD in those patients who possess at least a minimum of RRF. One of the great advantages of the CAPD modality is perhaps the longer preservation of this RRF. Commencing PD at an earlier stage of ESRD should further prolong the period where no great risk for inadequate dialysis and malnutrition is occurring.

We also believe that dose adaptation, in parallel with the decline in RRF, should be performed earlier in the follow-up of CAPD patients in order to maintain adequate dialysis for longer. In patients who do not have major contraindications to PD and who prefer a self-care, home treatment for a number of years, PD could be considered as an excellent first treatment. Based on our results obtained after conversion of treatment described earlier in this chapter, initial PD treatment does not compromise future applications of other dialysis modalities. The total length of dialysis treatment in a given patient can thus be prolonged.

A crucial moment in the PD treatment arrives when RRF completely disappears. Depending on the body size of the patient at that time, other means of treatment, whether it be HD, or one of its variants, or renal transplantation, should then be considered.

References

Acchiacardo, S., Kraus, A. P., and Jennings, B. R. (1989). Beta 2 microglobulin levels in patients with renal insufficiency. *American Journal of Kidney Diseases*, **13**, 70–4.

Ahlmen, J., Carlsson, L., and Schönborg, C. (1993). Well-informed patients with end-stage renal disease prefer peritoneal dialysis to hemodialysis. *Peritoneal Dialysis International*, **13** (Suppl. 2), S196–S197.

Alpert, M. A., Hüting, J., Twardowski, Z. J., Khanna, R., and Nolph, K. D. (1995). Continuous ambulatory peritoneal dialysis and the heart. *Peritoneal Dialysis International*, **15**, 6–11.

Amann, K., and Ritz, E. (1996). Cardiac structure and function in renal disease. *Current Opinion in Nephrology and Hypertension*, **5** 102–6.

Amici, G., Virga, G., Da Rin, *et al.* (1993). Serum beta-2 microglobulin level and residual renal function in peritoneal dialysis. *Nephron*, **65**, 469–71.

Bernardini, J., Holley, J. L., Johnston, J. R., *et al.* (1991). An analysis of 10-year trends in infections in adults on continuous ambulatory peritoneal dialysis (CAPD). *Clinical Nephrology*, **36**, 29–34.

Blagg, C. R., and Mailloux, L. U. (1996). Introduction: the case for home hemodialysis. *Advances in Renal Replacement Therapy*, **3**, 96–8.

Blagg, C. R., Liedtke, R. J., Batjer, J. D., *et al.* (1993). Serum albumin concentration—related health care financing administration quality assurance criterion is method-dependent: revision is necessary. *American Journal of Kidney Diseases*, **21**, 138–44.

Blake, P. G. (1996). Targets in CAPD and APD prescription. *Peritoneal Dialysis International*, **16**, S143–S146.

Bloembergen, W. E., Port, F. K., Mauger, E. A., and Wolfe, R. A. (1995). A comparison of mortality between patients treated with hemodialysis and peritoneal dialysis. *Journal of the American Society of Nephrology*, **6**, 177–83.

Blumberg, A., and Burgi W. (1987). Behaviour of β_2 microglobulin in patients with chronic renal failure undergoing hemodialysis, hemodiafiltration and continuous ambulatory peritoneal dialysis. *Clinical Nephrology*, **27**, 245–9.

Blumenkrantz, M. J., Wolfson, M., and Kopple, J. (1980). Nutritional status of patients on hemodialysis. *American Journal of Nutrition*, **33**, 1567–88.

Bonomini, V. (1987). Timing dialysis in chronic uraemic. *Life Support Systems*, **5**, 1–7.

Bonomini, V., Feletti, C., Scolari, M. P., Stefoni, S. (1984). Early dialysis. *Contributions to Nephrology*, **37**, 45–51.

Brunkhorst, R., Wrenger, E., Krautzig, S., Ehlerding, G., Mahiout, A., and Koch, K. M. (1994). Clinical experience with home automated peritoneal dialysis, *Kidney International*, **46** (Suppl. 48), S25–S30.

Burkart, J. M., and Nolph, K. D. (1996). Peritoneal dialysis In *The kidney* (5th edn) (ed. B. M. Brenner), pp. 2507–75. W. B. Saunders, Philadelphia.

Canadian Organ Replacement Register (1995). *1993 Annual Report*. Canadian Institute for Health Information, Don Mills, Ontario.

Caramelo, C., Alcazar, R., Gallar, P., *et al.* (1994). Choice of dialysis membrane does not influence the outcome of residual renal function in haemodialysis patients. *Nephrology, Dialysis, Transplantation*, **9**, 675–7.

Caro, J., Brown, S., Miller, O., Murray, T. G., and Erslev, A. J. (1979). Erythropoietin levels in uremic nephric and anephric patients. *Journal of Laboratory and Clinical Medicine*, **93**, 449–54.

Carpenter, C. B. (1995). Long-term failure of renal transplants: adding insult to injury. *Kidney International*, **48** (Suppl. 50), S40–S44.

Catizone, L., Cocchi, R., Fusaroli, M., and Zucchelli, P. (1993). Relationship between plasma β_2 microglobulin and residual diuresis in continuous ambulatory peritoneal dialysis and hemodialysis patients. *Peritoneal Dialysis International*, **13** (Suppl. 2), S523–S526.

Chandra, M., Clemons, G. K K., McVicar, M., Wilkes, B., and Mossey, R. T. (1988). Serum erythropoietin levels and hematocrit in end-stage renal disease: influence of the mode of therapy. *American Journal of Kidney Diseases*, **12**, 208–13.

Charra, B., Calemard, E., Ruffet, M., *et al.* (1992). Survival as an index of adequacy of dialysis. *Kidney International*, **41**, 1286–91.

Charra, B., Calemard, E., and Laurent, G. (1996). Importance of treatment time and blood pressure control in achieving long-term survival on dialysis. *American Journal of Nephrology*, **16**, 35–44.

Churchill, D. N. (1996a). Can peritoneal dialysis be equivalent to (or better than) optimal hemodialysis? *Seminars in Dialysis*, **9**, 240–1.

Churchill, D. N. (1996b). Indications for long term results and limitations of peritoneal dialysis. In *Replacement of renal function by dialysis* (4th edn) (Ed. C. Jacobs, C. M. Kjellstrand, K. M. Koch, and J. F. Winchester), pp. 603–18. Kluwer Academic, Dordrecht.

Churchill, D. N., Taylor, D. W., and Keshaviah, P. (1996). Adequacy of dialysis and nutrition in continuous peritoneal dialysis: association with clinical outcome. *Journal of the American Society of Nephrology*, **7**, 198–207.

Coles, G. A. (1995). Towards a more physiologic solution for peritoneal dialysis. *Seminars in Dialysis*, **8**, 333–5.

Culleton, B., and Parfrey, P. S. (1996). Cardiovascular risk in continuous ambulatory peritoneal dialysis. *Peritoneal Dialysis International*, **16**, 10–12.

Dasgupta, M. K. (1995). The role of new catheters in avoiding infections in peritoneal dialysis patients. *Seminars in Dialysis*, **8**, 362–6.

Davies, S. J., Bryan, J., Phillips, L., and Russel, G. I. (1996). The predictive value of KT/V and peritoneal solute transport in CAPD patients is dependent on the type of comorbidity present. *Peritoneal Dialysis International*, **16** (Suppl. 1), S158–S162.

De Fijter, C. W., Oe, L. P., Nauta, J. J., *et al.* (1994). Clinical efficacy and morbidity associated with continuous cyclic compared with continuous ambulatory peritoneal dialysis. *Annals of Internal Medicine*, **120**, 264–71.

Diaz-Buxo, J. A., and Suki, W. N. (1994). Automated peritoneal dialysis. In *The textbook of peritoneal dialysis* (ed.) R. Gokal and K. D. Nolph, pp. 399–418. Kluwer Academic, Dordrecht.

Dobbie, J. W. (1992). Pathogenesis of peritoneal fibrosing peritonitis in peritoneal dialysis. *Peritoneal Dialysis International*, **12**, 14–27.

Faller, B., and Lameire, N. (1994). Evolution of clinical parameters and peritoneal function in a cohort of CAPD patients followed over 7 years. *Nephrology, Dialysis, Transplantation*, **9**, 280–6.

Grantham, J. J., and Chonko, A. M. (1978). The physiologic basis and clinical use of diuretics. In *Contemporary issues in nephrology, sodium and water homeostasis*, (ed. B. M. Brenner and J. H. Stein), pp. 178–211, Churchill Livingstone, New York.

Heimburger, O., Waniewski, J., Werynski, A., Tranaeus, A., and Lindholm, B. (1990). Peritoneal transport in CAPD patients with permanent loss of ultrafiltration capacity. *Kidney International*, **38**, 495–506.

Heimburger, O., Bergstrom, J., and Lindholm, B. (1994). Is serum albumin an index of nutritional status in continuous ambulatory peritoneal dialysis patients? *Peritoneal Dialysis International*, **14**, 108–14.

Hiroshige, K., Yuu, K., Soejima, M., Takasugi, M., and Kuroiwa, A. (1996). Rapid decline of residual renal function in patients on automated peritoneal dialysis. *Peritoneal Dialysis International*, **16**, 307–15.

Iest, C. G., Vanholder, R. C., and Ringoir, S. M. (1989). Loss of residual renal function in patients on regular hemodialysis. *International Journal of Artificial Organs*, 12, 154–9.

Ikizler, T. A., Wingard, R. L., Breyer, J. A., Schulman, G., Parker, R. A., and Hakim, R. A. (1994). Short-term effects of recombinant human growth hormone in CAPD patients. *Kidney International*, 46, 1178–83.

Innes, A., Rowe, P. A., Burden, R. P., and Morgan, A. G. (1992). Early deaths on renal replacement therapy: the need for early nephrology referral. *Nephrology, Dialysis, Transplantation*, 7, 467–71.

Jindal, K. K. (1995). Avoiding technique failure in chronic peritoneal dialysis. *Seminars in Dialysis*, 8, 359–61.

Johnston, J. R., Bernardini, J., Holley, J., and Piraino, B. (1995). Effect of increasing exchange volume or frequency on CAPD efficiency. *Peritoneal Dialysis International*, 15, S41 (Abstract).

Jones, M. R. (1995). Intraperitoneal amino acids: a therapy whose times has come? *Peritoneal Dialysis International*, 15 (Suppl.), S67–S74.

Jongen, M. J. M., Van der Vijgh, W. S. F., Lip, P., and Netelenbos, J. C. (1984). Measurements of vitamin D metabolites in anephric subjects. *Nephron*, 36, 230–6.

Jörres, A., Gahl, G. M., and Frei, U. (1994). Peritoneal dialysis fluid biocompatibility: does it really matter? *Kidney International*, 48, S79–S86.

Kang, D. H., Lee, S. W., Kim, H. S., Choi, K. H., Lee, H. Y., and Han, D. S. (1994). Recombinant human growth hormone (rhGH) improves nutritional status of undernourished adult CAPD patients. *Journal of the American Society of Nephrology*, 5, 493 (Abstract).

Keshaviah, P. (1992). Adequacy of CAPD: a quantitative approach. *Kidney International*, 42 (Suppl. 38), S160–S164.

Keshaviah, P. (1996). Can peritoneal dialysis be equivalent to (or better than) optimal hemodialysis? *Seminars in Dialysis*, 9, 243–5.

Keshaviah, P. R., Nolph, K. D., and Van Stone, J. C. (1989). The peak concentration hypothesis: a urea kinetic approach to comparing the adequacy of continuous ambulatory peritoneal dialysis (CAPD) and hemodialysis. *Peritoneal Dialysis International*, 9, 257–60.

Keshaviah, P., Emerson, P. F., Vonesh, E. F., and Brandes, J. C. (1994). Relationship between body size fill volume, and mass transfer area coefficient in peritoneal dialysis. *Journal of the American Society of Nephrology*, 4, 1820–6.

Keshaviah, P., Ma, J., Thorpe, K., Churchill, D., and Collins, A. (1995). Comparison of 2 year survival on hemodialysis (HD) and peritoneal dialysis (PD) with a dose of dialysis matched using the peak concentration hypothesis. *Journal of the American Society of Nephrology*, 6, 540 (Abstract).

Koomen, G. C. M., van Straalen, J. P., Boeschoten, E. W., Gorgels, J. P. M. C., and Hoek, F. J. (1992). Comparison between dye binding methods and nephelometry for the measurement of albumin in plasma of peritoneal dialysis. *Peritoneal Dialysis International*, 12, S133 (Abstract).

Kumano, K., Manalaysay, M. T., Hyodo, T., Sakai, T., and Nakamura, K. (1994). Effects of advanced glycation end products of albumin on cell proliferation and protein synthesis in rat peritoneal mesothelial cells. *Journal of the American Society of Nephrology*, 5, 460 (Abstract).

Lameire, N. (1993). Cardiovascular risk factors and blood pressure control in continuous ambulatory peritoneal dialysis. *Peritoneal Dialysis International*, 13 (Suppl. 2), S394–S395.

Lameire, N. (1996). Referral pattern of ESRD patients and peritoneal dialysis. Presentation at the EDTNA meeting, Amsterdam, June 1996.

Lameire, N., and Faict, D. (1994). Peritoneal dialysis solutions containing glycerol and amino acids. *Peritoneal Dialysis International*, **14** (Suppl. 3), S145–S151.

Lameire, N., Matthys, D., Matthys, E., and Beheydt, R. (1988). Effects of long-term CAPD on carbohydrate and lipid metabolism. *Clinical Nephrology*, **30** (Suppl. 1), S53–S58.

Lameire, N., Vanholder, R., Vijt, D., Lambert, M. C., and Ringoir, S. (1992). A longitudinal five year survey of urea kinetic parameters in CAPD patients. *Kidney International*, **42**, 426–32.

Lameire, N., Bernaert, P., Lambert, M. C., and Vijt, D. (1994). Cardiovascular risk factors and their management in patients on continuous ambulatory peritoneal dialysis. *Kidney International*, **46** (Suppl. 48), S31–S38.

Lameire, N., Vanholder, R., Van Loo, A., *et al.* (1996*a*). Cardiovascular diseases in peritoneal dialysis patients—the size of the problem. *Kidney International* (In press).

Lameire, N., Lambert, M. C., Vijt, D., and Van Bockstaele, L. (1996*b*). Factors influencing the adequacy of peritoneal dialysis. *Saoudi Journal of Kidney Diseases and Transplantation*, **7** (Suppl.), S120–S126.

Locatelli, F., Marcelli, D., Conte, F., *et al.* (1995). 1983 to 1992: Report on regular dialysis and transplantation in Lombardy. *American Journal of Kidney Diseases*, **25**, 196–205.

Lysaght, M. J., Vonesh, E. F., Gotch, F., *et al.* (1991). The influence of dialysis treatment modality on the decline of remaining renal function. *American Society of Artificial Internal Organs Transactions*, **37**, 598–604.

Maiorca, R., and Cancarini, G. C., (1994). Outcome of peritoneal dialysis: comparative studies. In *The textbook of peritoneal dialysis* (ed. R. Gokal and K. D. Nolph), pp. 699–734, Kluwer Academic, Dordrecht.

Maiorca, R., Sandrini, S., Cancarini, G. C., *et al.* (1994). Kidney transplantation in peritoneal dialysis patients. *Peritoneal Dialysis International*, **14** (Suppl.), S162–S168.

Moncrief, J. W., Popovich, R. P., Dombros, N. V., Digenis, G. E., and Oreopoulos, D. G. (1994). Continuous ambulatory peritoneal dialysis. In *The textbook of peritoneal dialysis* (ed. R. Gokal and K. D. Nolph), pp. 357–97. Kluwer Academic, Dordrecht.

Montenegro, J., Martinez, I., Saracho, R., and Gonzalez, R. (1992). β2 Microglobulin in CAPD. *Advances in Peritoneal Dialysis*, **8**, 369–72.

Mulec, H., Blohmé, G., Kullenberg, K., Nyberg, G., and Björck, S. (1995). Latent overhydration and nocturnal hypertension in diabetic nephropathy. *Diabetologia*, **38**, 216–20.

Nissenson, A. R., Prichard, S. B., Cheng, I. K. P., *et al.* (1993). Non-medical factors that have impact on ESRD modality selection. *Kidney International*, **43** (Suppl. 40), S120–S127.

Nolph, K. D. (1990). Is residual renal function better preserved with CAPD than with hemodialysis? *American Kidney Foundation Nephrology Letters*, **7**, 1–7.

Nolph, K. D. (1994). Report at the Annual Peritoneal Dialysis Meeting, Baltimore.

Nolph, K. D., Twardowski, Z. J., and Keshaviah, P. R. (1992). Weekly clearances of urea and creatinine on CAPD and NIPD. *Peritoneal Dialysis International*, **12**, 298–303.

Nomoto, Y., Kawaguchi, Y., Kurokawa, K., *et al.* (1995). Carpal tunnel syndrome in patients undergoing CAPD. A collaborative study in 143 centers. *Peritoneal Dialysis International*, **15** (Suppl.), S86 (Abstract).

Parfrey, S., Harnett, J. D., and Foley, R. N. (1995). Heart failure and ischemic heart disease in chronic uremia. *Current Opinion in Nephrology and Hypertension*, **4**, 105–10.

Popovich, R. P., Moncrief, J. W., Decherd, J. F., Bomar, J. B., and Pyle, W. K. (1976). The definition of a novel portable/wearable equilibrium dialysis technique. *Transactions of the American Society of Artificial Internal Organs*, **5**, 64 (Abstract).

Prichard, S. (1996). Treatment modality selection in 150 consecutive patients starting ESRD therapy. *Peritoneal Dialysis International*, **16**, 69–72.

Ronco, C., Conz, P., Agostini, F., Bosch, J. P., Lew, S. Q., and La Greca, G. (1994). The concept of adequacy of peritoneal dialysis. *Peritoneal Dialysis International*, **14** (Suppl. 3), S93–S98.

Ronco, C., Conz, P., Bragantini, L., *et al.* (1996). Integration of peritoneal dialysis in active uremia. *Peritoneal Dialysis International*, **16** (Suppl. 1), S393–S397.

Rottembourg, J. (1993). Residual renal function and recovery of renal function in patients treated by CAPD. *Kidney International*, **43** (Suppl. 40), S106–S110.

Rottembourg, J., Issad, B., Gallego, J. L., *et al.* (1983). Evolution of residual renal function in patients undergoing maintenance hemodialysis or continuous ambulatory peritoneal dialysis. *Proceedings of the European Dialysis and Transplant Association*, **19**, 397–403.

Rottembourg, J., Allouache, M., Mussey, L., and Jacobs, C. (1987). Beta 2 microglobulin in dialyzed patients: hemodialysis versus continuous ambulatory peritoneal dialysis. *Nephrology, Dialysis, Transplantation*, **2**, 248–9.

Saldanha, L. F., Weiler, E., and Gonick, H. C. (1993). Effect of continuous ambulatory peritoneal dialysis on blood pressure control. *American Journal of Kidney Diseases*, **21**, 184–8.

Scalamogna, A., Imbasciati, E., Devecchi, A., *et al.* (1989). Beta 2 microglobulin in patients on peritoneal dialysis and hemodialysis. *Peritoneal Dialysis International*, **9**, 37–40.

Scarpioni, L., Ballochi, S., Bergonzi, G., Fontana, F., Poisetti, P., and Zanazzi, M. A. (1982). High dose diuretics in continuous ambulatory peritoneal dialysis. *Peritoneal Dialysis Bulletin*, **2**, 177–8.

Schulman, G. and Hakim, R. M. (1996). Improving outcomes in chronic hemodialysis patients: should dialysis be initiated earlier? *Seminars in Dialysis*, **9**, 225–9.

Selgas, R., Fdez-Reyes, M. J., Bosque, E., *et al.* (1994). Functional longevity of the human peritoneum: how long is continuous peritoneal dialysis possible? Results of a prospective medium long-term study. *American Journal of Kidney Diseases*, **23**, 64–73.

Selgas, R., Bajo, M. A., Del Peso, G., and Jimenez, C. (1995). Preserving the peritoneal membrane in long-term peritoneal dialysis patients. *Seminars in Dialysis*, **8**, 326–32.

Tattersall, J. E., Doyle, S., Greenwood, R. N., and Farrington, K. (1994). Maintaining adequacy in CAPD by individualizing the dialysis prescription. *Nephrology, Dialysis, Transplantation*, **9**, 749–52.

Tattersall, J., Greenwood, R., and Farrington, K. (1995). Urea kinetics and when to commence dialysis. *American Journal of Nephrology*, **15**, 283–9.

Thielemans, C., Dratwa, M., Bergmann, P., *et al.* (1988). Continuous ambulatory peritoneal dialysis versus haemodialysis: a lesser risk of amyloidosis. *Nephrology, Dialysis, Transplantation*, **3**, 291–4.

Twardowski, Z. and Nolph, K. D. (1996). Is peritoneal dialysis feasible once a large muscular patient becomes anuric? *Peritoneal Dialysis International*, **16**, 20–3.

Tzamaloukas, A. H., Saddler, M. C., Murata, G. H., *et al.* (1995). Symptomatic fluid retention in patients on continuous peritoneal dialysis. *Journal of the American Society of Nephrology*, **6**, 198–206.

Vanholder, R. and Lameire, N. (1996). Osmotic agents. *Kidney International* (In press).

Watson, P. E., Watson, I. D., and Batt, R. D. (1980). Total body water volumes for adult males and females estimated from simple anthropometric measurements. *American Journal of Clinical Nutrition*, **33**, 27–39.

Winchester, J. F., Rotellar, C., Goggins, M., *et al.* (1993). Transplantation in peritoneal dialysis and hemodialysis. *Kidney International*, **43** (Suppl. 40), S101–S105.

Worldwide Registry Update (1994). Baxter Healthcare Inc., Deerfield, IL.

Yamada, K., Miyahara, Y., Hamaguchi, K., *et al.* (1994). Immunohistochemical study of human advanced glycosylation end products (AGE) in chronic renal failure. *Clinical Nephrology*, **42**, 354–61.

Young, G. A., Kopple, J. D., Lindholm, B., *et al.* (1991). Nutritional assessment of continuous ambulatory peritoneal dialysis patients: an international study. *American Journal of Kidney Diseases*, **27**, 462–71.

Zappacosta, A. R., Caro, J., and Erslev, A. (1982). Normalization of hematocrit in patients with end-stage renal disease on CAPD. The role of erythropoietin. *American Journal of Medicine*, **72**, 53–7.

14

Avoiding hepatitis in patients on dialysis

Brian J. G. Pereira

Introduction

Patients on chronic dialysis are at increased risk of acquiring parenterally transmitted hepatitis viruses from blood product transfusions or nosocomial transmission in hemodialysis units (Knudsen *et al.*, 1993; Jadoul *et al.*, 1993; Irie *et al.*, 1994; Okuda *et al.*, 1994; Cendoroglo-Neto *et al.*, 1995). Biochemical abnormalities in liver function are seen in 10–44% of patients on chronic hemodialysis (Pereira and Levy, 1997). In the past, hepatitis B virus (HBV) was the major cause of parenterally transmitted viral hepatitis in dialysis patients, and the remaining cases were attributed to non-A, non-B hepatitis (NANBH). The discovery of new, parenterally transmitted hepatitis viruses such as hepatitis C (HCV) and GB virus (GBV)/hepatitis G (HGV) has shed light on the cause and clinical course of NANBH in patients on dialysis. Indeed, among dialysis patients serum markers of HBV, HCV, and GBV/HGV have been reported in 0.3–25.9%, 3.3–55%, and 3.1–55%, respectively (Anonymous, 1991; Mondelli *et al.*, 1992; Chaveau *et al.*, 1993; Dussol *et al.*, 1993; Geerlings *et al.*, 1994; Kohler, 1994; Tokars *et al.*, 1994; Valderrábano *et al.*, 1995).

The clinical consequences of parenterally transmitted viral hepatitides acquired during dialysis are especially manifest after renal transplantation (Parfrey *et al.*, 1985; Pereira *et al.*, 1995). Liver disease has been reported in 7–24% of transplant recipients, and liver failure is the cause of death in 8–28% of long-term survivors after renal transplantation (Sopko and Anuras, 1978; Ware *et al.*, 1979; LaQuaglia *et al.*, 1981; Parfrey *et al.*, 1985; Weir *et al.*, 1985; Harnett *et al.*, 1987; Boyce *et al.*, 1988; Debure *et al.*, 1988; Mahony, 1989; Braun, 1990). Indeed, patients with pretransplantation HBV or HCV infection are at increased risk of liver disease and death after transplantation. The advent of screening blood products for hepatitis B surface antigen (HBsAg) and anti-HCV has virtually eliminated the transmission of HBV and HCV infection by blood product transfusions (Donahue *et al.*, 1992). Consequently, the current debate is focused on other strategies to reduce the transmission of viral hepatitis among dialysis patients, and to lessen the consequences of liver disease among patients already infected (Pereira and Levey, 1997). The modes of transmission of HBV in dialysis units and strategies for control have been extensively reviewed (Jadoul, 1996; Pereira and Levey, 1997; Moyer 1990). On the other hand, information on the transmission and clinical consequences of GBV/HGV is just unfolding. Therefore, this review will primarily focus on the prevention and treatment of HCV in dialysis units.

Hepatitis C virus (HCV)

In 1989, the hepatitis C virus (HCV) was cloned, and identified as the major cause of parenterally transmitted NANBH (Choo *et al.*, 1989; Kuo *et al.*, 1989). The transmission of HCV by the transfusion of blood products and by needle-sharing among intravenous drug abusers has been unequivocally demonstrated (Alter *et al.*, 1989; Esteban *et al.*, 1990; Farci *et al.*, 1991). Horizontal transmission by sexual and/or household exposure and vertical transmission from mother to fetus have also been reported (Hess *et al.*, 1989; Giovannini *et al.*, 1990; Perez-Romero *et al.*, 1990; Riestra *et al.*, 1990; Calabrese *et al.*, 1991; Inoue *et al.*, 1991; Kiyosawa *et al.*, 1991; Thaler *et al.*, 1991; Okamoto *et al.*, 1992; Oymak *et al.*, 1994). Tests are now available that detect antibodies to multiple HCV antigens (anti-HCV), and the presence and titer of HCV RNA (Kuo *et al.*, 1989; Okamoto *et al.*, 1990*a*; Weiner *et al.*, 1990). These advances opened avenues to study the prevalence, transmission, and natural course of HCV infection in patients with ESRD (Pereira and Levey, 1997).

HCV genome

The hepatitis C virus is a small 40–60-nm virus with a lipid envelope and a single-stranded RNA viral genome comprising approximately 9400 nucleotides, and belongs to the Flaviviridae family (Choo *et al.*, 1989; Houghton *et al.*, 1991). The N-terminus encodes the basic nucleocapsid (C) followed by two glycoprotein domains, the envelope (E1) and second envelope/non-structural-1 (E2/NS1) regions (Houghton *et al.*, 1991). Downstream to this region are the non-structural genes NS2, NS3, NS4 and NS5, respectively. The 5′ non-coding region (5′NCR) represents the most conserved sequence, and the regions encoding the E1 and E2/NS1 are the most variable (Okamoto *et al.*, 1990*b*; Cha *et al.*, 1991; Han *et al.*, 1991; Hijikata *et al.*, 1991; Weiner *et al.*, 1991; Bukh *et al.*, 1992). Sequence analysis of the viral genome has identified a number of distinct HCV variants. Recently, a universal system for the nomenclature of hepatitis C viral genotypes has been proposed which has defined six major groups (1–6), designated as HCV *types* (Simmonds *et al.*, 1994). Each major type consists of one or more closely related variants, designated as *subtypes* and named *a*, *b*, *c*, etc. in order of discovery, and each subtype may consist of individual isolates.

Tests for HCV RNA

Polymerase chain reaction (PCR)

The detection of HCV RNA by reverse transcriptase polymerase chain reaction (PCR) has been used as the 'gold standard' to identify current HCV infection (Simmonds *et al.*, 1990; Ulrich *et al.*, 1990; Weiner *et al.*, 1990). Since the nucleotide sequence of the highly conserved 5′ end is shared by most HCV strains, 'universal' primers directed to this region are used to identify the presence or absence of the virus. In patients with post-transfusion NANBH, high levels of HCV RNA are detected in the circulation within a week, prior to the appearance of anti-HCV

(Weiner *et al.*, 1990; Farci *et al.*, 1991). Nonetheless, the reliability of this test is limited by false-positive and false-negative results. Imperfect handling and/or storage of blood samples can lead to a failure to detect HCV RNA in up to 40% of samples (Busch *et al.*, 1992). Also, due to the extreme sensitivity of the PCR, rigorous measures are required to prevent false-positive results due to even minor contamination (Kwok and Higuchi, 1989). Finally, performing PCR is labor intensive, protocols vary from laboratory to laboratory, and the test is available in only select clinical pathology laboratories (Wright, 1993). At the present time, PCR is not licensed for clinical use.

Quantitation of HCV RNA titers

The branched-chain DNA assay (bDNA assay) is a quantitative assay for HCV RNA in which the signal/probe rather than viral nucleic acid is amplified (Urdea *et al.*, 1991; Lau *et al.*, 1993*a*). The lower limit of detection of the bDNA assay is 350 000 molecules/ml (Lau *et al.*, 1993*a*) compared to 2000 molecules/ml for PCR (Lau *et al.*, 1993*b*). Although the bDNA assay is less sensitive than PCR, it is simple, automated, and is reproducible. Quantitative PCR has also been used to measure the level of HCV RNA in serum (Weiner *et al.*, 1990).

Tests for genotypes

Precise identification of the specific viral *type, subtype*, or *isolate* requires sequence analysis of the viral genome (Inoue *et al.*, 1991; Farci *et al.*, 1992; Feray *et al.*, 1992; Okamoto *et al.*, 1992; Weiner *et al.*, 1992; Widell *et al.*, 1994). However, this procedure is expensive, time-consuming and is fraught with the problem of mutations (Kurosaki *et al.*, 1993). Consequently, PCR using *subtype* specific primers (Okamoto *et al.*, 1992), restriction fragment length polymorphism (RFLP) analysis, and a line probe assay based on type-specific sequence variations in the 5′ untranslated region (Nakao *et al.*, 1991; Kurosaki *et al.*, 1993) have been used to identify HCV *subtypes*. Others have used an enzyme-linked immunosorbent assay (ELISA) that detects antibodies to serotype-specific immunodominant epitopes from the NS4 region of the HCV genome (Nagayama *et al.*, 1993; Stuyver *et al.*, 1993).

Tests for antibody to HCV (anti-HCV)

Tests for anti-HCV are the mainstay of the clinical diagnosis of HCV infection (Pereira and Levey, 1997). Enzyme-linked immunosorbent assays (ELISA) and recombinant immunoblot assays (RIBA) have been used to detect non-neutralizing antibodies. ELISA detects antibodies to specific HCV antigens in a standard ELISA plate, RIBA detects antibodies to HCV antigens on a strip that is read visually. While ELISAs have been used as screening tests, RIBAs have been considered confirmatory tests by virtue of their increased specificity. With the first-generation anti-HCV tests (which are now obsolete), the mean interval from transfusion with HCV-infected blood products to seroconversion was 16 weeks, but it could be as long as one year. Using these assays, anti-HCV was ultimately detected in 46–89% of patients (Esteban *et al.*, 1990; Aach *et al.*, 1991). The early stage in HCV infection, when HCV RNA is present but antibody response is not yet manifest, is defined as the 'window' period

(Farci *et al.*, 1991). The second generation tests incorporate c22 antigen from the nucleocapsid region and c200 which is a composite of c33 and c100-3 antigens from the NS3/NS4 region. RIBA2 uses four recombinant HCV antigens (c22, c33, c100, and 5-1-1). The use of a recombinant protein from the putative nucleocapsid region of the HCV genome could presumably reduce the window period between infection and seroconversion, since the antibody response against this capsid antigen occurs earlier than that against other HCV antigens (Nasoff *et al.*, 1991). Indeed, second generation tests can detect seroconversion as early as 4 weeks after exposure (Aach *et al.*, 1991). Recently, third generation anti-HCV tests have become available. Both, the ELISA3 and RIBA3 incorporate an additional recombinant antigen from the NS5 region, and the antigen corresponding to the NS3 region (c33) has been improved.

Difficulties in interpreting tests for HCV infection

Anti-HCV positive, but HCV RNA negative patients

The anti-HCV tests that are currently licensed for clinical use detect non-neutralizing antibodies to recombinant HCV antigens (Pereira and Levey, 1997). Thus, the presence of anti-HCV does not necessarily imply the presence of HCV RNA in the serum. Indeed, HCV RNA has been detected in only 52–93% of dialysis patients with anti-HCV (Dussol *et al.*, 1993; Pol *et al.*, 1993). Several possibilities could account for the presence of anti-HCV in the absence of HCV RNA:

1. HCV may be sequestered at sites other than the bloodstream such as the liver or peripheral blood mononuclear cells (Dussol *et al.*, 1993; Willems *et al.*, 1994).
2. Viremia could be intermittent and therefore HCV RNA may not be present in the plasma at the time of testing (Farci *et al.*, 1991).
3. The number of copies of HCV RNA may be below the limit of detection (Alter *et al.*, 1992).
4. Antibody to HCV may persist even after the viral RNA has disappeared. In this situation, anti-HCV positive but HCV RNA negative patients might represent a group that had been infected with the virus, but no longer harbor it, and for this reason they are no longer infective.
5. Anti-HCV may have been passively acquired from blood transfusions. In this situation, anti-HCV would disappear over the next few weeks in keeping with the half-life of IgG.
6. False-positive results can occur due to non-specific reactions, a problem which has been largely resolved with the current tests.

Anti-HCV negative, but HCV RNA positive patients

More than 90% of non-immunosuppressed, HCV-infected individuals test positive for anti-HCV (Alter *et al.*, 1992). Possible explanations for the presence of HCV RNA in the absence of anti-HCV include (Pereira and Levey, 1997):

1. The anti-HCV test may not be sensitive enough to detect existing anti-HCV antibody, either due to the low titer of antibody or because the antigen used in the assay

system cannot detect the serum antibody response to the particular genotype (Alter *et al.*, 1992; Nagayama *et al.*, 1993).

2. Various diseases or pharmacological immunosuppression could suppress or modify the anti-HCV response (Seelig *et al.*, 1994). Indeed, only 83% of HCV RNA positive dialysis patients test positive for anti-HCV, and 2.5–12% of anti-HCV negative dialysis patients test positive for HCV RNA (Sheu *et al.*, 1992; Bukh *et al.*, 1993; Chan *et al.*, 1993; Sakamoto *et al.*, 1993; Hayashi *et al.*, 1994).
3. The patient may be in the 'window' period between infection and seroconversion.
4. After anti-HCV antibody has persisted for a certain time, it can disappear despite the persistence of HCV RNA (Farci *et al.*, 1991).

In addition to the above, HCV RNA has been detected in peripheral blood mononuclear cells (PBMC) from HD patients without anti-HCV or HCV RNA in the serum (Oesterreicher *et al.*, 1995). The HCV RNA in these PBMC could serve as a viral reservoir and further frustrate efforts to identify HCV infection in HD patients.

Clinical features of HCV infection

Clinical course

Among patients with post-transfusion hepatitis C, HCV RNA is detected in the serum within 1–3 weeks after exposure, followed by elevated, serum alanine aminotransferase levels (ALT), several weeks later (Farci *et al.*, 1991). Seroconversion for anti-HCV begins at 4 weeks, but can take as long as 1 year (Esteban *et al.*, 1990; Aach *et al.*, 1991). Among patients with post-transfusion HCV infection, 50% have self-limited disease and 50% have persistently elevated serum alanine aminotransferase levels. Of those who undergo liver biopsy, 60% have chronic active hepatitis and 10–20% cirrhosis (Alter, 1989). Some of these patients progress to develop hepatocellular carcinoma (Colombo *et al.*, 1989; Kiyosawa *et al.*, 1990; Tanaka *et al.*, 1991). Nonetheless, the progression of liver disease is slow, and mortality among patients with post-transfusion NANBH followed for almost two decades was not significantly higher than that among patients without post-transfusion NANBH (Seeff *et al.*, 1992). It is possible that a longer follow-up may be required to reveal a difference in the mortality between the groups. This possibility is supported by Kiyosawa and colleagues (1990) who have shown that in patients with post-transfusion NANBH, the interval between the initial presentation and the onset of chronic hepatitis, cirrhosis, and hepatocellular carcinoma is 10, 21, and 29 years, respectively.

Relationship between serum ALT levels, HCV infection, and liver disease

Serum ALT levels are poor predictors of liver disease. Among HD patients, serum ALT levels are elevated in only 4–67% patients with anti-HCV, only 12–31% of patients with HCV RNA, and only one-third of those with biopsy-proven hepatitis (Jeffers *et al.*, 1990; Ayoola *et al.*, 1991; Roger *et al.*, 1991; Colombo *et al.*, 1992; Muller *et al.*, 1992; Vasile *et al.*, 1992; Pol *et al.*, 1993; Simon *et al.*, 1994). The discrepancy between serum ALT levels and the presence of anti-HCV is due to several reasons:

1. Chronic hepatitis C characteristically has a fluctuating course with multiple peaks and troughs in ALT levels (Farci *et al.*, 1991), and patients with normal ALT levels may have severe histological lesions.
2. HCV infection is not always associated with chronic liver disease. In fact, only 69% of anti-HCV positive symptom-free blood donors who underwent liver biopsy had histological evidence of chronic hepatitis, all of whom had HCV RNA in the serum (Alberti *et al.*, 1992). Therefore, a healthy carrier state can exist with viral replication occurring at extrahepatic sites.
3. As discussed earlier, some anti-HCV positive patients may have cleared the infection and anti-HCV may be the remnant of past infection.
4. Baseline ALT levels are depressed in patients on dialysis (Wolf *et al.*, 1972).

Interestingly, elevated ALT levels have also been observed in 4–23% of anti-HCV negative dialysis patients (Gilli *et al.*, 1990; Mondelli *et al.*, 1991; Colombo *et al.*, 1992; Vasile *et al.*, 1992; Pol *et al.*, 1993). These patients could be carriers of HCV infection in whom anti-HCV production is absent, or the liver disease might be due to a non-A, non-B virus other than HCV, or to non-viral causes. Consequently, liver biopsy remains the only reliable method of confirming the presence and assessing the severity of liver disease in patients with HCV infection. This is particularly true for patients who are being considered for renal transplantation, since liver histology at the time of initial presentation has been shown to be a good predictor of intermediate and long-term outcome after renal transplantation (Rao *et al.*, 1993). Over a mean follow-up of 6 years, progression to liver failure and death was rare in transplant recipients with mild histological abnormalities such as fat metamorphosis or chronic persistent hepatitis (Rao *et al.*, 1993). In contrast, 35% of recipients with early, chronic active hepatitis and 60% of recipients with advanced, chronic active hepatitis progressed to liver failure and death (Rao *et al.*, 1993).

Immunity

Humans exposed to HCV develop chronic infection despite the presence of antibodies to multiple regions of the HCV genome. The majority of these antibodies are non-neutralizing and hence do not represent immunity. Although neutralizing antibodies to the envelope regions of HCV have recently been characterized, their role in protective immunity has not been demonstrated (Zibert *et al.*, 1995). Indeed, studies in humans and animals with HCV infection have revealed a lack of protective immunity against reinfection (new infection after the previous infection has cleared) with the same or a different genotype (Farci *et al.*, 1992; Lai *et al.*, 1993) or superinfection (infection with a new genotype in the presence of a pre-existing infection) (Kao *et al.*, 1993). The newly introduced HCV genotype may either replace ('take over'), be eliminated, or coexist with the predecessor HCV genotype. The clinical implications of each of the these virological outcomes are currently unclear.

Prevalence of HCV infection and risk factors for infection in dialysis patients

Prevalence

The prevalence of anti-HCV among patients on dialysis is consistently higher than in healthy populations. Using ELISA1, the prevalence of anti-HCV among dialysis patients ranged from 8 to 36% in North America, 39% in South America, 1 to 54% in Europe, 17 to 51% in Asia, and 1.2 to 10% in New Zealand and Australia (Pereira and Levey, 1997). The advent of second generation tests has revealed an even higher prevalence of anti-HCV in HD patients (Blackmore *et al.*, 1992; Mondelli *et al.*, 1992; Sheu *et al.*, 1992; Niu *et al.*, 1993). Pooled data from studies in which dialysis patients were tested by both ELISA1 and ELISA2 revealed that ELISA2 identified more than twice the number of patients that tested positive by ELISA1 (Natov and Pereira, 1994). At the present time, there are insufficient comparative data with the new third generation anti-HCV tests. In addition to the wide range in the prevalence of HCV infection among different countries, there is also a wide variation in the prevalence of HCV infection among dialysis units within a single country. Among the 27 086 patients from dialysis centers participating in the National Surveillance of Dialysis Associated Diseases in the United States of America conducted by the Center for Disease Control and Prevention (CDC), the prevalence of anti-HCV by ELISA2 was 8.1%, with a range of 0 to 51% among centers with $\geq$ 40 patients (Tokars *et al.*, 1994). Likewise, the prevalence of HCV infection among HD units in Portugal ranged from 0 to 75.5%, and was lowest in the northern regions of the country and particularly high in the south and central regions (Loureiro *et al.*, 1995). Also, within Saudi Arabia, the prevalence of anti-HCV among HD units ranged from 15.4 to 94.7% (Huraib, 1995).

Trends

The incidence and prevalence of HCV infection among patients on dialysis is steadily declining. Among member nations in the European Dialysis and Transplant Association (EDTA), the prevalence of anti-HCV declined from 21% in 1992 to 17.7% in 1993 (Geerlings *et al.*, 1994; Valderrábano *et al.*, 1995). Nonetheless, the 0.4–15% incidence of anti-HCV in HD units continues to be a cause for concern (Niu *et al.*, 1993; Pascual *et al.*, 1992; Jadoul *et al.*, 1993; Lin *et al.*, 1993; Fabrizi *et al.*, 1994; Cendoroglo *et al.*, 1995). Among HD units in Portugal, the incidence of HCV infection declined from 11.2% in 1991 to 7.2% in 1992 and 6.5% in 1993 (Loureiro *et al.*, 1995). The initial decline could be attributed to a reduction in post-transfusion HCV infection. However, as discussed later, the subsequent decline in incidence probably reflects the implementation of infection-control measures to prevent nosocomial transmission within dialysis units.

Risk factors

The high incidence and prevalence of anti-HCV among patients on dialysis can be attributed to several risk factors.

Number of blood transfusions

Several studies in patients on dialysis prior to the advent of screening blood products for anti–HCV have shown that anti–HCV positive HD patients had received signifi - cantly more units of blood products than anti–HCV negative patients (Pereira and Levey, 1997). However, since the advent of screening blood products for anti–HCV, the risk of acquiring post-transfusion HCV infection has declined to less than one per 3000 units of blood products transfused (Donahue *et al.*, 1992), and future studies may not show the same association between anti–HCV and the number of blood products transfused.

Duration of ESRD

The interval since beginning dialysis was significantly longer among anti–HCV posi - tive patients compared to anti–HCV negative patients (Medici *et al.*, 1992), and the risk of acquiring HCV infection on HD has been estimated at 10% per year (Hardy *et al.*, 1992).

Mode of dialysis

Centers that compared the prevalence of anti–HCV in PD and HD patients have observed a consistently lower prevalence of anti–HCV among PD patients (Chan *et al.*, 1991; Brugnano *et al.*, 1992; Huang *et al.*, 1992; Barril and Traver, 1995; Cendoroglo *et al.*, 1995). In a group of 129 anti–HCV negative patients on chronic dialysis, the rate of seroconversion was 0.15/patient-year on HD compared to 0.03/patient-year on CAPD (Cendoroglo, 1995). Further, the majority of anti–HCV positive CAPD pa - tients may have acquired HCV infection while on HD. Indeed, Huang and colleagues (1992*a*) reported a 15.4% prevalence of anti–HCV among peritoneal dialysis patients. However, when patients with prior HD were excluded, the prevalence decreased to 5.9% (Huang *et al.*, 1992*a*). Factors that can account for the lower risk of HCV infection among PD patients include:

1. PD patients have a lower requirement for blood transfusion than HD patients (Chan *et al.*, 1991).
2. The absence of access site and extracorporeal blood circuit reduces the risk for parenteral exposure to the virus.
3. Because PD is primarily a home procedure, it offers a more isolated environment. Indeed, the prevalence of anti–HCV in patients receiving home-HD is also lower than in patients receiving center-HD (Bruguera *et al.*, 1990; Gilli *et al.*, 1990; Pas - cual *et al.*, 1992; Barril and Traver, 1995).

Prevalence of HCV infection in the dialysis unit

Patients treated in HD units with a high prevalence of HCV infection are at increased risk of acquiring infection (Jadoul *et al.*, 1993; Pinto dos Santos *et al.*, 1996). Indeed, a recent survey by the Portuguese Society of Nephrology showed that the incidence of HCV correlated directly with the prevalence of the infection in the HD units (Pinto dos Santos *et al.*, 1996). Amongst units with a prevalence of less than 19%, the annual incidence of seroconversion for anti–HCV was 2.5% compared with 35.3% amongst units with a prevalence greater than 60%. Indeed, several investigators have reported a relative homogeneity of HCV variants in patients receiving treatment in the same HD units (Corcoran *et al.*, 1994; Sampietro *et al.*, 1995).

Other factors

A history of previous organ transplantation is a risk factor for HCV infection in dialysis patients, possibly reflecting transmission from the organ donor (Cendoroglo, 1995). Intravenous drug abuse (IVDA) has been identified as an important risk factor for HCV infection in HD patients, and a history of IVDA was present in 30% of anti-HCV positive patients receiving HD at the Northwest Kidney Center, Seattle (DuBois *et al.*, 1994), and 73% in two urban HD units in Miami (Jeffers *et al.*, 1990). Males have been reported to have a higher prevalence of HCV infection than females (Alter *et al.*, 1990, 1992), and DuBois and colleagues (1994) observed that male HD patients infected with HCV had a significantly higher concentration of serum HCV RNA than females. However, there is currently no other data available regarding gender-related differences in the natural history of HCV infection.

Nosocomial transmission of HCV in hemodialysis units

Modes of transmission of HCV in hemodialysis units

The lower prevalence of HCV infection among PD and home HD patients, the correlation between the interval since beginning HD and the prevalence of anti-HCV, the relationship between the prevalence and incidence of anti-HCV in HD units, and the relative homogeneity of HCV variants in patients receiving treatment in the same HD strongly suggest patient-to-patient transmission of HCV in HD units (Pereira and Levey, 1997). Further, several studies have implicated a variety of potential modes of transmission.

Transmission of infection to dialysis staff by needlestick injury

The prevalence of anti-HCV among dialysis staff ranges from 0 to 6% and is comparable to that in blood donors (Pereira and Levey, 1997). In 1992, 10% of dialysis centers in the USA tested staff members for anti-HCV, and among the 2889 staff members tested, the prevalence of anti-HCV was 1.6% (range 0 to 6% among centers with ≥ 20 staff members (Tokars *et al.*, 1994). The risk of transmission of HCV from infected patients to medical staff, by needlestick injury, ranges from 2.7 to 10% (Kiyosawa *et al.*, 1991; Mitsui *et al.*, 1992). Indeed, genotype analysis has been used to prove that the viral strain acquired by the medical staff was the same as that in the index patient (Okamoto *et al.*, 1992).

Breakdown in standard infection-control practices

The implementation of universal precautions as well as measures to reduce the spread of HBV in dialysis units has resulted in a decline in the incidence of NANBH in dialysis units (Alter *et al.*, 1989). Consequently, strict adherence to standard infection-control practices would also be expected to prevent the transmission of HCV.

Indeed, several outbreaks of hepatitis C in HD units have been associated with a failure to enforce universal precautions and standard infection-control measures rigidly, such as sharing a multidose heparin vial between patients with and without HCV infection and a failure to change gloves between patients while performing HD treatments (Gilli *et al.*, 1990; Okuda *et al.*, 1994).

Physical proximity to an infected patient

In a multicenter study in Belgium, 38% of the HD patients who seroconverted had never been transfused and had no apparent risk factor for HCV infection (Jadoul *et al.*, 1993). Interestingly, clustering of seroconversion occurred only in dialysis units in which anti-HCV positive patients were being treated. Likewise, Da Porto and colleagues (1992) have found that anti-HCV positive HD patients were clustered in a group of patients who had never been transfused but who had been dialyzed in the same section of the unit. A Portuguese Society of Nephrology survey also found the lowest incidence of HCV infection among HD units that used isolated rooms to treat anti-HCV positive patients (Pinto dos Santos *et al.*, 1996). These data suggest that transmission of HCV may be enhanced by physical proximity.

Dialysis machines

Several reports have linked a high incidence of HCV infection among dialysis patients who shared dialysis machines in the HD unit (Brugnano *et al.*, 1992; Mitwalli *et al.*, 1992). Further, the use of dedicated machines and isolated areas for anti-HCV positive patients along with the strict enforcement of universal precautions was associated with a decrease in the incidence of seroconversion (Calabrese *et al.*, 1991; Vagelli *et al.*, 1992; Garcia-Valdescasas *et al.*, 1993). Likewise, a survey of HD units by the Portuguese Society of Nephrology found a significantly lower incidence of HCV infection among units that used dedicated machines for anti-HCV positive patients (Pinto dos Santos *et al.*, 1996).

Dialyzer membranes and hemodialysis ultrafiltrate

Theoretically, the passage of HCV through intact dialyzer membranes seems improbable as the viral particles have an estimated diameter of 35 nm, much higher than the pores of even the most permeable dialysis membrane (Yuasa *et al.*, 1991). However, any alteration in pore size or disruption of the membrane integrity, associated with the process of filter assembly, the dialysis session itself, or with dialyzer reuse, could hypothetically permit the passage of the virus into the dialysate compartment. In two recent studies it has been reported that neither low-flux (cellulose) nor high-flux (cellulose-diacetate, polysulfone, and polyacrilonitrile) dialyzers permit contamination of the dialysis ultrafiltrate with HCV RNA (Caramelo *et al.*, 1994; Hubmann *et al.*, 1995). In contrast, others have detected HCV RNA by PCR in the dialysate of apparently intact polyacrilonitrile membranes, but not cellulose membranes (Lombardi *et al.*, 1995). It is important to emphasize that detection of HCV RNA in the dialysate by PCR may only imply the presence of fragments of viral RNA, not the infective virus itself, a situation which may not lead to transmission of the infection. On the other hand, a negative PCR test does not absolutely rule out the presence of viral RNA in the dialysis ultrafiltrate as minimal amounts of HCV, below the detection threshold of the PCR assay, may have passed through the dialysis membrane. However, such a low viral load in the dialysis ultrafiltrate may represent only a negligible risk of transmission of HCV infection. To date, a higher prevalence of anti-HCV among HD patient has not been associated with any particular dialysis membrane (Gilli *et al.*, 1990; Muller *et al.*, 1992; Jadoul *et al.*, 1993; Lin *et al.*, 1993; Loureiro *et al.*, 1995).

Reprocessing the dialyzers

In a prospective study in 15 HD units in Belgium, Jadoul and colleagues (1993) did not find a higher incidence of HCV infection among patients treated in units that repro-cessed dialyzers compared with those that did not. Likewise, a Portuguese Society of Nephrology survey also found that the incidence of HCV infection among patients in HD units was not significantly different between those that did and did not reprocess dialyzers (Pinto dos Santos *et al.*, 1996). However, among units that did reprocess dia-lyzers, the lowest incidence was observed among patients in units that used separate rooms to reprocess dialyzers from anti-HCV positive and anti-HCV negative patients or which had a ban on reprocessing dialyzers from anti-HCV positive patients. These data suggest that contamination in the reprocessing room may be a vector for the transmission of HCV in HD units.

Strategies to control the transmission of HCV infection in hemodialysis units

The high prevalence of HCV infection among patients on HD, the limitations of current tests in identifying these patients, and uncertainty regarding the modes of transmission within dialysis units, have led to difficulty in formulating policies regarding HCV infection in HD units. The debate on the need for routine testing for anti-HCV, and the efficacy of patient isolation, dedicated machines, and a ban on the reuse of dialyzers in controlling transmission of HCV infection in HD units has not been resolved. Arguments in favor of such strategies in HD units include:

1. HCV is parenterally transmitted, and HD patients are at risk of nosocomial trans-mission.
2. Other parenterally transmitted viruses such as HBV have been shown to be trans-mitted within HD units and.
3. Similar strategies to reduce the transmission of HBV have resulted in a decrease in the incidence of HBV infection in HD units (Tokars *et al.*, 1990).

However, there are strong arguments against a policy of isolating anti-HCV posi-tive patients and their machines because:

1. HCV is not as infective as HBV, it circulates in low titers in infected serum and is rapidly degraded at room temperature (Bradley, 1990; Cuypers *et al.*, 1992). Indeed, chimpanzee transmission studies have shown that the viral titer of human non-A, non-B hepatitis sera is generally less than 10^2 chimpanzee-infective units (Yoshi-zawa *et al.*, 1982) compared to 10^8 chimpanzee-infective units for HBeAg-positive

sera (Shikata *et al.*, 1977) and 10^{11} chimpanzee-infective units for hepatitis D virus-infected sera (Ponzetto *et al.*, 1987).

2. Currently licensed anti-HCV tests detect non-neutralizing antibodies, do not distinguish between current and past infection, and a negative test does not exclude HCV infection. Consequently, isolation of anti-HCV positive patients does not eliminate the risk of transmission. Although the previous problem could potentially be circumvented by testing for HCV RNA by PCR, this test is not licensed for clinical use, is expensive, requires a specialized laboratory, and technical limitations can lead to false-positive and false-negative results.

3. Although isolation may protect uninfected patients, it might also increase the risk of superinfection in patients originally infected with a single strain (Farci *et al.*, 1992). Indeed, infection with two or more different HCV genotypes has been observed in HD patients and 13% of patients referred for renal transplantation (Okamoto *et al.*, 1992; Natov and Pereira, 1996). The clinical impact of such poly-genotype infections are currently undefined.

In view of the above debate, the Centers for Disease Control and Prevention in the USA does not recommend dedicated machines, patient isolation, or a ban on reuse in HD patients with HCV infection (Alter *et al.*, 1989). Meanwhile, strict adherence to 'universal precautions', careful attention to hygiene, and strict sterilization of dialysis machines is recommended (Pereira and Levey, 1997). Conventional cleansing and sterilization appear to be adequate to inactivate the virus (Gilli *et al.*, 1990; Jadoul *et al.*, 1993). Unfortunately, eliminating the spread of HCV infection in HD units may require the development of treatments to eradicate the virus or vaccines to prevent infection.

Effect of pretransplantation anti-HCV status on post-transplantation clinical outcomes

Among renal transplant recipients, the prevalence of pretransplantation anti-HCV is 11–49% (Ponz *et al.*, 1991; Huang *et al.*, 1992*b*; Fritsche *et al.*, 1993; Stempel *et al.*, 1993; Ynares *et al.*, 1993; Roth *et al.*, 1994; Pereira *et al.*, 1995; Roth, 1995). Pretransplantation anti-HCV is associated with an increased risk of post-transplant liver disease and is reported in 19–64% of recipients compared with 2–19% among recipients without anti-HCV (Fritsche *et al.*, 1993; Stempel *et al.*, 1993; Ynares *et al.*, 1993; Roth *et al.*, 1994; Pereira *et al.*, 1995). Indeed, studies from the New England Organ Bank have shown that for recipients with anti-HCV prior to transplantation, the relative risk of post-transplantation liver disease was 5.0 (95% confidence intervals of 2.4–10.5) (Pereira *et al.*, 1995). Among patients with pretransplantation HCV RNA in the serum, kidney transplantation was associated with a 1.8 to 30.3-fold increase in viral titer, suggesting that kidney transplantation is associated with proliferation of the hepatitis C virus. However, among patients with HCV RNA detected in the serum, the titer of HCV RNA did not differ between patients with and without post-transplantation liver disease. These data suggest that factors other than the viral load determine the risk of liver disease among transplant recipients with HCV infection.

Although pretransplantation anti-HCV is consistently associated with an increased risk of post-transplantation liver disease, post-transplantation patient survival was adversely affected in only some studies. While some studies failed to detect significant differences in patient survival between recipients with and without anti-HCV prior to renal transplantation (Stempel *et al.*, 1993; Ynares *et al.*, 1993; Roth *et al.*, 1994), others reported a lower patient survival among the anti-HCV positive recipients compared to anti-HCV negative controls (Fritsch *et al.*, 1993; Pereira *et al.*, 1995). Indeed, results from the New England Organ Bank study revealed that recipients with pretransplantation anti-HCV had a 3.3-fold higher risk of death (95% confidence intervals of 1.4–7.9) and a 9.9-fold higher risk of death due to sepsis (95% confidence intervals of 2.6–38.3) (Pereira *et al.*, 1995). Interestingly, infection rather than liver failure was the leading cause of death among anti-HCV positive recipients. However, it is not known whether survival for anti-HCV positive patients is greater with treatment by dialysis or transplantation. Preliminary results from a New England Organ Bank study, comparing survival between anti-HCV positive patients who underwent renal transplantation and anti-HCV positive patients referred for transplantation but who remained on dialysis, do not suggest that renal transplantation adversely affected survival (Natov *et al.*, 1996). Among anti-HCV positive patients awaiting transplantation between 1986 and 1990, the relative risk of death among those who received a transplant was 0.94 (95% confidence intervals, 0.55–1.59) compared to those who did not undergo transplantation. However, the wide confidence interval precludes definitive conclusions. In the absence of definite studies demonstrating worse outcomes after renal transplantation, we suggest that anti-HCV positive patients without evidence of liver disease should be allowed to make an informed choice of staying on dialysis or undergoing transplantation. However, as discussed earlier, patients on dialysis and transplant recipients can have histological evidence of liver disease in the absence of elevated serum ALT levels. Because the histological severity of liver damage is a strong predictor of liver failure and death after transplantation, there may be merit in a policy to perform liver biopsies on anti-HCV positive patients awaiting renal transplantation. In patients with histological evidence of liver disease, the decision to proceed with renal transplantation should be made cautiously, after taking into consideration the influence of immunosuppression on viral replication and possible exacerbation of liver disease.

GB virus (GBV)/hepatitis G virus (HGV)

Despite the development of reliable antibody assays and molecular probes for the detection of human hepatitis viruses A through E, the causative agents in about 10–20% of human hepatitis remains unexplained (Alter, 1994), suggesting the presence of other etiological agents. Indeed, in the USA, 25% of cases of presumed acute viral hepatitis are due to non-A, non-B hepatitis (NANBH), of which only 82% (or 20.5% of the total) are due to hepatitis C virus (Alter *et al.*, 1990). Consequently, in about 4.5% of patients with presumed acute viral hepatitis, the etiology remains unexplained. Further, the majority of non-A, non-B fulminant hepatic failure cases test negative for markers of HCV (Feray *et al.*, 1993; Koretz *et al.*, 1993). The search for etiological agents of hepatitis, for which the cause has thus far remained elusive, has been aided by the recent discovery of the GB group of viruses (GBV)/hepatitis G.

GBV/HGV

GB viruses are RNA viruses belonging to the Flaviviridae family (Muerhoff *et al.*, 1995). In the late 1960s, Deinhardt and colleagues (1967) demonstrated that an infective agent in plasma from a 34-year-old surgeon with acute hepatitis could be transmitted to marmosets, and described the histology of the liver lesions caused by this agent in animals. Subsequent cross-challenge studies from this plasma suggested that the infective agent was distinct from hepatitis A, B, C, D, and E (Holmes *et al.*, 1973; Deinhardt *et al.*, 1975; Tabor *et al.*, 1979, 1980; Feinstone *et al.*, 1980; Whittington *et al.*, 1983; Karayiannis *et al.*, 1989; Ticehurst, 1991; Purcell, 1993). More recently, using a subtractive polymerase chain reaction methodology known as representational difference analysis (RDA), Simons and colleagues (1995*a*) cloned two specific nucleotide sequences from the plasma of a tamarin that had been infected with pooled sera derived from serial passage in tamarins of the infective agent from the surgeon with hepatitis. These two agents were named GB virus-A (GBV-A) and GBV-B, after the initials of the surgeon from whom the infected serum was obtained. Subsequent studies on serum from a West African patient with antibody to GBV-A and -B, revealed the presence of a nucleotide sequence with a nucleotide homology of 59% with GBV-A, 47.9% with GBV-B, and 53.7% with HCV-1 (Simons *et al.*, 1995*b*). The same unique sequence was also identified in sera of some patients with non-A–E hepatitis (Simons *et al.*, 1995*b*). The nucleotide sequence of this virus, named GBV-C, has since been cloned and shown to contain the highly conserved RNA helicase domain characteristic of other members of the Flaviviridae family, including GBV-A, GBV-B, and HCV-1 (Leary *et al.*, 1996). In addition, Linnen and colleagues (1996) have recently identified an RNA virus from the plasma of a patient with chronic hepatitis and designated it as hepatitis G virus (HGV). HGV shows 95% amino-acid sequence identity to GBV-C (85% at the nucleotide level), suggesting that HGV and GBV-C are independent isolates of the same virus (Zuckerman, 1996), and hence the term HGV will be used hereafter.

Transmission of HGV

The prevalence of HGV RNA among volunteer blood donors varies from 0.9% in Japan (Masuko *et al.*, 1996) to 1.7% in the USA (Linnen *et al.*, 1996) and 3.2% in the UK (Jarvis *et al.*, 1996). Several lines of evidence suggest that HGV is a parenterally transmitted virus:

1. In animal experiments HGV has been unequivocally shown to be transmitted by inoculation of infected serum (Schlauder *et al.*, 1995), and the appearance of serum HGV RNA has been shown to coincide with transfusion-associated non-A–E hepatitis (Linnen *et al.*, 1996).
2. Among intravenous drug abusers the prevalence of antibodies to GBV-A and

GBV-B, and RNA of GBV-C/HGV is 3%, 11%, and 33.3%, respectively, compared with 0.3%, 1.2%, and 1.7%, respectively, among volunteer blood donors (Simons *et al.*, 1995*b*; Linnen *et al.*, 1996).

3. Among multitransfused anemic patients and hemophiliacs, the prevalence of HGV RNA was 18% and 18.3%, respectively (Linnen *et al.*, 1996).

4. Murthy and colleagues (1997*a*) have recently reported a high prevalence of HGV infection among cadaver organ donors, especially among those with serum markers of other parenterally transmitted viral infections. Indeed, the prevalence of HGV infection among anti–HCV positive donors (27.6%) was four times higher than that among anti–HCV negative donors (7.3%) (Murthy *et al.*, 1997*a*). Further, the prevalence of serum markers of HBV such as anti–HBs and anti–HBc antibodies was higher among donors with HGV infection than without infection.

5. Dialysis patients with HGV-C infection had received a higher number of blood transfusions and had a trend toward a longer duration of dialysis compared to patients without HGV infection (Murthy *et al.*, 1997*b*). These are both known risk factors for parenterally transmitted viral infections among dialysis patients (Jeffers *et al.*, 1990; Conway *et al.*, 1992; Dentico *et al.*, 1992; Oguchi *et al.*, 1992; Knudsen *et al.*, 1993).

These data suggest that HGV shares common modes of transmission with HBV and HCV, and hence is also a parenterally transmitted virus.

Prevalence and risk factors for HGV infection among hemodialysis patients

Among chronic hemodialysis patients, the prevalence of HGV RNA has been reported to be 3–55% in Asia (Masuko *et al.*, 1996; Tsuda *et al.*, 1996), 18–34% in the USA (Ashby *et al.*, 1996; Murthy *et al.*, 1997*b*), and 13–31% in Europe (Badalamenti *et al.*, 1996; Cabrrerizo *et al.*, 1996; Charrel *et al.*, 1996; Izopet *et al.*, 1996). The risk factors for HGV infection and the potential modes of transmission among hemodialysis patients are as yet incompletely defined. Increasing time on dialysis, higher number of blood product transfusions, and glomerulonephritides as the etiology of renal failure have been associated with an increased risk of HGV infection. Interestingly, most studies have failed to observe an increased prevalence of HGV infection among hemodialysis patients with HCV infection. Indeed, Murthy and colleagues (1997*b*) have reported that the 23% prevalence of HGV infection among anti–HCV positive dialysis patients was not significantly different from the 17% prevalence among anti–HCV negative patients. Likewise, Ashby and colleagues (1996) have reported that the 45% prevalence of HGV infection among anti–HCV positive dialysis patients was not significantly different from the 32% prevalence among anti–HCV negative patients. These data suggest that hemodialysis patients probably acquire HCV and HGV infection from different sources.

The reasons for the wide variation in the prevalence of HGV infection in different parts of the world are currently unclear. Possible explanations for these differences between different countries include: variations in the prevalence of HGV infection among blood donors (Linnen *et al.*, 1996; Masuko *et al.*, 1996); difference in the primers used for the detection of virus; and geographic differences in the prevalence of HGV due to differences in host susceptibility or virulence of different strains of HGV. The highest prevalence of HGV infection among hemodialysis patients reported thus far, 55%, was observed in Indonesia. However, this high prevalence is not surprising since the prevalence of anti-HCV (79%) among the same group of patients was also high— both infections are transmitted through the parenteral route. The high prevalence of these parenterally transmitted virus infections among hemodialysis patients in this unit possibly reflects suboptimal infection-control strategies in the dialysis units.

Effect of pretransplantation HGV status on post-transplantation clinical outcomes

The clinical impact of HGV infection acquired while on dialysis is currently unclear. Murthy and colleagues (1997*b*) did not find a statistically significant difference in the risk of post-transplantation liver disease in general, or NANBH specifically, between patients with or without pretransplantation HGV infection. However, the observed risks were higher (1.37 for post-transplantation liver disease and 2.09 for NANBH) in patients with pretransplantation HGV infection, but the confidence intervals were wide (0.55–3.40 and 0.64–6.79, respectively). Thus, they could not definitely exclude a role for HGV in post-transplantation liver disease. Nonetheless, if there is an effect of pretransplantation HGV infection on post-transplantation liver disease, it is much less than the effect of pretransplantation HCV infection. Indeed, in the same cohort of patients reported by Murthy and colleagues, patients with pretransplantation anti-HCV had a five-fold higher risk of post-transplantation liver disease compared to patients without pretransplantation anti-HCV (Pereira *et al.*, 1995). The role of HGV in post-transplantation liver disease needs to be further examined in a larger population.

Role of interferon-alpha (IFN-α) in the treatment of chronic hepatitis C infection in patients with ESRD

Treatment of acute hepatitis is not generally recommended in non-immunosuppressed patients. However, IFN-α has been used with a fair degree of success in patients with histological evidence of chronic hepatitis due to HBV, HCV, and hepatitis D infection (Davis *et al.*, 1989; Di Bisceglie *et al.*, 1989; Perrillo *et al.*, 1990; Korenman *et al.*, 1991; Shindo *et al.*, 1991; Black and Peters, 1992; Di Bisceglie, 1994; Farci *et al.*, 1994). The dose requirement and response to treatment differ among the three types of viral hepatitis. By the end of therapy (4 months for hepatitis B and D, and 6 months for hepatitis C), complete normalization of elevated liver enzymes and clearance of virus from the serum is observed in 30–40% of patients with chronic hepatitis D and 50% of patients with chronic hepatitis B or C (Davis *et al.*, 1989; Di Bisceglie *et al.*, 1989; Perrillo *et al.*, 1990; Korenman *et al.*, 1991; Shindo *et al.*, 1991; Farci *et al.*, 1994). The dose required to induce remission in chronic hepatitis C (3 million units administered three times a week) is threefold lower than that used in chronic hepatitis

B or D (9–10) million units administered three times a week). Remission is sustained in the majority of patients with chronic hepatitis B who demonstrate a response to interferon treatment (Perrillo *et al.*, 1990; Korenman *et al.*, 1991). In contrast, a sustained response to interferon treatment is observed in only 20–25% of patients with chronic hepatitis C or D. The efficacy of a longer period of treatment and higher doses are currently being evaluated (Di Bisceglie, 1994).

Among patients with chronic hepatitis C, the pretreatment clinical, biochemical, histological, and viral characteristics that predict the success of interferon treatment have been the subject of intense investigation. Patients with lower levels of viral RNA in the serum, and a lower concentration of HCV antigens in the liver are more likely to respond to interferon treatment (Di Bisceglie *et al.*, 1993). Preliminary results of a large European multicenter study suggest that age under 40 years, absence of cirrhosis, pretreatment ALT levels less than three times the upper limit of normal, post-transfusion rather than sporadic infection, and infection with the genotypes 1, 5, and 6, are predictors of a response to interferon treatment (Brouwer *et al.*, 1993). However, others have shown that patients infected with genotypes 2 and 3 have a better response to interferon than those infected with genotype 1 (Chemello *et al.*, 1994). Some of the differences in the relationship between HCV subtypes and response to interferon treatment could be related to the lack of uniformity in the viral nomenclature followed by different groups, and the different types of interferon used. Nevertheless, tailoring interferon treatment based on viral types promises to be an exciting possibility.

The initial response of dialysis patients to IFN-α treatment has been encouraging, with a majority of patients demonstrating a decrease in serum ALT levels and an improvement in liver histology (Harihara *et al.*, 1994; Koenig *et al.*, 1994; Casanovas *et al.*, 1995; Duarte *et al.*, 1995; Ozgur *et al.*, 1995; Pol *et al.*, 1995; Rao and Anderson *et al.*, 1995; Raptopoulou-Gigi *et al.*, 1995; Rostaing *et al.*, 1995). However, as in the case with non-renal patients, relapses are common after stopping treatment and long-term outcomes are not yet adequately defined (Pol *et al.*, 1995; Rostaing *et al.*, 1995). Further, although the disappearance of RNA from the serum is common, recurrence of viremia from extravascular sites remains a distinct possibility (Oesterreicher *et al.*, 1995; Rostaing *et al.*, 1995). Treatment with IFN-α is also associated with a 'flu-like' syndrome with asthenia, myalgia, headache as well as neutropenia, thrombocytopenia, and depression, and is partly related to the dose administered (Poynard *et al.*, 1995). Although the drop-out rate due to side-effects of IFN-α has been surprisingly low among non-renal patients (Poynard *et al.*, 1995), 0–54% of dialysis patients stopped IFN-α treatment due to side-effects (Koenig *et al.*, 1994; Casanovas *et al.*, 1995; Pol *et al.*, 1995; Rao *et al.*, 1995; Rostaing *et al.*, 1995). The reasons for this difference between non-renal and renal patients is currently unclear. More importantly, IFN-α therapy has been associated with a high incidence of acute rejection among transplant recipients with chronic hepatitis. This has led to the consideration that a safer, but probably less cost-effective strategy might be to treat dialysis patients with chronic hepatitis C prior to transplantation. Indeed, two recent studies in patients with chronic hepatitis C who were treated with IFN-α while on dialysis did not observe a recurrence of liver disease or an increased risk of rejection after subsequent transplantation (Casanovas *et al.*, 1995; Duarte *et al.*, 1995). Controlled studies will be required to evaluate the long-term effects of this strategy on the course of liver disease, rates of transplantation, and graft and patient survival.

References

Aach, R. D., Stevens, C. E., Hollinger, F. B., *et al.* (1991). Hepatitis C virus infection in post-transfusion hepatitis. *New England Journal of Medicine*, **325**, 1325–9.

Alberti, A., Morsica, G., Chemello, L., *et al.* (1992). Hepatitis C viraemia and liver disease in symptom-free individuals with anti-HCV. *Lancet*, **340**, 697–8.

Alter, H. J. (1989). Chronic consequences of non-A, non-B hepatitis. In *Current perspectives in hepatology* (ed. L. B. Seeff and L. J), Plenum Medical, New York, pp. 83–97.

Alter, H. J. (1994). Transfusion transmitted hepatitis C and non-A, non-B, non-C. *Vox Sanguinis*, **67**, 19–24.

Alter, H. J., Purcell, R. H., Shih, J. W., Melpolder, J. C., Houghton, M., and Choo, Q.-L. (1989). Detection of antibody to hepatitis C virus in prospectively followed transfusion recipients with acute and chronic non-A, non-B hepatitis. *New England Journal of Medicine*, **321**, 1494–500.

Alter, M., Hadler, S. C., Judson, F. N., *et al.* (1990). Risk factors for acute non-A, non-B hepatitis in the United States and association with hepatitis C virus infection. *Journal of the American Medical Association*, **264**, 2231–5.

Alter, M. J., Favero, M. S., Moyer, L. A., and Bland, L. A. (1991). National surveillance of dialysis-associated diseases in the United States, 1989. *American Society of Artificial Internal Organs*, **37**, 97–109.

Alter, M. J., Margolis, H. S., Krawczynski, K., *et al.* (1992). The natural history of community-acquired hepatitis C in the United States. The Sentinel Countries Chronic non-A, non-B Hepatitis Study Team. *New England Journal of Medicine*, **327**, 1899–905.

Anonymous. (1991). Combined report on regular dialysis and transplantation in Europe, XXI, 1990. *Nephrology, Dialysis, Transplantation*, **6**, 5–29.

Ashby, M., de Medina, M., Schluter V., *et al.* (1996). Prevalence of hepatitis G infection in chronic hemodialysis patients. *Journal of the American Society of Nephrology*, **7**, 1471 (Abstract).

Ayoola, E. A., Huraib, S., Arif, M., *et al.*(1991). Prevalence and significance of antibodies to hepatitis C virus among Saudi haemodialysis patients. *Journal of Medical Virology*, **35**, 155–9.

Badalamenti, S., Sampietro, S., Corbetta, N., *et al.* (1996). High prevalence of HCV, a novel hepatitis virus, among hemodialysis patients. *Journal of the American Society of Nephrology*, **7**, 1472 (Abstract).

Barril, G., and Traver, J. A. (1995). Prevalence of hepatitis C virus in dialysis patients in Spain. *Nephrology, Dialysis, Transplantation*, **10** (Suppl. 6), 78–80.

Black, M. and Peters, M. (1992). Alpha-interferon treatment of chronic hepatitis C: need for accurate diagnosis in selecting patients. *Annals of Internal Medicine*, **116**, 86–8.

Blackmore, T. K., Maddocks, P., Stace, N. H., and Hatfield, P. (1992). Prevalence of antibodies to hepatitis C virus in patients receiving renal replacement therapy, and in the staff caring for them. *Australian and New Zealand Journal of Medicine*, **22**, 353–7.

Boyce, N. W., Holdsworth, S. R., Hooke, D., Thomson, N. M., and Atkins, R. C. (1988). Non-hepatitis B-related liver disease in a renal transplant population. *American Journal of Kidney Diseases*, **11**, 307–12.

Bradley, D. W. (1990). Hepatitis non-A, non-B viruses become identified as hepatitis C and E viruses. *Progress in Medical Virology*, **37**, 101–35.

Braun, W. E. (1990). Long-term complications of renal transplantation. *Kidney International*, (Nephrology Forum), **37**, 1363–78.

Brouwer, J. T., Nevens, F., Kleter, G. E. M., Elewaut, A., Adler, M., and Brenard, R. ea. (1993). Treatment of chronic hepatitis C: efficacy of interferon dose and analysis of factors predictive of response. Interim report of 350 patients treated in a Benelux multicenter study. *Hepatology*, **18**, 110 A.

Brugnano, R., Francisci, D., Quintaliani, G., *et al.* (1992). Antibodies against hepatitis C virus in hemodialysis patients in the central Italian region of Umbria: evaluation of some risk factors. *Nephron*, **61**, 263–5.

Bruguera, M., Vidal, L., Sanchez-Tapias, J. M., Costa, J., Revert, L., and Rodes, J. (1990). Incidence and features of liver disease in patients on chronic hemodialysis. *Journal of Clinical Gastroenterology*, **12**, 298–302.

Bukh, J., Purcell, R. H., and Miller, R. H. (1992). Importance of a primer selection for the detection of hepatitis C virus RNA with the polymerase chain reaction assay. *Proceedings of the National Academy of Sciences, USA*, **89**, 187–91.

Bukh, J., Wantzin, P., Krogsgaard, K., ea. (1993). High prevalence of hepatitis C virus (HCV) RNA in dialysis patients: failure of commercially available antibody tests to identify a significant number of patients with HCV infection. *Journal of Infectious Diseases*, **168**, 1343–8.

Busch, M. P., Wilber, J. C., Johnson, P. J., Tobler, L., and Evans, C. S. (1992). Impact of specimen handling and storage on detection of hepatitis C virus RNA. *Transfusion*, **32**, 420–5.

Cabrerizo, M., Bartolome, J., Bello, E., *et al.* (1996). Hepatitis g virus (HGV) infection in hemodialysis patients. *Journal of the American Society of Nephrology*, 7, 1478. (Abstract).

Calabrese, G., Vagelli, G., Guaschino, R., and Gonella, M. (1991). Transmission of anti-HCV within the household of hemodialysis patients. *Lancet*, **338**, 1466.

Cantu, P., Mangano, S., Masini, M., Limido, A., Crovetti, G., Defilippo, C. (1992). Prevalence of antibodies against hepatitis C virus in a dialysis unit. *Nephron*, **61**, 337–8.

Caramelo, C., Navas, S., Alberola, M. L., ea. (1994). Evidence against transmission of hepatitis C virus through hemodialysis ultrafiltrate and peritoneal fluid. *Nephron*, **66**, 470–3.

Casanovas, T. T., Baliellas, C., Sese, E., *et al.* (1995). Interferon may be useful in hemodialysis patients with hepatitis C virus chronic infection who are candidates for kidney transplant. *Transplantation Proceedings*, **27**, 2229–30.

Cendoroglo, M. N., Manzano, S. I., Canziani, M. E. *et al.* (1995). Environmental transmission of hepatitis B and hepatitis C viruses within the hemodialysis unit. *Artificial Organs*, **19**, 251–5.

Cha, T. A., Kolberg, J., Irvine, B., ea. (1991). Use of a signature nucleotide sequence of hepatitis C virus for detection of viral RNA in human serum and plasma. *Journal of Clinical Microbiology*, **29**, 2528–34.

Chan, T. M., Lok, A. S. F., and Cheng, I. K. P. (1991). Hepatitis C infection among dialysis patients: a comparison between patients on maintenance haemodialysis and continuous ambulatory peritoneal dialysis. *Nephrology, Dialysis, Transplantation*, **6**, 944–7.

Chan, T. M., Lok, A. S. F., Cheng, I. K. P., and Chan, R. T. (1993). Prevalence of hepatitis C virus infection in hemodialysis patients: a longitudinal study comparing the results of RNA and antibody assays. *Hepatology*, **17**, 5–8.

Charrel, R., de Lamballerie, X., Dussol, B., *et al.* (1996). Prevalence of hepatitis G virus (HGV) infection among 32 transplant recipients. *Journal of the American Society of Nephrology*, **7**, 1904 (Abstract).

Chauveau, P., Couroucé, A. M., Lemarec, N., ea. (1993). Antibodies to hepatitis C virus by second generation test in hemodialyzed patients. *Kidney International*, **43** (Suppl. 41), S149–S152.

Chemello, L., Alberti, A., Rose, K., and Simmonds, P. (1994). Hepatitis C serotype and response to interferon therapy. *New England Journal of Medicine*, **330**, 143.

Choo, Q., Kuo, G., Weiner, A. J., Overby, L. R., Bradley, D. W., and Houghton, M. (1989). Isolation of a cDNA clone derived from a blood-borne non-A, non-B viral hepatitis genomen. *Science*, **244**, 358–62.

Colombo, M., Kuo, G., Choo, Q. L., ea. (1989). Prevalence of antibodies to hepatitis C virus in Italian patients with hepatocellular carcinoma. *Lancet*, **2**, 1006–8.

Colombo, P., Filiberti, O., Porcu, M., *et al.* (1992). Prevalence of hepatitis C infection in a hemodialysis unit. *Nephron*, **61**, 326–7.

Conway, M., Catterall, A. P., Brown, E. A., *et al.* (1992). Prevalence of antibodies to hepatitis C in dialysis patients and transplant recipients with possible routes of transmission. *Nephrology, Dialysis, Transplantation*, **7**, 1226–9.

Corcoran, G. D., Brink, N. S., Millar, C. G., ea. (1994). Hepatitis C virus infection in hemodialysis patients: a clinical and virological study. *Journal of Infectious Diseases*, **28**, 279–85.

Cuypers, H. T. M., Bresters, D., Winkel, I. N., ea. (1992). Storage conditions of blood samples and primer selection affect the yield of cDNA polymerase chain reaction products of hepatitis C virus. *Journal of Clinical Microbiology*, **30**, 3220–4.

Da Porto, A., Adami, A., Susanna, F., *et al.* (1992). Hepatitis C virus in dialysis units: a multicenter study. *Nephron*, **61**, 309–10.

Davis, G. L., Balart, L. A., Schiff, E. R., *et al.* (1989). Treatment of chronic hepatitis C with recombinant interferon alfa. A multicenter randomized, controlled trial. Hepatitis Interventional Therapy Group. *New England Journal of Medicine*, **321**, 1501–6.

Debure, A., Degos, F., Pol, S., ea. (1988). Liver disease and hepatic complications in renal transplant patients. *Advances in Nephrology*, **17**, 375–400.

Deinhardt, F., Holmes, A. W., Capps, R. B., and Popper, H. (1967). Studies on the transmission of disease of human viral hepatitis to marmoset monkeys, I: transmission of disease, serial passage and description of liver lesions. *Journal of Experimental Medicine*, **125**, 673–87.

Deinhardt, F., Peterson, D., Cross, G., Wolfe, L., and Holmes, A. W. (1975). Hepatitis in marmosets. *American Journal of the Medical Sciences*, **270**, 73–80.

Dentico, P., Buongiorno, R., Volpe, A., *et al.* (1992). Prevalence and incidence of hepatitis C virus (HCV) in hemodialysis patients: study of risk factors. *Clinical Nephrology*, **61**, 49–52.

Di Bisceglie, A. M. (1994). Interferon therapy for chronic viral hepatitis. *New England Journal of Medicine*, **330**, 137–8.

Di Bisceglie, A. M., Martin, P., Kassianides, C., *et al.* (1989). Recombinant interferon alfa therapy for chronic hepatitis C. A randomized, double-blind, placebo-controlled trial. *New England Journal of Medicine*, **321**, 1506–10.

Di Bisceglie, A. M., Hoofnagle, J. H., and Krawczynski, K. (1993). Changes in hepatitis C virus antigen in liver with antiviral therapy. *Gastroenterology*, **105**, 858–62.

Donahue, J. G., Muñoz, A., Ness, P. M., *et al.* (1992). The declining risk of post-transfusion hepatitis C virus infection. *New England Journal of Medicine*, **327**, 369–73.

Duarte, R., Huraib, S., Said, R., *et al.* (1995). Interferon-alpha facilitates renal transplantation in hemodialysis patients with chronic viral hepatitis. *American Journal of Kidney Diseases*, **25**, 40–5.

DuBois, D. B., Gretch, D., dela Rosa, C., *et al.* (1994). Quantitation of hepatitis C viral RNA in sera of hemodialysis patients: gender-related differences in viral load. *American Journal of Kidney Diseases*, **24**, 795–801.

Dussol, B., Chicheportiche, C., Cantaloube, J. F., *et al.* (1993). Detection of hepatitis C infection by polymerase chain reaction among hemodialysis patients. *American Journal of Kidney Diseases*, **22**, 574–80.

Dussol, B., Berthezene, P., Brunet, P., Berland, Y. (1995). Hepatitis C virus infection among chronic dialysis patients in the south-east of France. *Nephrol Dial Transplant*, **10**, 477–8.

Esteban, J. I., Gonzales, A., Hernandez, J. M., *et al.* (1990). Evaluation of antibodies to hepatitis C virus in a study of transfusion-associated hepatitis. *New England Journal of Medicine*, **323**, 1107–12.

Fabrizi, F., Lunghi, G., Guarnor, I. *et al.*. (1994). Incidence of seroconversion for hepatitis C virus in chronic haemodialysis patients. A prospective study. *Nephrology, Dialysis, Transplantation*, **9**, 1611–15.

Farci, P., Alter, H. J., Wong, D., *et al.* (1991). A long-term study of hepatitis C virus replication in non-A, non-B hepatitis. *New England Journal of Medicine*, **325**, 98–104.

Farci, P., Alter, H. J., Govindarajan, S., *et al.* (1992). Lack of protective immunity against reinfection with hepatitis C virus. *Science*, **258**, 135–40.

Farci, P., Mandas, A., Coiana, A., *et al.* (1994). Treatment of chronic hepatitis D with interferon alfa-2a. *New England Journal of Medicine*, **330**, 88–94.

Feinstone, S. M., Alter, H. J., Dienes, H. P., *et al.* (1980). Non-A, non-B hepatitis in chimpanzees and marmosets. *Journal of Infectious Diseases*, **144**, 588–98.

Feray, C., Samuel, D., Thiers, V., *et al.* (1992). Reinfection of liver graft by hepatitis C virus after liver transplantation. *Journal of Clinical Investigation*, **89**, 1361–5.

Feray, C., Gigou, M., Samuel, D., *et al.* (1993). Hepatitis C virus RNA and hepatitis B virus DNA in serum and liver of patients with fulminant hepatitis. *Gastroenterology*, **104**, 549–55.

Fritsche, C., Brandes, J. C., Delaney, S. R., *et al.* (1993). Hepatitis C is a poor prognostic indicator in black kidney transplant recipients. *Transplantation*, **55**, 1283–7.

Garcia-Valdescasas, J., Bernal, M. C., Cerezo, S., Garcia, F., and Pereira, B. J. G. (1993). Strategies to reduce the transmission of HCV infection in hemodialysis (HD) units. *Journal of the American Society of Nephrology*, **4**, 347.

Geerlings, W., Tufveson, G., Ehrich, J. H. H., ea. (1994). Report on the management of renal failure in Europe, XXIII. *Nephrology, Dialysis, Transplantation*, **9**, 6–25.

Gilli, P., Moretti, M., Soffritti, S., *et al.* (1990). Non-A, non-B hepatitis and anti-HCV antibodies in dialysis patients. *International Journal of Artificial Organs*, **13**, 737–41.

Giovannini, M., Tagger, A., Ribero, M. L., *et al.* (1990). Maternal–infant transmission of hepatitis C virus and HIV infections: a possible interaction. *Lancet*, **335**, 1166.

Han, J. H., Shyamala, V., Richman, K. H., ea. (1991). Characterization of the terminal regions of hepatitis C viral RNA: identification of conserved sequences in the 5′ untranslated region and poly(A) tails at the 3′ end. *Proceedings of the National Academy of Sciences, USA*, **88**, 1711–15.

Hardy, N. M., Sandroni, S., Danielson, S., and Wilson, W. J. (1992). Antibody to hepatitis C virus increases with time on dialysis. *Clinical Nephrology*, **38**, 44–8.

Harihara, Y., Kurooka, Y., Yanagisawa, T., Kuzuhara, K., Otsubo, O., and Kumada, H. (1994). Interferon therapy in renal allograft recipients with chronic hepatitis C. *Transplantation Proceedings*, **26**, 2075.

Harnett, J. D., Zeldis, J. B., Parfrey, P. S., ea. (1987). Hepatitis B in dialysis and transplant patients. *Transplantation*, **44**, 369–76.

Hayashi. J., Nakashima, K., Yoshimura, E., Kishihara, Y., Ohmiya, M., and Hirata, M. (1994). Prevalence and role of hepatitis C viraemia in haemodialysis patients in Japan. *Journal of Infection*, **28**, 271–7.

Hess, G., Massing, A., Rossol, S., Schütt, H., Clemens, R., Meyer zum Buschenfelde, K.-H. (1989). Hepatitis C virus and sexual transmission. *Lancet*, **ii**, 987.

Hijikata, M., Kato, N., Ootsuyama, Y., ea. (1991). Hypervariable regions in the putative glycoprotein of hepatitis C virus. *Biochemical and Biophysical Research Communications*, **175**, 220–8.

Holmes, A. W., Deinhardt, F., Wolfe, L., *et al.* (1973). Specific neutralization of human hepatitis type A in marmoset monkeys. *Nature*, **243**, 419–20.

Houghton, M., Weiner, A., Han, J., Kuo, G., and Choo, Q. L. (1991). Molecular biology of the hepatitis C viruses: implications for diagnosis, development and control of viral disease. *Hepatology*, **14**, 381–8.

Huang, C. C., Wu, M. S., Lin, D. Y., and Laiw, Y. F. (1992*a*). The prevalence of hepatitis C virus antibodies in patients treated with continuous ambulatory peritoneal dialysis. *Peritoneal Dialysis International*, **12**, 31–3.

Huang, C.-C., Liaw, Y.-F., Lai, M.-K., ea. (1992*b*). The clinical outcome of hepatitis C virus antibody-positive renal allograft recipients. *Transplantation*, **53**, 763–5.

Huraib, S., Al-Rasheed, R., Aldrees, A. *et al.*. (1995). High prevalence of and risk factors for hepatitis in haemodialysis patients in Saudi Arabia: A need for new dialysis strategies. *Nephrology, Dialysis, Transplantation*, **10**, 470–74.

Hubmann, R., Zazgornik, J., Gabriel, C., ea. (1995). Hepatitis C virus—does it penetrate the haemodialysis membrane? PCR analysis of haemodialysis ultrafiltrate and whole blood. *Nephrology, Dialysis, Transplantation*, **10**, 541–2.

Inoue, Y., Miyamura, T., Unayama, T., and Takahashi, K. (1991). Maternal transmission of HCV. *Nature*, **353**, 609.

Irie, Y., Hayashi, H., Yokozeki, K., ea. (1994). Hepatitis C infection unrelated to blood transfusion in hemodialysis patients. *Journal of Hepatology*, **20**, 557–9.

Izopet, J., Rostaing, L., Sandres, K., *et al.* (1996). Impact of HGV infection in hemodialysis patients. *Journal of the American Society of Nephrology*, **7**.

Jadoul, M., Cornu, C., Van Ypersele de Strihou, C., the UCL Collaborative Group. (1993). Incidence and risk factors for hepatitis C seroconversion in hemodialysis: a prospective study. *Kidney International*, **44**, 1322–6.

Jadoul, M. (1996). Transmission routes of HCV infection in dialysis. *Nephrology, Dialysis, Transplantation*, **11**, [suppl 4], 36–8.

Jarvis, L. M., Davidson, F., Hanley, J. P., Yap, P. L., Ludlam, C. A., and Simmonds, P. (1966). Infection with hepatitis G virus among recipients of plasma products. *Lancet*, **348**, 1352–5.

Jeffers, L. J., Perez, G. O., de Medina, M. D., *et al.* (1990). Hepatitis C infection in two urban hemodialysis units. *Kidney International*, **38**, 320–2.

Jonas, M. M., Zilleruelo, G. E., Larue, S. I., Abitbol, C., Strauss, J., Lu, Y. (1992). Hepatitis C infection in pediatric dialysis population. *Pediatrics*, **89**, 707–9.

Kao, J. H., Chen, P. J., La, M. Y., ea. (1993). Superinfection of heterologous hepatitis C virus in a patient with chronic type C hepatitis. *Gastroenterology*, **105**, 583–7.

Karayiannis, P., Petrovic, L. M., Fry, M., *et al.* (1989). Studies on the GB hepatitis agent in tamarins. *Hepatology*, **9**, 186–92.

Kiyosawa, K., Sodeyama, T., Tanaka, E., ea. (1990). Interrelationship of blood transfusion, non-A, non-B hepatitis and hepatocellular carcinoma: analysis by detection of antibody to hepatitis C virus. *Hepatology*, **12**, 671–5.

Kiyosawa, K., Sodeyama, T., Tanaka, E., *et al.* (1991). Hepatitis C in hospital employees with needlestick injuries. *Annals of Internal Medicine*, **115**, 367–9.

Knudsen, F., Wantzin, P., Rasmussen, K., *et al.* (1993). Hepatitis C in dialysis patients: relationship to blood transfusions, dialysis and liver disease. *Kidney International* **43**, 1353–6.

Koenig, P., Vogel, W., Umlauft, F., Weyrer, K., Prommegger, R., and Lhotta, K. (1994). Interferon treatment for chronic hepatitis C virus infection in uremic patients. *Kidney International*, **45**, 1507–9.

Kohler, H. (1994). Hepatitis B immunization in dialysis patients—is it worthwhile? (Editorial comment). *Nephrology, Dialysis, Transplantation*, **9**, 1719–20.

Korenman, J., Baker, B., Waggoner, J., Everhart, J. E., Di Bisceglie, A. M., and Hoofnagle, J. H. (1991). Long-term remission of chronic hepatitis B after alpha-interferon therapy. *Annals of Internal Medicine*, **114**, 629–34.

Koretz, R. L., Brezina, M., Polito, A. J., *et al.* (1993). Non-A, non-B posttransfusion hepatitis: comparing C and non-C hepatitis. *Hepatology*, **17**, 361–5.

Kuo, G., Choo, Q. L., Alter, H. J., *et al.* (1989). An assay for circulating antibodies to a major etiologic virus of human non-A, non-B hepatitis. *Science*, **244**, 362–4.

Kurosaki, M., Enomoto, N., Marumo, F., and Sato, C. (1993). Rapid sequence variation of the hypervariable region of hepatitis C virus during the course of chronic infection. *Hepatology*, **18**, 1293–9.

Kwok, S. and Higuchi, R. (1989). Avoiding false positives with PCR. *Nature*, **339**, 237–8.

Lai, M. E., Mazzoleni, A. P., Argiolu, F., ea. (1993). Hepatitis C virus in multiple episodes of acute hepatitis in polytransfused thalassaemic children. *Lancet*, **343**, 388–90.

LaQuaglia, M. P., Tolkoff-Rubin, N. E., Dienstag, J. L., *et al.* (1981). Impact of hepatitis on renal transplantation. *Transplantation*, **32**, 504–7.

Lau, J. Y. N., Davis, G. L., Kniffen, J., *et al.* (1993*a*). Significance of serum hepatitis C virus RNA levels in chronic hepatitis C. *Lancet*, **341**, 1501–4.

Lau, J. Y. N., Davis, G. L., Orito, E., Qian, K. P., and Mizokami, M. (1993*b*). Significance of antibody to the host cellular gene derived epitope GOR in chronic hepatitis C virus infection. *Journal of Hepatology*, **17**, 253–7.

Leary, T. P., Muerhoff, A. S., Simons, J. N., *et al.* (1996). Sequence and genomic organization of GBV-C: a novel member of the Flaviviridae associated with human non-A–E hepatitis. *Journal of Medical Virology*, **48**, 60–7.

Lin, D. Y., Lin, H. H., Huang, C. C., and Liaw, Y. F. (1993). High incidence of hepatitis C virus infection in hemodialysis patients in Taiwan. *American Journal of Kidney Diseases*, **21**, 288–91.

Linnen, J., Wages, J. Jr., Zhang-Keck, Z. Y., *et al.* (1996). Molecular cloning and disease association of hepatitis G virus: a transfusion-transmissible agent. *Science*, **271**, 505–8.

Lombardi, M., Cerrai, T., Dattolo, P., ea. (1995). Is the dialysis membrane a safe barrier against HCV infection? *Nephrology, Dialysis, Transplantaion*, **10**, 578–9.

Loureiro, A., Pinto dos Santos, J., Schmid, C. S., ea. (1995). Trends in incidence of hepatitis C (HCV) infection in hemodialysis (HD) units. *Journal of the American Society of Nephrology*, **6**, 547.

McIntyre, P. G., McCruden, E. A., Dow, B. C., *et al.*. (1994). Hepatitis C virus infection in renal dialysis patients in Glasgow. *Nephrol Dial Transplant*, **9**, 291–5.

Mahony, J. F. (1989). Long-term results and complications of renal transplantation: the kidney. *Transplantation Proceedings*, **21**, 1433–4.

Masuko, K., Mitsui, T., Iwano, K., *et al.* (1996). Infection with hepatitis GB virus C in patients on maintenance hemodialysis. *New England Journal of Medicine*, **334**, 1485–90.

Medici, G., Depetri, G. C., and Mileti, M. (1992). Anti-hepatitis C virus positivity and clinical correlations in hemodialyzed patients. *Nephron*, **61**, 363–4.

Mitsui, T., Iwano, K., Masuko, K., ea. (1992). Hepatitis C virus infection in medical personnel after needlestick accident. *Hepatology*, **16**, 1109–14.

Mitwalli, A., Al-Mohaya, S., Al-Wakeel, J., *et al.* (1992). Hepatitis C in chronic renal failure patients. *American Journal of Nephrology*, **12**, 288–91.

Mondelli, M. U., Smedile, V., Piazza, V., *et al.* (1991). Abnormal alanine aminotransferase activity reflects exposure to hepatitis C virus in haemodialysis patients. *Nephrology, Dialysis, Transplantation*, **6**, 480–3.

Mondelli, M. U., Cristina, G., Pazza, V., Cerino, A., Villa, G., and Salvadeo, A. (1992). High prevalence of antibodies to hepatitis C virus in hemodialysis units using a second generation assay. *Nephron*, **61**, 350–1.

Moyer, L. A., Alter, M. J., Favero, M. S. (1990). Hemodialysis-associated hepatitis B: Revised recommendations for serological screening. *Semin Dal*, **3**, 201–4.

Muerhoff, A. S., Leary, T. P., Simons, J. N., *et al.* (1995). Genomic organisation of GB viruses A & B: two new members of the Flavi-viridae associated with GB agent hepatitis. *Journal of Virology*, **69**, 5621–30.

Muller, G. Y., Zabaleta, M. E., Arminio, A., *et al.* (1992). Risk factors for dialysis-associated hepatitis C in Venezuela. *Kidney International*, **41**, 1055–8.

Murthy, B. V. R., Muerhoff, A. S., Desai, S. M., *et al.* (1997*a*). GB hepatitis agent among cadaver organ donors and their recipients. *Transplantation a*, **63**, 346–51.

Murthy, B. V. R., Muerhoff, A. S., Desai, S. M., *et al.* (1997*b*). Impact of pre-transplantation GB virus-C (GBV-C) infection on the outcome of renal transplantation. *Journal of the American Society of Nephrology*, **8**, 1164–73.

Nagayama, R., Tsuda, F., Okamoto, H., ea. (1993). Genotype dependence of hepatitis C virus antibodies detectable by the first generation enzyme-linked immunosorbent assay with C100-3 protein. *Journal of Clinical Investigation*, **92**, 1529–33.

Nakao, T., Enomoto, N., Takada, N., ea. (1991). Typing of hepatitis C virus genomes by restriction fragment length polymorphism. *Journal of General Virology*, **72**, 2105–12.

Nasoff, M. S., Zebedee, S. L., Inchauspé, G., ea. (1991). Identification of an immunodominant epitope within the capsid protein of hepatitis C virus. *Proceedings of the National Academy of Sciences*, USA, **88**, 5462–6.

Natov, S. N., and Pereira, B. J. G. (1994). Hepatitis C infection in patients on dialysis. *Seminars in Dialysis*, **7**, 360–8.

Natov, S. N. and Pereira, B. J. G. (1997). Transmission of disease by organ transplantation. In *Organ and tissue donation for transplantation* (ed. J. R. Chapman, M. Deierhoi and C. Wight), pp.120–51. . Edward Arnold, London.

Natov, S. N., Bouthot, B. A., Ruthazer, R., Schmid, C. H., Levey, A. S., and Pereira, B. J. G. (1996). Effect of renal transplantation on patient survival in anti-HCV positive patients. *XV Annual Meeting of the American Society of Transplant Physicians*, Dallas, May 26–29.

Niu, M. T., Alter, M. J., Kristensen, C., Margolis, H. S. (1992). Outbreak of hemodialysis-associated non-A, non-B hepatitis and correlation with antibody for hepatitis C virus. *Am J Kid Dis*, **19**, 345–52.

Niu, M. T., Coleman, P. J., Alter, M. J. (1993). Multicenter study of hepatitis C virus infection in chronic hemodialysis patients and hemodialysis center staff members. *American Journal of Kidney Diseases*, **22**, 568–73.

Oesterreicher, C., Hammer, J., Koch, U., *et al.* (1995). HBV and HCV genome in peripheral blood mononuclear cells in patients undergoing hemodialysis. *Kidney International*, **48**, 1967–71.

Oguchi, H., Miyasaka, M., Tokunaga, S., *et al.* (1992). Hepatitis virus infection (HBV and HCV) in eleven Japanese hemodialysis units. *Clinical Nephrology*, **38**, 36–43.

Okamoto, H., Okada, S., Sugiyama, T., ea. (1990*a*). Detection of hepatitis C virus RNA by a two-stage polymerase chain reaction with two pairs of primers deduced from the 5'-noncoding region. *Japanese Journal of Experimental Medicine*, **60**, 215–22.

Okamoto, H., Okada, S., Sugiyama, Y., ea (1990*b*). The 5′-terminal sequence of the hepatitis C virus genome. *Japanese Journal of Experimental Medicine*, **60**, 167–77.

Okamoto, H., Sugiyama, Y., Okada, S., *et al.* (1992). Typing hepatitis C virus by polymerase chain reaction with type-specific primers: application to clinical surveys and tracing infectious sources. *Journal of General Virology*, **73**, 673–9.

Okuda, K., Hayashi, H., Yokozeki, K., ea. (1994). Mode of nosocomial HCV infection among chronic hemodialysis patients and its prevention. *Hepatology*, **19**, 293.

Oymak, O., Akpolat, T., Arik, N., ea. (1994). Horizontal transmission of hepatitis C virus to the spouses of patients on renal replacement therapy. *Nephron*, **66**, 246–7.

Ozgur, O., Boyacioglu, S., Telatar, H., and Haberal, M. (1995). Recombinant alpha-interferon in renal allograft recipients with chronic hepatitis C. *Nephrology, Dialysis, Transplantation*, **10**, 2104–6.

Parfrey, P. S., Forbes, R. D. C., Hutchinson, T. A., ea. (1985). The impact of renal transplantation on the course of hepatitis B liver disease. *Transplantation*, **39**, 610–15.

Pascual, J., Teruel, J. L., Mateos, M., ea. (1992). Nosocomial transmission of hepatitis C virus (HCV) infection in a hemodialysis (HD) unit during two years of prospective follow-up. *Journal of the American Society of Nephrology*, **3**, 386.

Pereira, B. J. G. and Levey, A. S. (1997). Hepatitis C virus infection in dialysis and renal transplantation. *Kidney International*, **51**, 981–99.

Pereira, B. J. G., Wright, T. L., Schmid, C. H., Levey, A. S., for the New England Organ Bank Hepatitis C Study Group. (1995). The impact of pretransplantation hepatitis C infection on the outcome of renal transplantation. *Transplantation*, **60**, 799–805.

Pereira, B. J. G., Natov, S. N., Bouthot, B. A., *et al.* (1998). Effect of hepatitis C infection and renal transplantation on survival in end-stage renal disease. *Kidney International*, **53**, 1374–81.

Perez-Romero, M., Sanchez-Quijano, A., and Lissen, E. (1990). Transmission of hepatitis C virus. *Lancet*, **336**, 411.

Perrillo, R. P., Schiff, E. R., Davis, G. L., *et al.* (1990). A randomized, controlled trial of interferon alfa-2b alone and after prednisone withdrawal for the treatment of chronic hepatitis B. The Hepatitis Interventional Therapy Group. *New England Journal of Medicine*, **323**, 295–301.

Pinto dos Santos, J., Loureiro, A., Cendoroglo, M., and Pereira, B. J. G. (1996). Impact of dialysis room and reuse strategies on the incidence of HCV infection in HD units. *Nephrology, Dialysis, Transplantation*, **11**, 2017–22.

Pol, S., Romeo, R., Zins, B., *et al.* (1993). Hepatitis C virus RNA in anti-HCV positive hemodialyzed patients: significance and therapeutic implications. *Kidney International*, **44**, 1097–100.

Pol, S., Thiers, V., Carnot, F., *et al.* (1995). Efficacy and tolerance of alpha-2b interferon therapy on HCV infection of hemodialyzed patients. *Kidney International*, **47**, 1412–18.

Ponz, E., Campistol, J. M., Barrera, J. M., *et al.* (1991). Hepatitis C virus antibodies in patients on hemodialysis and after transplantation. *Trasnplantation Proceedings*, **23**, 1371–2.

Ponzetto, A., Hoyer, B. H., Popper, H., Engle, R., Purcell, R. H., and Gerin, J. L. (1987). Titration of the infectivity of hepatitis D virus in chimpanzees. *Journal of Infectious Diseases*, **155**, 122–8.

Poynard, T., Bedrossa, P., Chevallier, M., *et al.* (1995). A comparison of three interferon alpha-2b regimens for the long-term treatment of chronic non-A, non-B hepatitis. *New England Journal of Medicine*, **332**, 1457–62.

Purcell, R. H. (1993). The discovery of hepatitis viruses. *Gastroenterology*, **104**, 955–63.

Rao, V. K., and Anderson, W. R. (1995). Clinical and histological outcome following interferon treatment of chronic viral hepatitis, in uremic patients, before and after renal transplantation. ASTP Abstract 99.

Rao, K. V., Anderson, R. W., Kasiske, B. L., and Dahl, D. C. (1993). Value of liver biopsy in the evaluation and management of chronic liver disease in renal transplant recipients. *American Journal of Medicine*, **94**, 241–50.

Raptopoulou-Gigi, M., Spaia, S., Garifallos, A., *et al.* (1995). Interferon-alpha-2b treatment of chronic hepatitis C in haemodialysis patients. *Nephrology, Dialysis, Transplantation*, **10**, 1834–7.

Riestra, S., Suarez, A., and Rodrigo, L. (1990). Transmission of hepatitis C virus. *Lancet*, **336**, 411.

Roger, S. D., Cunningham, A., Crewe, E., and Harris, D. C. (1991). Hepatitis C virus infection in haemodialysis patients. *Australian and New Zealand Journal of Medicine*, **21**, 22–4.

Rostaing, L., Izopet, J., Baron, E., *et al.* (1995). Preliminary results of treatment of chronic hepatitis C with recombinant interferon alpha in renal transplant patients. *Nephrology, Dialysis, Transplantation*, **10**, 93–6.

Roth, D., (1995). Hepatitis C virus: the nephrologist's view. *American Journal of Kidney Diseases*, **25**, 3–16.

Roth, D., Zucker, K., Cirocco, R., *et al.* (1994). The impact of hepatitis C virus infection on renal allograft recipients. *Kidney International*, **45**, 238–44.

Sakamoto, N., Enomoto, N., Marumo, F., ea. (1993). Prevalence of hepatitis C virus infection among long-term hemodialysis patients: detection of hepatitis C virus RNA in plasma. *Journal of Medical Virology*, **39**, 11–15.

Sampietro, M., Badalamenti, S., Salvadori, S., ea. (1995). High prevalence of a rare hepatitis C virus in patients treated in the same hemodialysis unit: evidence for nosocomial transmission of HCV. *Kidney International*, **47**, 911–17.

Schlauder, G. G., Dawson, G. J., Simons, J. N., *et al.* (1995). Molecular and serological analysis in the transmission of the GB hepatitis agents. *Journal of Medical Virology*, **46**, 81–90.

Seeff, L. B., Buskell-Bales, Z., Wright, E. C., *et al.* (1992). Long-term mortality after transfusion-associated non-A, non-B hepatitis. The National Heart, Lung, and Blood Institute Study Group. *New England Journal of Medicine*, **327**, 1906–11.

Seelig, R., Renz, M., Bottner, C., ea. (1994). Hepatitis C virus infection in German dialysis units: prevalence of HCV-RNA and antibodies to HCV recombinant antigens. *Annals of Medicine*, **26**, 45–52.

Selgas, R., Martinez-Zapico, R., Bajo, M. A., *et al.* (1992). Prevalence of hepatitis C antibodies (HCV) in dialysis population at one centre. *Perit Dial Int*, **12**, 28–30.

Sheu, J. C., Lee, S. H., Wang, J. T., Shih, L. N., Wang, T. H., and Chen, D. S. (1992). Prevalence of anti-HCV and HCV viremia in hemodialysis patients in Taiwan. *Journal of Medical Virology*, **37**, 108–12.

Shikata, T., Karasawa, T., Abe, K., ea. (1977). Hepatitis B e antigen and infectivity of hepatitis B virus. *Journal of Infectious Diseases*, **136**, 571–6.

Shindo, M., Di Bisceglie, A. M., Cheung, L., *et al.* (1991). Decrease in serum hepatitis C viral RNA during alpha-interferon therapy for chronic hepatitis C. *Annals of Internal Medicine*, **115**, 700–4.

Simmonds, P., Zhang, L. Q, Watson, H. G., *et al.* (1990). Hepatitis C quantification and sequencing in blood products, hemophiliacs, and drug users. *Lancet*, **336**, 1469–71.

Simmonds, P., Alberti, A., Alter, H. J., ea. (1994). A proposed system for the nomenclature of hepatitis C virus genotypes. *Hepatology*, **19**, 1321–24.

Simon, N., Couroucé, A. M., Lemarrec, N., ea. (1994). A twelve year natural history of hepatitis C virus infection in hemodialyzed patients. *Kidney International*, **46**, 504–11.

Simons, J. N., Pilot-Matias, T. J., Leary, T. P., *et al.* (1995*a*). Identification of two flavivirus-like genomes in the GB hepatitis agent. *Proceedings of the National Academy of Sciences, USA*, **92**, 3401–5.

Simons, J. N., Leary, T. P., Dawson, G. J., *et al.* (1995*b*). Isolation of novel virus-like sequences associated with human hepatitis. *Nature Medicine*, **1**, 564–9.

Sopko, J. and Anuras, S. (1978). Liver disease in renal transplant recipients. *American Journal of Medicine*, **64**, 139–46.

Stempel, C. A., Lake, J., Kuo, G., and Vincenti, F. (1993). Hepatitis C—its prevalence in end-stage renal failure patients and clinical course after kidney transplantation. *Transplantation*, **55**, 273–6.

Stuyver, L., Rossau, R., Wyseur, A., ea. (1993). Typing of hepatitis C virus isolates and characterization of new. *Journal of General Virology*, **74**, 1093–102.

Tabor, E., Seef, L. B., and Gerety, R. J. (1979). Lack of susceptibility of marmosets to human non-A, non-B hepatitis. *Journal of Infectious Diseases*, **140**, 794–7.

Tabor, E., Peterson, D. A., April, M., Seef, L. B., and Gerety, R. J. (1980). Transmission of human non-A, non-B hepatitis to chimpanzees following failure to transmit GB agent hepatitis. *Journal of Medical Virology*, **5**, 103–8.

Tanaka, K., Hirohata, T., Koga, S., ea. (1991). Hepatitis C and hepatitis B in the etiology of hepatocellular carcinoma in the Japanese population. *Cancer Research*, **51**, 2842–7.

Thaler, M. M., Par, C.-K., Landers, D. V., ea. (1991). Vertical transmission of hepatitis C virus. *Lancet*, **338**, 17–18.

Ticehurst, J. (1991). Identification and characterization of hepatitis E virus. In *viral hepatitis and liver disease* (ed. F. Hollinger, S. M. Lemon, and H. S. Margolis, pp. 501–13. Williams and Wilkins, Baltimore.

Tokars, J., Alter, M. J., Favero, M. S., Moyer, L. A., and Bland, L. E. (1993). National surveillance of hemodialysis associated diseases in the United States. *American Society of Artificial Internal Organs Journal*, **39**, 71–80.

Tokars, J., Alter, M. J., Favero, M. S., ea. (1994). National surveillance of hemodialysis associated diseases in the United States, 1992. *American Society of Artificial Internal Organs Journal*, **40**, 1020–31.

Tsuda, F., Hadiwandowo, S., Sawada, N., *et al.* (1996). Infection with GB virus C (GBV-C) in patients with chronic liver disease or on maintenance hemodialysis in Indonesia. *Journal of Medical Virology*, **49**, 248–52.

Ulrich, P. P., Romeo, J. M., Lane, P. K., Kelly, I., Danial, L. J., and Vyas, G. N. (1990). Detection, semiquantitation, and genetic variation in hepatitis C virus sequences amplified from the plasma of blood donors with elevated alanine aminotransferase. *Journal of Clinical Investigation*, **86**, 1609–14.

Urdea, M. S., Horn, T., Fultz, T. J., ea. (1991). Branched DNA amplication multimers for the sensitive, direct detection of human hepatitis viruses. Nucleic Acids Research Symposium Series Oxford: Oxford University Press, **24**, 197–200.

Vagelli, G., Calabrese, G., Guaschino, R., and Gonella, M. (1992). Effect of HCV+ patients isolation on HCV infection incidence in a dialysis unit. *Nephrology, Dialysis, Transplantation*, **7**, 1070.

Valderrábano, F., Jones, E. H. P., and Mallick, N. P. (1995). Report on management of renal failure in Europe, XXIV, 1993. *Nephrology, Dialysis, Transplantation*, **10** (Suppl. 5), 1–25.

Vasile, A., Allegra, V., Canciani, D., Forchi, G., and Mengozzi, G. (1992). Prospective and retrospective assessment of clinical and laboratory parameters in maintenance hemodialysis patients with and without HCV antibodies. *Nephron*, **61**, 318–19.

Ware, A. J., and Luby, J. P., Hollinger, B., ea. (1979). Etiology of liver disease in renal transplant recipients. *Annals of Internal Medicine*, **91**, 364–71.

Weiner, A. J., Kuo, G., Bradley, D. W., *et al.* Detection of hepatitis C viral sequences in non-A, non-B hepatitis. *Lancet*, **335**, 1–3.

Weiner, A. J., Brauer, M. J., Rosenblatt, J., ea. (1991). Variable and hypervariable domains are found in the regions of HCV corresponding to the flavivirus envelope and NSI proteins and the pestivirus envelope glycoproteins. *Virology*, **180**, 842–8.

Weiner, A. J., Geysen, H. M., Christopherson, C., *et al.* (1992). Evidence for immune selection of hepatitis C virus (HCV) putative envelope glycoprotein variants: potential role in chronic HCV infections. *Proceedings of the National Academy of Sciences, USA*, **89**, 3468–72.

Weir, M. R., Kirkman, R. L., Strom, T. B., and Tilney, N. L. (1985). Liver disease in recipients of long-surviving renal allografts. *Kidney International*, **28**, 839–44.

Whittington, R. O., Decker, R. H., Ling, C. M., and Overby, L.R. (1983). Viral and Immunological Diseases in Nonhuman Primates. In (ed. S. S. Kalter) pp. 221–4. Liss, New York.

Widell, A., Shev, S., Mansson, S., ea. (1994). Genotyping of hepatitis C virus isolates by a modified polymerase chain reaction assay using type specific primers: epidemiological applications. *Journal of Medical Virology*, **44**, 272–9.

Willems, M., Peerlinck, K., Moshage, H., *et al.* (1994). Hepatitis C virus-RNAs in plasma and in peripheral blood mononuclear cells of hemophiliacs with chronic hepatitis C: evidence for viral replication in peripheral blood mononuclear cells. *Journal of Medical Virology*, **42**, 272–8.

Wolf, P. L., William, D., Coplon, N., ea. (1972). Low aspartate transaminase activity in serum of patients undergoing chronic hemodialysis. *Clinical Chemistry*, **18**, 567–73.

Wright, T. L. (1993). Hepatitis C virus infection and organ transplantation. *Progress in Liver Diseases*, **11**, 215–30.

Ynares, C., Johnson, H. K., Kerlin, T., Crowe, D., MacDonell, R., and Richie, R. (1993). Impact of pretransplant hepatitis C antibody status upon long-term patient and renal allograft survival—a 5- and 10- year follow-up. *Transplantation Proceedings*, **25**, 1466–8.

Yoshida, C. F. T., Takahashi, C., Gaspar, A. M. C., Schatzmayr, H. G., Ruzany, F. (1992). Hepatitis C virus in chronic hemodialysis patients with non-A, non-B hepatitis. *Nephron*, **60**, 150–3.

Yoshizawa, H., Otoh, Y., Iwakiri, K., Tanaka, A., and Tachibana, T. (1982). Non-A, non-B (type 1) hepatitis agent capable of inducing tubular structures in the hepatocyte cytoplasm of chimpanzees: inactivation by formalin and heat. *Gastroenterology*, **82**, 502–6.

Yuasa, T., Ishikawa, G., Manabe, S., Sekiguchi, S., Takeuchi, K., and Miyamura, T. (1991). The particle size of hepatitis C virus estimated by filtration through microporous regenerated cellulose fibre. *Journal of General Virology*, **72**, 2021–4.

Zibert, A., Schreier, E., and Roggendorf, M. (1995). Antibodies in human sera to hypervariable region 1 of hepatitis C virus can block viral atttachment. *Virology*, **208**, 653–61.

Zuckerman, A. J. (1996). Alphabet of hepatitis viruses. *Lancet*, **347**, 558–9.

INDEX

Note to index: page numbers in **bold** refer to tables.